Soda Politics

Soda Politics

Taking on Big Soda (and Winning)

MARION NESTLE

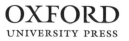

OXFORD
UNIVERSITY PRESS

Oxford University Press is a department of the
University of Oxford. It furthers the University's objective
of excellence in research, scholarship, and education
by publishing worldwide.

Oxford   New York
Auckland   Cape Town   Dar es Salaam   Hong Kong   Karachi
Kuala Lumpur   Madrid   Melbourne   Mexico City   Nairobi
New Delhi   Shanghai   Taipei   Toronto

With offices in
Argentina   Austria   Brazil   Chile   Czech Republic   France   Greece
Guatemala   Hungary   Italy   Japan   Poland   Portugal   Singapore
South Korea   Switzerland   Thailand   Turkey   Ukraine   Vietnam

Oxford is a registered trade mark of Oxford University Press
in the UK and certain other countries.

Published in the United States of America by
Oxford University Press
198 Madison Avenue, New York, NY 10016

Library of Congress Cataloging-in-Publication Data
Nestle, Marion.
Soda politics : taking on big soda (and winning) / Marion Nestle.
p. ; cm.
Includes bibliographical references and index.
ISBN 978-0-19-026343-0 (hardback : alk. paper)
I. Title. [DNLM: 1. Carbonated Beverages.   2. Consumer Advocacy.
3. Dietary Sucrose—adverse effects.   4. Food Industry.
5. Marketing.   6. Politics. WA 695]
TP630
663'.62—dc23
2015018561

9 8 7 6 5 4 3 2
Printed in the United States of America
on acid-free paper

Contents

"Hardball" Tactics: Defending Turf, Attacking Critics

Advocacy: Soda Caps, Taxes, and More

Foreword

Mark Bittman

No one who knows the field would make a list of the five most important people in the fight for good food in the United States over the last couple of decades and leave off the name of Marion Nestle. This would probably be true even if she had retired after publishing her groundbreaking and still relevant work *Food Politics*. That book was a revelation to just about everyone who read it, a brilliant description of how Big Food methodically manipulates both individuals and our so-called representatives.

As those of us who rely on or simply follow her know well, she did not stop there. At least two of the books she's published in the last ten years have been equally important. (You can judge which two; all of her books are worth reading.)

With *Soda Politics*, Marion sharpens her focus to lay bare the rapacious and despicable marketing practices used by the producers of soda (and, of course, the other sugar-sweetened beverages that are equally harmful) to push their worse-than-useless products on an increasingly obese country and, indeed, world.

I'll leave it to her to tell that story, which involves not only the twin tragedies of obesity and diabetes but also sad stories of water use, land grabs, and exploitation of the poor, undereducated, and illiterate, as well as the targeting of children.

This last is ultra-important, because the "get 'em while they're young" strategy works: as anyone over the age of thirty knows, it's hard to change the style of eating you developed before you reached adolescence. And as long as pushers of soda and other junk food have their way with kids, we have to look twenty years down the road to really begin to solve our dietary problems.

The parallels between the marketing of cigarettes and that of soda have only recently become generally known. (Again, Marion has played a large part in this.) Cigarettes remain a threat, but the damage from sugar-sweetened beverages is among the great public health challenges of the twenty-first century. One can say with accuracy that the targeting of children by junk food marketers—and soda purveyors lead this pack—is among the greatest concerns of both public health advocates and those advocating good food.

One great thing about Marion is that she is not a pure academic: she does not merely describe problems, although she does that with unerring accuracy and wit. To (partially) quote her, she does "everything possible to discourage the marketing, promotion, and political protection of sugary drinks." To her, soda is not just an "interesting" marketing phenomenon; it's a concrete threat to our public health, and she is here not only to describe that threat but to help us figure out how to combat it.

She's uniquely equipped to do so. There is not a better-educated (and I'm talking not only about school learning but also about daily reading, writing, and other ongoing hard work) and more principled person in her field.

If the consumption of soda has declined in the last few years (it has), it's in no small part thanks to her advocacy. If purveyors of sugar-sweetened beverages are looking at falling profits (and they are), it's precisely because a movement has grown around principles that were largely first presented to the public by Marion.

I personally am deeply in Marion Nestle's debt; my guess is you'll feel that way too by the time you finish reading this book.

Abbreviations

ABA	American Beverage Association
AHA	American Heart Association
ALEC	American Legislative Exchange Council
AND	Academy of Nutrition and Dietetics (formerly American Dietetic Association)
ASN	American Society for Nutrition
BIHW	Beverage Institute for Health and Wellness (of Coca-Cola)
CARU	Children's Advertising Review Unit
CCF	Center for Consumer Freedom
CDC	Centers for Disease Control and Prevention
CORE	Center for Organizational Research and Education
CRA	Corn Refiners of America
CSPI	Center for Science in the Public Interest
CSR	Corporate social responsibility
DMFT	Decayed, missing, or filled teeth (adults)
dmft	Decayed, missing, or filled teeth (children)
DPS	Dr Pepper Snapple
EBT	Electronic Benefit Transfer
FAO	Food and Agriculture Organization
FCC	Federal Communications Commission
FDA	Food and Drug Administration
FRAC	Food Research and Action Center
FTC	Federal Trade Commission
GMA	Grocery Manufacturers of America

GMOS	Genetically modified organisms
HFCS	High-fructose corn syrup
IOM	Institute of Medicine
IWG	Interagency Working Group
LGBT	Lesbian, gay, bisexual, and transgender
NAACP	National Association for the Advancement of Colored People
NAFLD	Nonalcoholic fatty liver disease
NANA	National Alliance for Nutrition and Activity
NHANES	National Health and Nutrition Examination Survey
PAHO	Pan American Health Organization
PPPS	Public-private partnerships
RWJF	Robert Wood Johnson Foundation
SEC	U.S. Securities and Exchange Commission
SSB	Sugar-sweetened beverage
SNA	School Nutrition Association
SNAP	Supplemental Nutrition Assistance Program (formerly the Food Stamp Program)
USDA	U.S. Department of Agriculture
WHO	World Health Organization
WIC	Special Supplemental Nutrition Program for Women, Infants, and Children
WWF	World Wildlife Fund

Soda Politics

Introduction

I can't remember when my literary agent, Lydia Wills, along with another of her clients, the physician, writer, and television producer Neal Baer, first suggested that I write a book about advocacy for reducing soda consumption, but I do remember my reaction: this was one terrific idea. Sodas are astonishing products. Little more than flavored sugar water, these drinks cost practically nothing to produce or buy, yet have turned their makers—principally Coca-Cola and PepsiCo—into multibillion-dollar industries with global recognition, distribution, and political power.

I have spent the last twenty years or so teaching, speaking, and writing books about how food companies encourage people to eat more and to gain weight as a result. My research aims to explain how—as part of the normal course of doing business—food companies use marketing, lobbying, partnerships, and philanthropy to promote sales, regardless of how their products might affect health. And affect health they do, none more than the sugar-sweetened, carbonated beverages familiarly known as Coke and Pepsi. Today, it is so well established that sodas and other sugary drinks contribute to higher calorie intake, weight gain, obesity, and type 2 diabetes that stopping drinking them is the first line of defense against any of these conditions. Many people can lose weight, keep it off, and reduce or eliminate symptoms of diabetes by doing nothing more than removing sugary drinks from their daily diets.

I have been acutely conscious of the particular role of sodas in health since the early 1990s. Soon after starting my job as a nutrition professor at New York University, I was invited to speak at a conference on behavioral risk factors—cigarette smoking and diet—sponsored by the National Cancer

Institute. Most of the speakers were international physicians and scientists whose research focused on anti-smoking advocacy. In that pre-PowerPoint era, their lectures featured slide shows of cigarette marketing throughout the world, from the jungles of Africa to the high Himalayas, much of it aimed at children.

The talks were a revelation. I was well aware that cigarette marketing induced young people to start smoking, and I had seen plenty of advertisements featuring Joe Camel, the cartoon cigarette character expressly designed to entice kids to smoke. But I had never paid much attention to these ads. Cigarette advertising was ubiquitous—part of the normal landscape of everyday life. The speakers demonstrated how cigarette companies deliberately created their ads to blend into the surroundings and to slip below the radar of conscious notice or critical thought. I left that meeting convinced that those of us who care about diet and health ought to follow the lead of anti-smoking advocates and pay that same kind of close critical attention to the marketing of Coke and Pepsi.

Of course, Coca-Cola, PepsiCo, and the other makers of sweetened drinks are much more complicated targets of public health advocacy than cigarette companies. For one thing, they are among the top-ranked, most recognized, and most admired brands in the world. Sodas are not cigarettes. An occasional sugary drink is hardly a health concern. But many Americans—especially those who are young, members of minority groups, and poor—habitually drink large volumes of soda on a daily basis at great harm to their health. It is hardly a coincidence that soda marketers single out precisely those groups as prime targets for marketing efforts.

Having done my share of international travel, I've seen the reach of soda companies into the most remote and poverty-stricken areas of the world. Viewed from this perspective, the marketing practices of cigarette and soda companies seem eerily similar. Both aim to sell as much of their products as possible, regardless of health consequences. Both encourage consumption with massive amounts of advertising, much of it aimed at children and low-income groups. Both use philanthropy to community organizations as a means to create goodwill and build brand loyalty. Both lobby Congress and government agencies and spend fortunes to head off unfavorable regulation. Both forge alliances with health organizations and researchers to make the science appear confusing and to silence criticism.

By this time, it seems clear that everyone interested in health should be taking a closer look at how, when, where, and to whom soda companies are selling their products, and doing everything possible to discourage the marketing, promotion, and political protection of sugary drinks. "Everything possible" means advocacy—encouraging individuals, private and public groups, and government agencies to discourage consumption of sugary drinks and replace them with healthier drinks.

I live in New York City, where health advocacy is part of a long civic tradition dating back to the earliest years of the twentieth century. In recent years, city officials, alarmed by the high prevalence of obesity and its related diseases, created a series of subway poster campaigns to discourage soda consumption, and attempted to tax sodas, prevent their purchase with food stamps, and limit the size of drinks that could be sold. I witnessed how the soda industry spared no expense to oppose these health initiatives and, ultimately, to defeat them.

Despite these setbacks, health advocates continue to press for regulatory and social changes to discourage soda consumption. They start by asking some basic questions: How did products containing absurdly inexpensive ingredients—sugar and water and not much else—become multibillion-dollar industries and international brand icons? How did products that are essentially candy in liquid form come to be considered acceptable for children as well as adults to drink as a substitute for water? What do soda companies do, overtly and covertly, to discourage legislators and health officials from focusing on their products as targets of "drink less" messages? How do these companies promote brand loyalty so intense that customers will take to the streets to protect their inalienable right to consume as much soda as they want? And how do soft drink companies use their own version of the science to promote their products as essential for well-being and happiness? This book addresses these questions from the standpoint of advocacy—what those of us who care about such issues, individually and collectively, can do to counter soda marketing and create a healthier food environment for ourselves and our children.

I wrote *Soda Politics* to address such questions. Why, you may wonder, is such a book needed, and why now? Doesn't everyone know that sodas are bad for health? This is hardly the first book to take a critical look at soda companies. Indeed, as I explain in Appendix 3, an entire library can be filled with books about Coca-Cola and PepsiCo, their history, and their leaders, as well as their effects on health and society. But I view the soda situation in the United States as having reached a tipping point. Sodas are worth reading about for two reasons: health and advocacy. By now, research overwhelmingly links soda consumption to overweight, poor health, and type 2 diabetes, and demonstrates that these illnesses pose critical problems not only for the people who have these conditions but also for society as a whole. The cost of obesity alone, in treatment and lost productivity, runs to hundreds of billions of dollars annually.

As for advocacy, sodas are, in public health jargon, "low-hanging fruit"—easy targets. The drinks contain sugars but nothing else of redeeming nutritional value. This explains in part why sodas are so useful an example of *successful* advocacy. Soda consumption is falling in the United States. We are not buying Coke and Pepsi the way we used to, and we are only partially replacing these products with other sugary drinks. This did not happen accidentally. As any soda company executive will tell you, health advocacy has become the single greatest threat to company profits. Advocates, with far fewer resources than soda companies, have used their democratic rights as citizens—and time-honored methods for promoting social change—to counter soda industry marketing, lobbying, and public relations. Advocates are gaining increasing public support and scoring wins, with all signs pointing to more to come. I argue in this book that declining soda sales are a result of effective food advocacy, and that this example provides lessons readily applicable to other advocacy targets. This book, unlike other books about the soda industry, explains why advocacy is so badly needed and how food and health advocacy can best be used to promote desirable social changes.

In *Soda Politics*, I focus primarily on one particular category of sugary drinks, the carbonated beverages variously known as sodas, pop, or soda pop—drinks mainly produced by Coca-Cola and PepsiCo. Although sugary drinks collectively account for fully half—yes, half—of all sugar consumed in the United States, sodas alone account for a third. And although many companies manufacture such drinks, Coca-Cola and PepsiCo thoroughly dominate the market. These companies are better established and their history and business practices are better studied than those of most other producers of sugary beverages or food products. They exemplify companies willing to spend vast fortunes to market their products, to protect their marketing practices against government regulation, and to promote sales to children and other vulnerable populations in developing countries as well as in industrialized nations. To my mind, the standard operating practices of these companies demand the same kind of close scrutiny as has been given to cigarette companies, and for many of the same reasons.

Soda Politics provides information, ideas for strategies, and resources for anyone who cares enough about the current dietary practices of adults and children to want to improve the environment of food choice. I wrote it to encourage efforts to counter the soda industry's use of marketing, public relations, and manipulation of the political system to protect sales and profits at the expense of public health. I wrote it for parents who wish restaurants would not serve sodas with kids' meals, schools would not offer sodas for sale, and soda companies would not advertise to their kids—and want such practices to stop. I wrote it for teenagers who want to take control of their own food environments. I wrote it for African and Hispanic Americans who are tired of being special targets of soda marketing and want to promote the health of their communities. I wrote it for elected officials who care about the health of their constituents but feel that their jobs depend on financial contributions from soda and other food companies. And, professor that I am, I wrote it for students who want to work for a healthier and more sustainable food environment but do not know how or where to start. My explicit purpose in writing this book is to inspire readers to join the food movement and become advocates for healthier food systems.

TO BEGIN WITH, SOME DEFINITIONS

In this book, I use the terms for sodas and other such drinks in specific ways. To avoid confusion, it's best to know what they are right from the start.

- *Soft drinks.* This is the generic term for nonalcoholic beverages other than plain water and 100 percent fruit juices. Soft drinks may be carbonated or noncarbonated, unsweetened or sweetened with sugar, high-fructose corn syrup (HFCS), or artificial sweeteners.
- *Sugar-sweetened beverages (SSBs) or their less formal synonym, sugary drinks.* This term refers to any soft drink, carbonated or noncarbonated, sweetened with sugar or HFCS. The universe of SSBs includes sodas but also juice drinks, fruit drinks, fruit ades, teas and coffees, sports drinks, energy drinks, tonic water, vitamin waters, and any other drink containing sugars or HFCS.
- *Sodas (also known as pop or soda pop).* In this book, these terms mean carbonated soft drinks—mostly colas, and mostly produced

by the Coca-Cola and PepsiCo companies—sweetened with sugars or HFCS. The industry refers to these drinks as "regular" sodas, to distinguish them from artificially sweetened diet sodas, and I do too, occasionally.

- **Diet sodas.** These are carbonated soft drinks made with one or more artificial sweeteners such as aspartame, acesulfame potassium, or stevia. They contain no or very little sugar and provide no or very few calories.

Because Coca-Cola and PepsiCo so heavily dominate the soft drink industry in all categories, this book is mainly about how to advocate for curbing the practices of these two companies and their trade association, the American Beverage Association (ABA). Despite declining sales, sodas still dominate the soft drink market. Sales of diet sodas are also in sharp decline, but I will have much less to say about them, mainly because they do not contain sugars and their effects on health are less certain. And although many of the issues discussed in this book apply to sugary beverages other than sodas, I also do not say much about them even though their consumption is increasing and many of their brands are owned by Coca-Cola or PepsiCo. Despite their rising importance, their sales do not yet come close to those of these companies' flagship carbonated cola products.

A QUICK OVERVIEW

I present the material in this book in eight sections. The first (Chapters 1–3) provides the background for understanding what sodas are and why anyone should care about their effects. The second (Chapters 4–6) deals with the health implications of sodas: dietary recommendations and the research that links soda consumption to health problems. This section also includes the first of the chapters that focus on advocacy, in this instance to prevent the most widespread of soda-induced health problems—dental disease. Section Three (Chapters 7–9) introduces the soda industry, its response to the rising prevalence of obesity and diabetes, and its marketing practices. In Section Four (Chapters 10–13), I delve into the vexing issues of marketing directed at children. I present specific examples of how advocates have attempted to regulate marketing to children, remove sodas from schools, and teach kids to take matters into their own hands. Section Five (Chapters 14–16) examines the complicated history and current politics of the ways soda companies target marketing to African and Hispanic Americans and low-income groups in the United States and in the vast populations of developing countries.

In Sections Six and Seven I take on the soda industry's "softball" marketing methods, those disguised as philanthropy or social responsibility—methods similar to those used by cigarette companies to neutralize critics and keep government regulators at bay. Like cigarette companies, soda companies use corporate social responsibility to win friends and neutralize critics through "healthwashing," investment in communities, support of health professional organizations and research (Chapters 17–20), and promotion of environmental protection (Chapters 21–22).

Chapters 23 and 24 examine the industry's "hardball" tactics, those that take place behind the scenes where soda companies lobby Congress, donate to election campaigns, and use public relations and front groups to head off regulation and gain public support. The last section (Chapters 25–28) illustrates these tactics and shows how advocates are working to counter them by limiting soda portion sizes and taxing sodas in the United States and internationally.

Finally, the concluding chapter and Appendices 1 and 2 describe the groups most active in this kind of advocacy, along with the methods they have developed to achieve their goals. Neal Baer contributes an afterword explaining how to access the electronic materials he has developed to support advocacy for healthier diets.

At this point, I should say something about the notes. Because much of what I discuss in this book can be construed as critical of one or another food company or marketing practice, I provide extensive (sometimes ridiculously extensive) source notes. I do this to encourage you to do your own research and to form your own opinion of what it means. In the course of researching this book, I came across many videos, films, and other illustrative material that might prove useful to advocates. I post this material on my website, www.foodpolitics.com, on the page devoted to this book.

My hope is that *Soda Politics* will inspire you not only to reduce your own consumption of sugary drinks but also to advocate for actions and policies to promote healthier food choices for everyone. I'd like you to think of this book as a guide and set of tools for making healthier foods more available, accessible, and affordable—in the United States and through-out the world—and for connecting with others interested in pursuing the same goals.

Enjoy!

And take action.

—Marion Nestle, May 2015

What Is Soda? Why Advocacy Is Needed

1

Sodas

Inside Those Containers

In this book, I use the word *sodas* to mean carbonated, sugar-sweetened drinks, usually colas, dispensed from fountains into cups or sold in bottles, cans, or jugs. Depending on where you live, you may refer to them as pop, soda pop, fizzy drinks, or tonic, or call them by their brand nicknames—Coke or Pepsi, for example.[1] No matter what you call them, all sodas share three characteristics in common: they are carbonated, contain sugars of one kind or another, and are flavored. These features distinguish soda pop from noncarbonated but just as sugary or almost as sugary sports drinks, energy drinks, juice drinks, and waters. They also distinguish sodas from waters, flavored waters, and diet drinks that are not sugar-sweetened or that contain artificial sweeteners.

From my nutritionist's standpoint, sodas have only two ingredients that count: water and sugars. The others—sodium, caffeine, and color and flavor additives—are present in amounts too small to make much nutritional difference even when some of these chemicals occasionally raise health concerns. In the United States, the sizes of soda containers range from 7.5 to 64 ounces (2 liters), but let's begin our examination of these drinks by taking a look at the contents of 12-ounce cans of Pepsi and Coca-Cola—the standard serving size proposed for a soda by the U.S. Food and Drug Administration (FDA) in 2014.[2] These are shown in Figure 1.1.

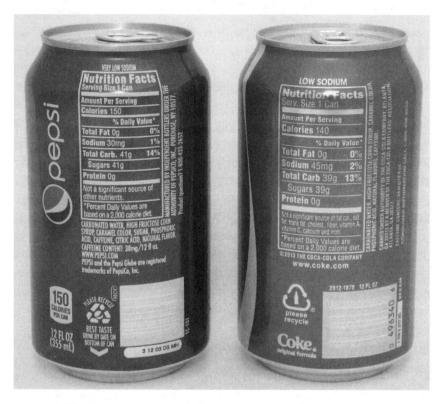

FIGURE 1.1 The Nutrition Facts panels from 12-ounce cans of regular (sugar-sweetened) Pepsi and Coke in 2014. That year, the FDA proposed to raise the standard serving size for a soft drink from 8 to 12 ounces, and to include information about added sugars on the Nutrition Facts panel. At the time this book went to press, 12 ounces meant 1.5 servings. Photo courtesy of Charles Nestle.

SODAS: NUTRITION FACTS

The Nutrition Facts portion of the label tells you how much water, sugar, sodium, and caffeine—and how many calories—these drinks contain. A 12-ounce Pepsi contains 41 grams of carbohydrates, all from sugars, and 30 milligrams of sodium. The sugars provide 150 calories. That's it. In slight contrast, a 12-ounce Coca-Cola provides 10 fewer calories, a bit less sugar (39 grams), and a bit more sodium (45 milligrams), but these differences are too small to matter much. Even 45 milligrams of sodium makes only a small contribution to diets that typically contain 3,500 milligrams a day, which is why the labels say "very low sodium."[3] Sodium is not a nutrition issue for sodas. Sugars are the issue, and a big one. A 12-ounce Coke or Pepsi contains *ten* teaspoons.

Sugars are carbohydrates. On average, each gram of carbohydrate provides 4 calories. But soda companies use the more precise 3.7 calories per gram as the basis of their calorie estimations, explaining why the 12-ounce Pepsi lists 150 calories on the label rather than 164. Yes, this minimizes the apparent calorie content, but the difference is too small to worry about. You can take the calorie numbers listed on the labels at face value.

No matter the number, soda calories—all of them from the sugars—are "empty." Beyond calories, they have no nutritional value. As I explain in Chapter 5, the health implications of sodas depend almost entirely on their sugar content. To a much smaller extent, the health effects also depend on how much caffeine the drink contains, and on what the flavoring and coloring substances might do, which takes us to considerations of the ingredient list.

SODA INGREDIENTS

Both Coca-Cola and Pepsi make a big deal about keeping the formulas for their products deep trade secrets. Historically, Coca-Cola referred to its ingredients as "merchandises." The company listed Merchandise No. 1 as sugar, No. 2 as caramel, No. 3 as caffeine, No. 4 as phosphoric acid, and No. 5 as a blend of three parts coca and one part cola. Beyond that, the historical information became vague.[4]

Today, the FDA makes keeping such secrets somewhat difficult. It requires food and beverage companies to list all ingredients on product labels in order of decreasing weight, although, as I will explain, it makes an exception for caffeine. The can of Pepsi contains, from most to least, carbonated water, high-fructose corn syrup (HFCS), caramel color, sugar, phosphoric acid, caffeine, citric acid, and natural flavor. Coca-Cola's ingredients are almost the same: carbonated water, high-fructose corn syrup, caramel color, phosphoric acid, natural flavors, and caffeine. The differences between Coke and Pepsi are mainly in the order of ingredients. Pepsi—but not Coke—lists sugar as well as HFCS; it also contains citric acid. Although the ingredients in Coke and Pepsi have not changed much for a century or more, nearly everything in them has caused controversy at one time or another, some ingredients quite recently. Let's take a look at the ingredients, starting from the top.

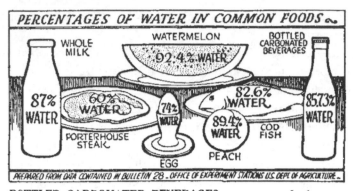

PERCENTAGES OF WATER IN COMMON FOODS

BOTTLED CARBONATED BEVERAGES are composed of sugar, plus pure flavoring ingredients, plus carbonated water. Nearly all foods contain high percentages of water as shown in chart.

FIGURE 1.2 Percentages of water in common foods, 1950. Then, sodas were 85.73 percent water. If so, they must have been sweeter than they are now. Current USDA food composition figures show colas to be 89.62 percent water. The illustration is from *Food and Nutritional Values of Carbonated Beverages, 1950*, a pamphlet produced by the American Bottlers of Carbonated Beverages, the forerunner of today's American Beverage Association.

Carbonated Water

Carbonated water, according to Coca-Cola, is "water with carbon dioxide bubbles added to provide fun and refreshment," and many people do enjoy the feel and "bite" of carbonation. Water comes first on the list because, as the soda industry has long explained (Figure 1.2), its products—like many foods—are mostly water.[5]

Sugars: High-Fructose Corn Syrup and Sucrose

In both Coke and Pepsi, the sugars largely come from HFCS. American sodas used to be sweetened entirely with sucrose from cane or beet sugar. In some countries, like Mexico, they still are, although bottlers even in that country are increasingly replacing sucrose with the less expensive HFCS.[6] For political reasons, the European Union favors sucrose. Its countries grow sugar beets rather than corn, and several of its former colonies grow sugar cane.

In the 1970s, U.S. corn refiners developed HFCS as a cheaper alternative to cane and beet sugars. Coca-Cola permitted HFCS to be used in all of its products—except classic Coke—beginning in 1974, but did not actually use much until 1981, when Congress raised the minimum price for sugar as part of its support program for domestic producers of sugar cane and sugar beets. Federal quotas and tariffs pushed the price of cane and beet sugar above that of world market levels, whereas subsidies on corn reduced the price of HFCS.[7] The result was that cane and beet sugar became three times more expensive than HFCS. To save on costs, Coca-Cola authorized the use of corn sweeteners in about 75 percent of its products. Pepsi did too and allowed HFCS to replace up to 50 percent of the sugars in bottled and canned drinks, and up to 80 percent in fountain drinks.

Sales did not suffer. On the contrary, blind taste tests proved that few soda drinkers could tell whether a soda was made with HFCS or sucrose. On that basis, both companies went 100 percent HFCS in 1984. At the time, business analysts estimated that the switch would save Coke about $28 million annually and Pepsi about $60 million.[8]

By the early 2000s, however, the public had begun to associate HFCS with cheap food and to view it as less desirable than sucrose. Because corn crops were increasingly diverted to production of ethanol fuels, the price differential between HFCS and sucrose narrowed. When Pepsi announced in 2014 that it was replacing HFCS with "real sugar" in some of its products, this move was widely understood as a strategy to reverse declining soda sales.[9]

One reason why the drinks taste much the same is that sucrose and HFCS contain the same two sugars—glucose and fructose—in similar amounts, even though the sweeteners are produced from different crops using different methods. Sucrose is extracted and crystallized from watery extracts—the "juice"—of sugar cane and sugar beets. It is a double sugar: its glucose and fructose are held together by chemical bonds that must be split by an enzyme before they can be used in the body, an action that happens quickly in the small intestine.

In contrast, corn refiners make HFCS by extracting the starch from field corn and treating it with enzymes to release glucose. They use other enzymes to convert about half the glucose to fructose. The result is liquid syrup containing the two single sugars in the proportion 45 percent glucose and 55 percent fructose, although the fructose percentage can be higher in some drinks.[10] In slight contrast, sucrose is always 50 percent glucose and 50 percent fructose. Whether the difference in the percentage of glucose and fructose has any biological significance is a matter of some debate, but for the purposes of this discussion I think we can consider the two sources of glucose and fructose to be roughly equivalent.

The trade associations that represent these sweeteners, however, strongly disagree with this view. The Sugar Association represents producers of cane and beet sugar. It insists that the singular noun *sugar* should refer *only* to sucrose. Indeed, when you see sugar mentioned halfway down the Pepsi ingredient list, it means sucrose. But the Corn Refiners Association, which represents HFCS producers, wishes that you would call its product "corn sugar." Never mind. Sucrose and HFCS are both sources of the sugars (plural) glucose and fructose. These sugars, whether from sucrose, HFCS, or both, are present in sodas at a concentration of ten teaspoons per 12-ounce drink, meaning that every ounce of soda contains just under a teaspoon of a mixture of glucose and fructose sugars.

Let's pause and consider what it means to put ten teaspoons of sugar into a 12-ounce drink. You can do the experiment at home. Measure 12 ounces of water into a glass. Now add ten teaspoons of table sugar or ten restaurant sugar packets or cubes to the water, one at a time. Stir until dissolved. Drink. The purpose of the other soda ingredients now becomes clear: they are there to mask the cloying sweetness.

Caramel Color

Pepsi says it adds this coloring agent "to correct natural variations in the color of our ingredients or simply to make our products more appealing or fun." Coca-Cola helpfully explains that the caramel color "is made by a process involving the heating of corn or cane sugar and other carbohydrates to achieve the desired color."[11] Nobody worried much about caramel color until someone noticed that producing it in the presence of ammonia creates a potential carcinogen, 4-methylimidazole (4-MeI). Advocates petitioned soda companies to eliminate this chemical.

When testing showed that amounts of 4-MeI exceeded California's strict standards for carcinogens, Coca-Cola completely switched to another process. Pepsi also made the switch, but only in California. As companies often do in such situations, Pepsi said that "the safety of our products is PepsiCo's top priority" and "we abide by the regulatory guidelines everywhere we do business." It promised to meet California standards throughout the rest of its supply chain by February 2014. That month, however, testing by *Consumer Reports* identified high levels of 4-MeI in Pepsi One (a diet drink), although levels in the sugar-sweetened drinks were low or undetectable. *Consumer Reports* continued to pressure soda companies to remove 4-MeI from caramel color, as did class-action lawsuits, and the companies promised to comply with California's standards, although they did not say by when.[12] When they finally do, chalk this up as a victory for advocates.

The Minor Ingredients

To end any speculation: you do not see cocaine listed as an ingredient in Coke and Pepsi because neither drink has any. Coca leaves, which contain cocaine, were basic ingredients in the original Coca-Cola, but the company now processes out all traces of the drug and has done so for more than a century.[13] Let's move right along to the other, perhaps less interesting ingredients.

Phosphoric and citric acids

The acids reduce microbial growth and impart a tangy flavor made even more pleasurable by the addition of all that sugar. These functions, according to the litigious, make phosphoric and citric acids undisclosed flavoring and preservative agents. A class-action lawsuit filed in 2014 argues that Coca-Cola is illegally misbranded because it neither identifies the function of phosphoric acid on its label nor discloses the presence of chemical preservatives.[14] I leave it to the courts to decide this case, viewing issues related to other ingredients as worth more attention. Consider caffeine, for example.

Caffeine

The FDA does not require soda companies to list caffeine or its amounts on labels, but both Coca-Cola and PepsiCo have done so voluntarily since 2007. Twelve ounces of Pepsi and Coca-Cola contain 38 and 34 milligrams of caffeine, respectively. These amounts are low. To reach the 100 to 200 mg of caffeine in one typical cup of coffee, you would have to drink three to six cans.

The caffeine is low for a reason. The historian of caffeine Murray Carpenter argues that once the cocaine was out, caffeine became the entire point of sodas. In 1909, Coca-Cola contained three times as much caffeine as it now has—120 milligrams in 12 ounces—making these sodas "high technology caffeine delivery systems more than enough to create and sustain addiction in people who drink them regularly."[15] Whether today's lower amounts do so is debatable.

A century ago, the idea that so much caffeine might be consumed by children troubled Harvey Wiley, then head of the USDA's Bureau of Chemistry, the forerunner of today's FDA. Wiley thought Coca-Cola promoted addiction, undermined moral fiber, and ruined health. Adding caffeine to cola drinks, he said, constituted adulteration and violated the Pure Food and Drug Act of 1906. He took the company to court. Coca-Cola's defense? Caffeine was not an "additive"; it was an *essential* component of the drink. The case dragged on for nine years but was settled when Coca-Cola agreed to reduce the amount of caffeine to about its present level. Using the same logic, Coca-Cola also headed off congressional efforts to require caffeine to be listed on food labels.[16]

Attempts to require caffeine labeling continued throughout the twentieth century, but company lobbying succeeded in blocking them. In 1958, soda companies induced the FDA to declare the amounts of caffeine in soft drinks as generally recognized as safe (GRAS). When, in the early 2000s, some beverage companies began adding much more caffeine to energy and sports drinks, consumer groups petitioned the FDA to require caffeine labeling. The American Academy of Pediatrics, alarmed by the possibility that high levels of caffeine could cause physical and psychological harm, warned that caffeine and other stimulants in energy drinks have no place in the diets of children and adolescents. It advised physicians and parents to discourage consumption of any level of caffeine by children. To stave off further demands for regulation, soda companies volunteered to label caffeine as an ingredient and to state the amount they were adding to drinks.[17]

Natural flavors

These, of course, are the big trade secrets. All Coke will say is that the flavors "are derived from the essential oils or extracts of spices, fruits, vegetables and herbs." Mark Pendergrast's history of the company, *For God, Country, and Coca-Cola*, provides a recipe for the "sacred formula" based on personal records of Coca-Cola's inventor, John Pemberton. Bob Stoddard's official history of Pepsi reproduces a letter revealing the formula that had been submitted during the company's 1923 bankruptcy proceedings.[18] Internet sites also give versions. Nearly all list tiny amounts of a fluid extract of leaves of the coca plant, citric acid, lime juice, vanilla, and alcohol extracts of the oils of orange, lemon, nutmeg, cinnamon, coriander, neroli (bitter orange), and cinnamon. Given that the amounts of flavoring agents are so small, the secret recipes don't appear to differ much.

In short, with only small differences, Coke, Pepsi, and other cola sodas contain much the same ingredients, are virtually identical products, and can be lumped together for the purposes of this book.

BUT SURELY COKE AND PEPSI DON'T TASTE THE SAME?

I can hear your objections. You insist you can taste the difference between Coke and Pepsi, so much so that you greatly prefer (fill in the blank). Much as soda companies wish this were true, hardly anyone can tell Coke and Pepsi apart in blind taste tests. This is so easy to prove that even junior high school students can do it, as I described in my book *Food Politics*. As a science fair project, the eighth-grade daughter of some friends of mine asked her classmates to say whether they preferred Coke, Pepsi, or a store brand of cola. About half said they preferred Pepsi and the other half said they preferred Coke. None picked the store brand. Then she asked them to taste the three colas in unmarked cups. Many preferred the store brand, and hardly any could identify the cola they said they preferred. You are still skeptical? More sophisticated tests using brain scans to evaluate taste preferences come to the same conclusion. Brain scans also demonstrate that the most important factors in cola taste perception are the package type (cans hold the carbonation better) and the brand. If you are convinced that you prefer one over the other, you tend to like it better.[19]

To repeat: Coke and Pepsi are, for all practical purposes, virtually identical products. Or, as has been remarked since the 1950s, "the plural of Coca-Cola is Pepsi-Cola."[20] The two drinks have roughly the same sugar content, calories, ingredients, and flavor profile. The only difference that matters is that they are made by different companies with different brand names, corporate cultures, and marketing practices. Otherwise, they are two sides of the same coin—sodas.

Fountain Drinks: Pouring Money

Soda fountains were a quintessential part of the American landscape from the 1800s on, when they became ubiquitous parts of drugstores, ice cream parlors, department stores, and train stations. They evolved as community centers where neighbors could meet, parents could take children, and young people could flirt. Soda fountains began to disappear in the 1950s

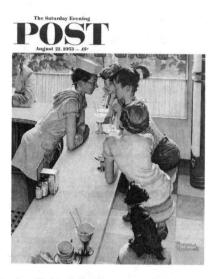

FIGURE 1.3 Norman Rockwell's "Soda Jerk" cover to the August 22, 1953, *Saturday Evening Post*. Soda fountains were centers of community life, not least for teenagers. In the 1960s, they were the sites of the lunch counter sit-ins that sparked the civil rights movement (see Chapter 14). Illustration provided by SEPS. All rights reserved.

with the advent of full-service drugstores and the increased ownership of personal automobiles. Their last vestiges remain in gas stations, movie theaters, and restaurants. Today they evoke nostalgia for an earlier era in American life, as Figure 1.3 recalls.

Until now, we have been talking about the nutritional implications of soft drinks based on package labels. But the sodas you buy in movie theaters do not carry Nutrition Facts labels. They are drinks delivered from "soft-drink dispensing systems," mixed on-site and poured over ice into cups of various sizes. The more ice, the less of both the sugars and the calories. Ice pleases nutritionists, but it also pleases soda sellers. The flavored syrup is their most expensive ingredient. Ice dilutes the ingredients and reduces the cost of the drinks.

Fountain drinks begin with deliveries of carbon dioxide cylinders and "bag-in-the-box" containers of flavored syrup. These vary according to the size of the dispenser and the volume of sales. In general, the dispensing machines work like this:

- A carbonator blows carbon dioxide into tap water to produce carbonated water.

- A refrigeration unit cools the carbonated water on its way to the dispensing valve.
- The refrigeration unit also cools the syrup.
- The dispensing valve mixes the carbonated water and syrup in the correct proportions and delivers the drink at a temperature equal to or less than 40°F.[21]

Next comes the ice. Ice performs four critical functions: it chills the drink, improves the taste, dilutes the ingredients, and reduces the retailer's cost. If you pack ice to the brim, less than half the volume of your drink comes from the soda mix.[22]

All of this makes fountain sodas famously profitable. According to one industry source, the flavored syrup cost retailers a bit more than 30 cents for each 16-ounce drink in 2012. The carbon dioxide costs less than 1 cent per serving. But all this is *before* the addition of ice. Once ice is added, these ingredients are so diluted that the final cost of fountain drinks to the seller— including the cup, lid, and straw—comes to just over 1 cent per ounce.[23] This explains why many places are so generous with free refills. Even though refills usually have less ice than the initial drink and end up costing the seller more, they are still highly profitable. Convenience stores, restaurants, sports facilities, and movie theaters make so much money on fountain sodas that they can well be generous: a typical return is more than 80 cents on the dollar.

DIET SODAS

Before moving on to dealing with sugar-sweetened sodas and what to do about them, I had best make a few comments about diet drinks. These are carbonated but contain no sugars. Instead, they are artificially sweetened with aspartame, acesulfame K (potassium), sucralose, stevia, or other non-nutritive chemicals. Because they are sugar-free, diet sodas provide no or very few calories.

The FDA says all non-nutritive sweeteners are safe at current levels of use, particularly when consumed, as they usually are, in extremely small amounts. Others disagree and argue that frequent consumption fools the body into behaving as if it were dealing with sugars, inappropriately stimulates insulin release, and raises the risk of obesity and type 2 diabetes.

At least one study suggests that several kinds of artificial sweeteners alter the microbial composition of the mouse and human intestinal tracts in ways—as yet unexplained—that promote glucose intolerance. These contentions remain to be confirmed by further research. What is thoroughly evident, however, is that diet drinks do not help most people control weight, perhaps because it is so easy to compensate for reduced calories by eating more food.[24]

Nevertheless, soda companies view diet drinks as an important strategy for sales growth. In 2005, as part of a deliberate effort to appeal to male customers, Coca-Cola introduced Coca-Cola Zero ("zero calories, zero carbs, zero sugar, zero color, and zero caffeine") in a rugged-looking black can. PepsiCo introduced Sierra Mist Free. Both are sweetened with aspartame and acesulfame K.[25] In part because of the introduction and marketing of these products, diet sodas now account for 30 percent of carbonated soft drink sales in the United States, considerably more than in most other countries. Even so, as discussed in later chapters, their U.S. sales are declining, and so are sales in other countries.

This book is mainly devoted to health and advocacy issues related to the remaining 70 percent—sugar-sweetened or "regular" sodas. The sugars and other ingredients in sodas would be of little interest if nobody consumed more than the standard 12 ounces or so per week. But, as Chapter 2 explains, moderation is not a term that applies to many soda drinkers.

2

Soda Drinkers

Facts and Figures

If sodas were an occasional treat, I would not be writing this book. But they are produced, sold, and consumed in vast quantities. How vast? To decide whether soda drinking is a problem and, if so, how much of a problem, you need to know the average amount consumed, how much is consumed by men, women, and children of different ages, and the proportion of light and heavy soda drinkers, both in the United States and throughout the world.

How I wish I could push a button and have this information instantly available, preferably in understandable units of 12-ounce servings. No such luck. Getting reliable and useful data on soda consumption takes effort, time, a calculator, and sometimes money. The difficulty of getting this information is a story in itself. This chapter is about how much soda is consumed by whom, and how such information is known. Bear with me as I walk you through all this.

Sodas are manufactured, sold, and consumed. Not all of those produced are necessarily sold, and sodas that are sold may not be completely consumed. But for such information, only two sources of data exist: industry and government. The industry provides numbers on soda *production* and assumes that production equals sales. Government surveys give numbers for amounts reported as *consumed* by individuals. Both data sets are frustratingly difficult to interpret, not least because they—and the graphs and tables derived from them—are presented inconsistently in units of gallons, liters, or cases of 8-ounce servings per population or individual, per day or per year.

The soda industry considers its production figures to be proprietary and does not share them with government agencies or make them public. I bought one industry research report and have access to others at university libraries. These reports provide equally inconsistent numbers, sometimes for the same item. They also do not consistently distinguish between carbonated and noncarbonated beverages, colas and non-colas, sugar-sweetened and diet sodas, or those sold in bottles, in cans, or from fountains. I did the best I could with all of this, but you cannot take the numbers presented here too literally. They are best considered approximations.

The complexity of the soda retail market explains some of the inconsistencies. Sodas are sold in multiple locations, which the industry divides into two categories, unhelpfully called "scanner" (or "off-trade") and "non-scanner" (or "on-trade"). Scanner/off-trade channels are large grocery chains, drugstores, and mass merchandise retail stores—except for Walmart. These account for about 35 percent of total soda sales. Non-scanner/on-trade channels account for the 65 percent majority and include food service, vending machines, convenience stores, and gas stations, as well as Walmart—on its own, the largest single source of U.S. soda sales.

I soon gave up on finding reliable sales figures, although occasionally they are reported by brand, making it possible to create illustrations such as the clever one shown in Figure 2.1.[1] The soda industry is able to control inventory so tightly that it sells virtually all of what it produces. It considers production and sales to be equivalent. You and I might as well do the same.

Production or sales figures are often used as proxies for consumption, but both overestimate intake. People do not always finish their drinks, and some soda is undoubtedly wasted or thrown away. In contrast, dietary surveys invariably underestimate soda intake. Even the most carefully conducted survey depends on self-reports from individuals who may not be able to recall precisely how much soda they consume, especially from fountain drinks. This makes production data better to use for estimating the amount of soda available and for following trends. On the other hand, dietary intake data work better for answering questions about who drinks sodas. Let's start with production figures for the United States.

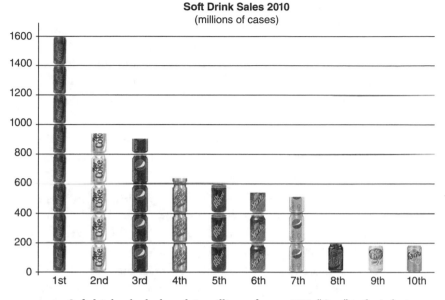

FIGURE 2.1 Soft drink sales by brand, in millions of cases, 2010. "Case" is the industry term for twenty-four 8-ounce cans or bottles (the volume equivalent of sixteen 12-ounce servings). Coca-Cola leads soda sales by a substantial margin. Sales of Diet Coke surpassed Pepsi for the first time in 2010 but again fell to third place in 2015. The chart is by TimWit, based on figures from *Beverage Digest*, posted at timwit.wordprcss.com on March 25, 2011. Used with TimWit's permission.

SODA PRODUCTION: UNITED STATES

Here is one reason the "how much" question is so hard to answer. Every year, from 1947 until 2003, the USDA published estimates of the number of gallons of carbonated soft drinks—total, regular (sugar-sweetened), and diet—available for consumption per capita. These estimates were averages. They applied to everyone in the population regardless of age, from newborn babies to the oldest old, no matter how much soda anyone actually consumed. To obtain these numbers, the USDA took data from industry sources on billions of gallons of soda produced and divided this number by the population of the United States on July 1. Because the USDA collected and dealt with this information every year in the same way, its numbers revealed trends in production and gave an authoritative estimate of the maximum volume of carbonated beverages available for consumption by the population.

But this data set stops cold in 2003. After that, the Beverage Marketing Corporation (BMC), the industry trade association that used to give this information to the USDA, refused to allow its proprietary data to be released to the public. This forced the USDA to discontinue its historical data set.[2] The BMC, however, still publishes the figures annually. With the help of a small grant, I bought its 2013 report on carbonated beverages—at the discounted cost to academics of $5,795.

The report provides tables that list annual production from 1984 to 2012—in billions of gallons—of total, regular, and diet sodas.[3] Based on these tables, Figure 2.2 illustrates the trends.

Soda production—for both regular and diet drinks—increased rapidly from the early 1980s to the early 2000s, leveled off, and then declined. I show Figure 2.2 to illustrate such trends, but also to emphasize the enormous amount of sugar-sweetened soda produced in the United States. Even with the decline, more than 9 billion gallons—meaning more than 95 billion 12-ounce servings—were available for consumption and, presumably, consumed by Americans in 2012.

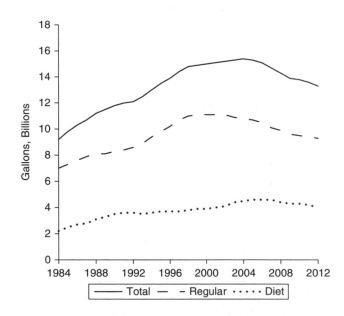

FIGURE 2.2 Trends in production of total, diet, and regular (sugar-sweetened) carbonated soft drinks, United States, 1984 to 2012, in billions of gallons. A gallon is nearly 11 (10.7) 12-ounce servings. Data are from Beverage Marketing Corporation, *Carbonated Soft Drinks in the U.S.*, 2013: Exhibit 3.20.

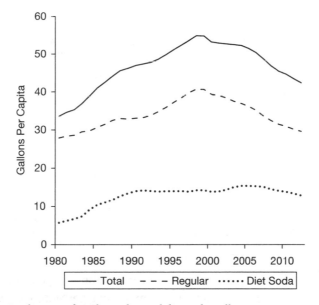

FIGURE 2.3 Production of total, regular, and diet soda, gallons per capita, 1980 to 2012, United States. Data are from Beverage Marketing Corporation, *Carbonated Soft Drinks in the U.S.*, 2013: Exhibits 1.2 and 3.20.

Translating soda production into the amounts available per capita—per person, regardless of age or consumption patterns—requires dividing the billions of gallons produced by Census Bureau estimates of the U.S. population on July 1 of each year. The population on July 1, 2012, for example, was 313.9 million. By using other tables in the report, I could calculate per capita production of regular and diet sodas from 1980 to 2012, as shown in Figure 2.3.[4]

Peak soda production occurred in the late 1990s and in total amounted to more than 50 gallons a year per capita, of which nearly 40 gallons were sugar-sweetened. Since then, production of both regular and diet sodas has declined. In 2012, companies produced enough regular soda to supply every single person in America, regardless of age, with nearly 30 gallons for the year—a decline of about 20 percent since the peak year.

Drawing on all sources available, we can look at longer-term trends. In Table 2.1, I show per capita production of total, diet, and regular sodas at ten-year intervals from 1952 to 2012, and translate regular sodas into units of 12-ounce servings.

The table shows that per capita production of carbonated soft drinks—regular plus diet—rose from 11.5 gallons in 1952 to 42.4 gallons in 2012. In

TABLE 2.1 Production of sodas per capita, 1952 to 2012*

YEAR	TOTAL, GALLONS	DIET, GALLONS	REGULAR, GALLONS	REGULAR, 12-OUNCE SERVINGS PER YEAR
1952	11.5	0	11.5	123
1962	15.1	0.7	14.5	155
1972	26.2	2.3	23.9	256
1982	35.3	5.5	29.8	319
1992	47.8	14.0	33.8	362
2002	52.7	14.4	38.4	411
2012	42.4	12.8	29.6	317

* Data from 1952 to 1982 are from USDA. Later amounts are from the 2013 Beverage Marketing Corporation report, but the two data sets do not overlap consistently. One gallon provides nearly 11 (10.7) 12-ounce servings.

1952, all sodas were sugar-sweetened. Once diet sodas were invented in the early 1960s, they began to account for an increasing percentage of the total—at least 25 percent since 1985, and at least 30 percent since 2005. The peak year for diet soda production occurred in 2006—15.3 gallons per capita. Since then, production of diet sodas has declined and continues to decline in a trend widely attributed to health concerns about artificial sweeteners.[5]

But for the purposes of this book, it's the regular sodas that count. In 1952, manufacturers produced the equivalent of 123 standard 12-ounce servings per capita, or about 4 ounces of soda per capita per day. According to the 2013 Beverage Marketing Corporation report, per capita production of regular sodas reached its highest level in 1998—40.7 gallons (not shown in table). This came to 434 standard 12-ounce servings, or 14 ounces per day. But by 2012, production had declined to the 317 standard 12-ounce servings of regular sodas shown in the table. These numbers, the best I can find, indicate that production of sugar-sweetened sodas amounted to about 10 ounces per capita per day in 2012, a decline of 4 ounces since 1998.

If you will grant me a slight exaggeration, we can assume that enough sugary soda is produced in America to provide every person—from newborn babies to the oldest old—with about one 12-ounce can or bottle every day.

Chalk up the decline since the late 1990s to effective health advocacy. Health-conscious Americans have increasingly replaced sugary drinks with less sugary sports drinks and bottled water, as shown in Figure 2.4. While one regular soda a day may not sound like much, it is still more than twice

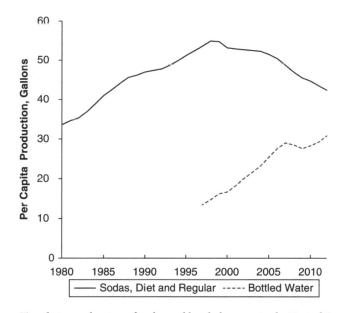

FIGURE 2.4 Trends in production of sodas and bottled waters in the United States, 1980 to 2012, gallons per capita. Total sodas include both regular and diet. The proportion of diet sodas ranged from 25 percent to 30 percent during this period. A gallon is nearly 11 (10.7) 12-ounce servings. Data are from Beverage Marketing Corporation, *Carbonated Soft Drinks in the U.S.*, 2013.

the amount in the 1950s and 1960s. And even the more precise 10 daily ounces represents the average consumption of children and adults. The intake of individuals may range from no soda at all to liters a day.

SODA PRODUCTION: INTERNATIONAL

The decline in sales in the United States has induced soda companies to turn their attention to international markets. For international production figures, we must go to yet another data source, Euromonitor International.[6] This research firm collects beverage production figures from companies in many countries throughout the world. It reports amounts in liters. Since all of the numbers are estimates anyway, let's round them off.

- One gallon is nearly 4 liters (3.8, actually).
- One liter is nearly 34 ounces (33.8, actually).

TABLE 2.2 Total sodas (regular plus diet) sold in selected
countries and percent diet soda, 2012

COUNTRY	TOTAL SODA, LITERS PER CAPITA[a]	PERCENT DIET SODA[b]
U.S.A.	160	20[c]
Argentina	145	15
Mexico	142	7
Norway	101	33
Germany	97	23
Australia	93	24
Saudi Arabia	87	4
United Kingdom	81	29
Bulgaria	74	3
Venezuela	63	2
Japan	34	18
Egypt	20	3
China	9	2
Indonesia	4	5
India	3	1

[a] Liters per capita are from Euromonitor International, 2013, rounded off. A
liter is nearly 3 (2.8) 12-ounce servings.
[b] Estimates of percent diet sodas are from Credit Suisse, 2013.
[c] The Credit Suisse estimate for diet soda in the United States is 10 percent
below that reported by the Beverage Marketing Corporation, for unknown
reasons.

Euromonitor reports that the soda industry produced 220 billion liters
of carbonated beverages, diet and regular, throughout the world in 2012.
The world's population reached 7 billion that year, giving about 31 liters per
person. This translates to 87 standard 12-ounce servings per capita, an
amount that includes *both* sugar-sweetened and diet drinks. But, according
to Euromonitor, diet drinks account for 21 percent of total worldwide soda
production. Therefore, the average production of regular soda is 69 standard 12-ounce servings per capita per year for the entire world. Another
source, the banking firm Credit Suisse, has published estimates of the percentage of diet drinks sold and consumed in various countries. As might be
expected, the percentages vary widely from country to country, from about
1 percent in India to 33 percent in Norway.[7] Table 2.2 gives some examples.

The United States leads the world in total soda sales, followed by Argentina, Mexico, Norway, and Germany. But because the percentage of diet
sodas sold in various countries differs so widely, I thought it would help to
calculate the amounts for regular sodas, and to translate those figures into
12-ounce servings per person, as shown in Table 2.3.

TABLE 2.3 Regular sodas available for consumption in selected countries, 12-ounce servings per capita, 2012*

COUNTRY	REGULAR SODA, 12-OUNCE SERVINGS PER CAPITA
Mexico	372
United States	360
Argentina	347
Saudi Arabia	235
Germany	211
Bulgaria	202
Australia	199
Norway	191
United Kingdom	185
Venezuela	123
Japan	79
Egypt	56
China	24
Indonesia	10
India	9

* Figures in this table are calculated from the percentages of diet sodas in Table 2.2. If, as reported by the Beverage Marketing Corporation, diet sodas actually account for 30 percent of U.S. production, the number of regular soda servings for the United States would be 315, which is close to the 317 shown in Table 2.1.

When it comes to regular sodas, Mexico beats the United States with an average availability of more than one 12-ounce serving a day. U.S. residents have access to slightly less than one 12-ounce daily serving per capita. Next come consumers in Argentina, Saudi Arabia, and Germany. As a general rule, soda sales closely follow economic development and higher income, but some countries, such as Mexico and Argentina, consume more than expected, as does the United States.[8] Figure 2.5 shows this relationship. More soda is consumed in industrialized countries, and less in those that are resource-poor. The Chinese, for example, have access to just 24 standard 12-ounce servings per year, while even less is available to the population of India (9 per year). Mexico and Argentina are outliers: they are relatively low-income countries with high soda sales. In contrast, several relatively wealthy countries in Asia have very low soda sales. These low numbers— and their sharp contrast with the much higher amounts available in Mexico and Argentina—make it clear why developing countries in Asia, the Indian subcontinent, and Africa are prime targets for expansion of soda marketing, as I discuss in Chapter 15.

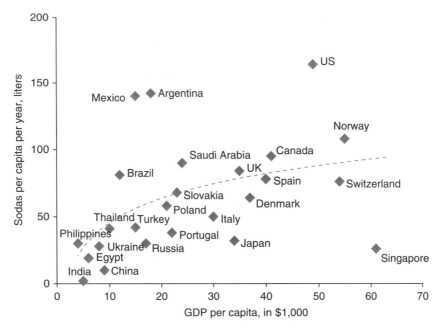

FIGURE 2.5 Annual global soda production versus gross domestic product (GDP). The GDP is an index of economic development. The dotted line gives an approximate estimation of the trend toward higher soda production with higher economic development. The figure is based on data from a report from the Credit Suisse Research Institute, *Sugar Consumption at a Crossroads*, September 2013.

SODAS CONSUMED

In contrast to production figures, those for dietary intake depend on self-reports from individuals. To assess your soda intake, a researcher might ask you to record or recall what you ate or drank, usually during one 24-hour period. Such methods are famously inaccurate. Consciously or unconsciously, almost everyone overreports consumption of healthier foods and underreports foods thought to be less healthful, and hardly anyone can correctly recall or estimate portion sizes. As a result, dietary records typically underreport amounts actually consumed, often by a factor of 30 to 40 percent.[9]

To repeat: the production of regular sodas in the United States is about one 12-ounce serving per person per day. This estimate is for the entire population and includes individuals who never drink sodas. For people who do drink sodas, the production numbers seriously underestimate actual intake.

In the United States, information on self-reported dietary intake comes from the ongoing National Health and Nutrition Examination Surveys (NHANES), conducted by the Centers for Disease Control and Prevention (CDC). Since the 1970s, these surveys have used trained interviewers to do in-person interviews with a statistically representative sample of the population and ask probing, cross-cutting questions about eating, drinking, and other health habits. Government and private researchers analyze the responses. They too are interested in how consumption of sugary drinks might affect health. Researchers analyzing NHANES data have come to several reasonably consistent conclusions.[10]

The first conclusion: only half the population drinks sodas on any given day. Of NHANES respondents who do report drinking sodas, one-quarter say they drink more than one 12-ounce cola a day, one-fifth report drinking more than four a day, and 5 percent say they drink even more. Figure 2.6 illustrates the overall distribution of soda intake.[11]

Another conclusion: children drink sodas from a remarkably early age, as shown in Table 2.4. Even very young children are given measurable amounts of soda to drink. Calories from sugary drinks increase with age during childhood, whereas those from chocolate milk decrease. Sodas account for an increasing proportion of sugary drink calories. Children ages 2–5, 6–11, and 12–19 are reported to consume 2, 5, and 12 ounces a day, respectively. High as these amounts may seem, they are likely to be underestimated. By one analysis, 5 percent of young children, 16 percent of adolescents, and 20 percent of young adults consume more than 500 calories a day from sodas (the equivalent of about 40 ounces).[12]

As for adults, those who report drinking sodas say they consume an average of 155 calories a day from that source—the equivalent of about 13 ounces. This is only slightly more than the average production figure. But if only half the population drinks sodas, this amount is also grossly underestimated.[13]

All age groups report drinking less soda now than they did in the late 1990s, a trend that reflects replacement of carbonated, sugar-sweetened sodas with sports drinks, teas, diet drinks, and bottled waters. This means that sugar consumption from sodas has also gone down. Even so, the combined category of sodas, energy drinks, and sports drinks continues to be the fourth-leading source of total calories in the diets of adults, and the third-leading calorie source for children.[14]

The calories in sodas come from the sugars. According to the surveys, sodas alone account for one-third of total sugar intake. When you add in

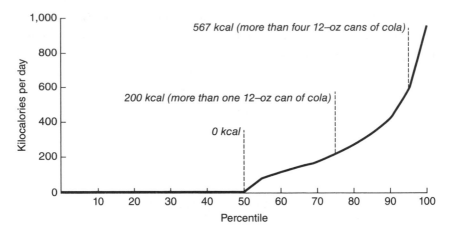

FIGURE 2.6 Percent of Americans, age 2 and over, who report consuming sugar-sweetened cola drinks. Half the population reports consuming none at all on any given day. But 10 percent report consuming more than four 12-ounce colas a day, for a total of 567 soda calories. Source: National Center for Health Statistics, 2011.

TABLE 2.4 Calories consumed by American children from sugary drinks and sodas, 2005–2008

AGE RANGE	ALL SUGARY DRINKS	SODAS	FRUIT DRINKS	FLAVORED MILK	OTHER*
2–5	91	25	40	21	5
6–11	157	66	55	22	14
12–19	245	145	49	7	44

* Energy and sports drinks and sweetened teas

sweetened juice drinks, teas, coffees, and milk, sugary drinks account for fully half of all sugar intake. The conclusion is inescapable: some segments of the population, children and adults, consume far more soda and other sugar-sweetened beverages than can possibly be good for their health.

But which segments? Researchers can mine NHANES demographic data to find out who drinks sodas and how much. Health advocates need this information as a basis for designing policy and program interventions. But the soda industry also wants this kind of information as a basis for creating advertising messages. To that end, the Beverage Marketing Corporation collects information about soda consumers from its own sources. In this instance, the information from government, academic, and industry

TABLE 2.5 Demographic characteristics of regular (sugar-sweetened) soda consumers, by index (consumption relative to average)*

POPULATION SEGMENT	DEMOGRAPHIC INDEX
Adults	
Males	106
Females	94
Age	
18–24	124
45–54	95
65+	79
Marital status	
Single	114
Married or partnered	95
Education	
Some high school	118
Graduated from college	83
Income, per year	
< $10,000	116
> $75,000	88
Occupation	
Blue collar	115
White collar	95
Ethnicity	
Hispanic	121
African-American	113
White	94
Asian	89
Region	
South	108
Midwest	101
West	99
Northeast	86

* Examples: an index of 115 indicates a 15 percent greater-than-average likelihood of consuming regular sodas. An index of 88 indicates 12 percent less likelihood. Data are from Beverage Marketing Corporation, Carbonated Beverages in the U.S., 2013: adapted from Exhibit 13.

sources is similar. I particularly like the way the Beverage Marketing Corporation summarizes its findings in a "demographic index." The corporation defines average soda intake in the overall population as an index of 100. Higher-than-average soda consumption gives an index higher than 100. An index below 100 indicates lower-than-average consumption. Table 2.5 summarizes some of these results.

From Table 2.5, we can see that the soda-drinking half of the population is more likely to be male, young, single, poorly educated, low-income, blue-collar, Hispanic or African American, and living in the South or Midwest. Data from the CDC's Behavioral Risk Factor Surveillance System confirm these observations. Let me add one more comparison based on NHANES observations: soda drinkers are also slightly more likely to be overweight.[15]

In contrast, the half of the population that does not drink sodas is more likely to be female, older, married or partnered, educated, higher-income, white-collar, white or Asian, living in the West or Northeast, and of normal weight.

Soda drinking, therefore, is an indicator of class and hence of socioeconomic and educational inequities. Consuming sugary drinks may be a health issue, but it is an issue complicated by class, race, and ethnicity. It is also complicated by soda industry marketing targeted specifically to low-income and minority groups, as I discuss in later chapters.

Is soda drinking a problem? For heavy users, it most definitely is. Soda drinkers are precisely the groups most at risk for obesity and the other health conditions covered in Chapter 5. But before we get to that, let's take a closer look at the main causes of the health effects: the sugars and calories in sodas.

3

The Sugar(s) Problem

More Facts and Figures

Sugars are the most important ingredient in sodas. They are the source of its calories and most of the nutritional concerns. I use the plural, *sugars*, because sodas are made with sucrose, common table sugar, but also with high-fructose corn syrup (HFCS). Both are at the forefront of current health debates. On one extreme are the people who view sugars as toxic, addictive, and directly responsible for obesity, type 2 diabetes, and numerous other health conditions. On the other are those who believe that sugars are harmless, natural, and healthful, and that they greatly add to the pleasure of eating. The truth, as is often the case with nutrition issues, lies someplace in between. Sugar is neither a poison nor entirely harmless. Because its effects depend on how much is consumed, this particular debate is not easily resolved. Sugars are indeed delicious, and even their severest critics are not concerned about small amounts. But as we saw in the previous chapter, many children and adults consume far more sugar than is recommended, much of it from sodas and other sugary drinks. Here let's examine the ways in which the sugars in sodas might affect health: their amounts, but also their calories, liquid form, content of HFCS, content of fructose, and what happens when they are accompanied by caffeine and flavoring ingredients. This chapter focuses specifically on sugars. Chapter 5 takes up the closely related matter of how sugar-sweetened beverages specifically affect health.

Let me begin with some basic observations. A substantial body of research correlates excessive consumption of sugars—of any type and from any source—to obesity. Cutting down on sugar is associated with a decrease in body weight. Eating more sugar is associated with weight gain. Excessive sugar intake, either mediated through overweight and obesity or perhaps on its own, is linked to a higher risk for type 2 diabetes, heart disease, stroke, and other such conditions.[1]

At issue is the meaning of "excessive." In the United States, children are said to consume an average of 16 percent of their daily calories from sugars added to foods and drinks, and adults 13 percent. Such percentages alarm health officials. The risk of heart disease death, for example, begins to rise when 15 percent of calories derives from added sugars, and risks increase sharply above that percentage. Dr. Robert Lustig, a pediatric endocrinologist concerned about the effects of sugars on children's health, calls sugar a poison, although one directly related to dose. A dose of up to 50 grams a day, he says, poses little risk. It accounts for 200 sugar calories, amounting to 10 percent of a 2,000-calorie daily diet. But, he insists, twice that much is *toxic*.[2]

Dr. Lustig's 100-gram toxic dose is close to the upper level of nutritional safety—25 percent of total calories—proposed in 2002 by the Institute of Medicine (IOM), a branch of the National Academies of Science.[3] In Chapter 4, I explain how the IOM fully intended that percentage as an upper safety limit, not a recommendation. Instead, most health authorities recommend consuming no more than 10 percent of calories from added sugars per day, an amount consistent with Dr. Lustig's zone of sugar safety. But for now, let's deal with the question of how much sugar Americans actually consume.

AMOUNTS: TOO MUCH

No nutritionist or government official is the slightest bit concerned about the sugars and 90 calories in an occasional 7.5-ounce can of soda. But this size is now the smallest available. For decades, Coca-Cola was sold in 6.5-ounce bottles. Although Pepsi came out with a 12-ounce size—"twice as much for a nickel"—in the late 1930s, Coca-Cola did not start competing using larger sizes until the mid-1950s.[4] In 2014, I did a quick inventory of the sizes of sodas sold in local drugstores and supermarkets. These presented a bewildering array of options, ranging from 7.5-ounce cans to 2-liter bottles, as shown for Coca-Cola in Table 3.1. The table demonstrates the effects on sugars and calories from sodas when the sizes increase. For Pepsi, you must add 1 or 2 grams of sugars and another 5 or 10 calories to the amounts shown.

TABLE 3.1 The sizes of Coca-Cola cans and bottles available early in 2014

VOLUME, OUNCES	SUGAR, GRAMS	SUGAR, TEASPOONS*	CALORIES
7.5	25	6	90
8	26	7	100
12	39	10	140
16	54	13	200
20	65	16	240
24	81	20	300
34 (1 liter)	117	30	420
40 (1.25 liters)	135	34	500
64 (2 liters)	216	54	800

* Teaspoons are estimated at 4 grams each and rounded to the nearest whole number. Grams and calories are derived from Coca-Cola labels or websites and apply to cans or bottles with Nutrition Facts labels, but not to fountain cups that contain varying amounts of ice. Sugar is commonly assumed to provide about 4 calories per gram, but Coca-Cola uses the more precise 3.7, and also rounds off calories to the nearest 10.

Fountain drinks fall somewhere in this range but provide less sugar and fewer calories for their cup size because the ice dilutes both. If you want to estimate the sugars and calories in fountain drinks, you have to measure the volume of the drink in the cup, subtract the volume of the ice, and see how much drink remains.

If I could convey one message about soda sizes, it is this: larger sodas have more sugar and provide more calories. I say this because most people have only the vaguest idea about the amount of sugars in sodas. By market-place standards, the FDA's decades-long definition of a soda serving—8 ounces—is small compared to most sizes sold as well as to average consumption levels, which is why the agency proposed raising the standard portion size to 12 ounces in 2014.[5]

If you do the sugar-in-water experiment suggested in Chapter 2, you must add ten teaspoons of sugar or ten sugar cubes—nearly 40 grams—to 12 ounces of water. Figure 3.1 shows the number of cubes of sugar that went into a 12-ounce can (10), a 20-ounce vending machine bottle (16+), and a 1-liter bottle (30+).

To keep the soda market humming, companies come out with new sizes occasionally. In 2014, Coca-Cola introduced a 19.2-ounce can to be sold in convenience stores alongside liter bottles. Why? These are "just the thing to keep the momentum going!...designed to maximize immediate sales by offering the 'gas and go' customer a value price and an all-star allure."[6] The marketing materials do not mention the nearly 65 grams of sugars (16 teaspoons) and 240 calories in each can.

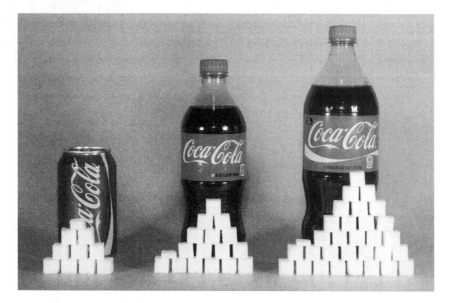

FIGURE 3.1 The sugar in 12-ounce, 20-ounce, and 1-liter sodas. The larger the soda size, the more sugar it contains. These sizes require at least 10, 16, and 30 cubes of sugar, respectively. One cube is 4 grams. Display and photo courtesy of Charles Nestle, based on models by Sugar Stacks (sugarstacks.com).

Fountain drinks promote large sizes as normal. Fast-food restaurants offer 12-ounce sodas as the child's portion, and the smallest adult size is 16 ounces. Movie theaters give a whole new meaning to the concept of "small"; theirs can be 32 ounces (as shown later in Table 9.7). Most people buy medium fountain drinks. Medium means 21 ounces at McDonald's, but 44 ounces at some movie houses. Depending on how much ice it contains, this last size can exceed Dr. Lustig's cutoff point for toxicity all on its own.

I repeat: the larger the soda, the more sugar and calories it contains, even if diluted with ice. But larger sizes do more than that. First, they encourage greater consumption. Researchers find that people consume more from large containers than from small ones, even when they leave the drink unfinished. Second, large portions confuse size estimations. People given larger servings tend to underestimate how much they are eating to a much greater extent than when given smaller portions.[7] This makes smaller sugary drinks healthier for three reasons: they provide less sugar and fewer calories, they discourage excessive intake, and they promote more realistic estimates of the amounts consumed.

SUGAR TRENDS: FALLING, BUT NOT ENOUGH

Sugars of one kind or another are ingredients in three-quarters of packaged foods in America, but regular sodas contribute a third of the total sugar in American diets. Obviously, trends in sugar availability look just like trends in soda availability, as shown in Figure 3.2. In 2011, the U.S. sugar supply—

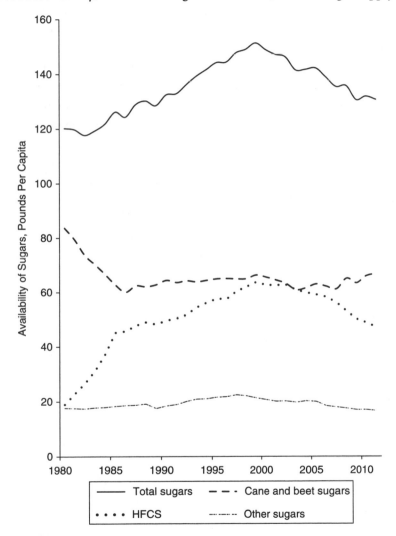

FIGURE 3.2 Trends in the availability of added sugars in the U.S. food supply: total sugars, cane and beet sugars (sucrose), high-fructose corn syrup (HFCS), and other caloric sweeteners, pounds per capita by year. Virtually all of the increase in sugar availability between 1980 and the early 2000s can be accounted for by the rise in HFCS. Source: USDA's food availability (per capita) data system.

the amount produced domestically, less exports, plus imports—provided an average of nearly 132 pounds per capita: 67 pounds of cane and beet sugars (sucrose), 47 pounds of high-fructose corn syrup (HFCS), and the rest from honey, maple syrup, and other such sources.[8]

Sugars added to the U.S. food supply began to rise from about 120 pounds per capita in 1980 to a peak of 151 pounds in 1999. After that, the supply declined, but there are still 12 more pounds of sugars available per person per year than there were in 1980. The 132 pounds in 2012 works out to an availability of 164 grams (41 teaspoons) per day per capita—well over the 100-gram daily upper safety limit for added sugars. Because a third of added sugar intake comes from sodas, sodas alone could contribute as much as 54 grams (13 teaspoons) of sugars a day per capita—220 calories. But those are food supply figures. If you ask Americans how much sugar they eat, they report an average of 120 grams of total sugars a day, an amount that includes added sugars as well as those intrinsically in food. This amount undoubtedly underestimates true intake but still comes to 30 teaspoons a day, of which 10 come from sodas—just the amount in one 12-ounce drink, the per capita daily average.[9]

In Chapter 2 and in this one, I use 1980 as the baseline for trends in sugar and soda production and consumption. The early 1980s marked the beginning of a sharp rise in the prevalence of obesity, as shown in Figure 3.3.

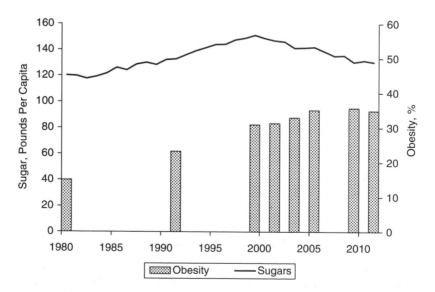

FIGURE 3.3 The availability of total sugars in the food supply tracks closely with trends in the prevalence of obesity.

From then until the late 1990s, obesity rose in parallel to the increasing production of sugars in the food supply. The subsequent decline in sugar availability is consistent with the recent leveling off in obesity prevalence.[10]

This figure compares total sugars to obesity, even though—as shown in Figure 3.2—only trends in production of HFCS parallel those in obesity prevalence. As I explained in Chapter 1, I remain to be convinced that there is anything unique about HFCS that could cause weight gain, as opposed to the effects of the sucrose in cane and beet sugars. HFCS and sucrose yield the same two sugars in the body, glucose and fructose, and their calories are the same. Sugars of any kind are associated with obesity.[11] The effects of liquid calories and fructose intake, as I soon explain, also are common to both sugar sources. But because HFCS is popularly believed to be worse for health than sucrose, the Corn Refiners Association, the trade association for producers of HFCS, funded a weight loss study. This was a randomized, prospective, double-blind clinical trial—the gold standard for nutrition research—that compared the effects of diets formulated to contain 10 or 20 percent of calories as either HFCS or sucrose. In this industry-funded study of people living on their own in the community, weight loss occurred at the same rate regardless of sugar type.[12] Although I am not surprised by this result, I would feel more confident about it if the study had been funded by an independent agency. Funding has a strong tendency to introduce biases into research, as I discuss in Chapter 19.

SUGAR TRENDS: FALLING BUT UNDERESTIMATED, DELIBERATELY

Even if sugar is produced and available, it is not necessarily consumed. How much sugar do people really eat? As noted in the previous chapter, food availability data overestimate actual intake, but dietary surveys underestimate it. The true value lies in between those values. The USDA wanted to get at the "in between." Its researchers adjusted the food supply data for losses that occur in transportation, at retail stores, and at home and in restaurants.[13] They reported loss-adjusted amounts as "consumption," in teaspoons per capita per day, as shown in Figure 3.4. The quotation marks are a reminder that the USDA did not measure sugar intake directly or ask people how much they ate but instead estimated intake based on the loss adjustments.

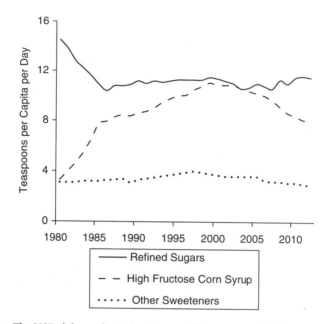

FIGURE 3.4 The USDA's loss-adjusted estimates of "consumption" of sugars, HFCS, and other caloric sweeteners in teaspoons per person per day, 1980 to 2012. In 2012, the total added up to nearly 23 teaspoons a day—about 97 grams. By USDA's definition, a teaspoon is 4.2 grams of sugars.

In 2012, according to the USDA's estimates, the average American consumed nearly 12 teaspoons of cane and beet sugars, 8 teaspoons of HFCS, and 3 teaspoons of other sugars, for a total of nearly 23 teaspoons every day. This amount, which comes to nearly 100 grams, is a bit more than half of the 41 teaspoons of total sugars available in the food supply (Figure 3.2).

Half? How is that possible? If 23 teaspoons per day is correct, it means that nearly half the sugars produced and available are wasted, an amount that hardly seems possible. This result is especially unlikely because dietary surveys say that people consume 120 grams a day (30 teaspoons), and even that amount is probably underestimated.

I am not alone in having doubts about the reliability of the USDA's loss-adjusted estimates. In 2012, the Center for Science in the Public Interest (CSPI), the venerable consumer advocacy group based in Washington, D.C., filed a Freedom of Information Act request to find out how the USDA arrived at its estimates. This led to a surprising—and disturbing—discovery. The USDA had "adjusted" its methods to minimize the amount of sugar consumption. It seems that sugar industry trade groups had lobbied the

USDA to alter its adjustment methods so that Americans would appear to be consuming less sugar. As reported in the *New York Times*:

> "We perceive it to be in our interest to see as low a per-capita sweetener consumption estimate as possible," Jack Roney, director of economics and policy analysis at the American Sugar Alliance, wrote in an e-mail on March 30, 2011. Mr. Roney said in a telephone interview that he was pleased to have "more accurate" information about sugar consumption available. "The extent to which caloric sweeteners are in the public's eye as a possible source or cause of increasing obesity in this country is huge," he said. "If folks are assuming there is much greater consumption than there really is, then we are misleading the public unnecessarily."[14]

These are the kinds of problems that make the more objective data on sugar production more reliable, at least when looking at trends. But whatever the correct figure for average sugar consumption, it is uncomfortably close to—or above—what many consider to be the upper limit of safe intake. Americans would be healthier consuming fewer sugars of any kind.

SUGAR CALORIES: EMPTY AND LIQUID

In effect, sodas are a method for rapid delivery of large amounts of sugars into the bloodstream. Because sugars have no nutrients, their calories are "empty"—devoid of nutritional value. People consuming large amounts—25 percent or more of calories, according to the IOM—are at risk of nutritional deficiencies and need to choose the rest of the diet more carefully to compensate for the missing nutrients. On this basis alone, health authorities for decades have issued advice to consume less sugar. Because sodas contribute so much sugar to daily diets, they raise the same concerns as sugars alone. But the sugars in soft drinks raise an additional concern—an important one, as it turns out. Soda sugars are consumed in liquid form. Sodas and other sugary drinks, says CSPI, are "liquid candy" (see Figure 3.5).[15]

In experiments using rats and mice, consuming sugars as liquids rather than solid foods bypasses the physiological regulatory systems that control appetite and food intake. Some studies of human eating behavior support this idea: the more sugary drinks people consume, the more calories they

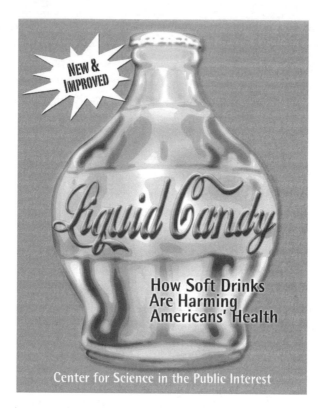

FIGURE 3.5 The Center for Science in the Public Interest (CSPI) refers to sodas as "liquid candy." CSPI began campaigning vigorously for a reduction in soda consumption with the first edition of this report in 1998. This "new & improved" edition appeared in 2005. Courtesy of Michael Jacobson.

consume from any source. Sugar alone or in solid foods does not have this effect; even people eating jelly beans tend to compensate for the calories they take in from candy. Neither do liquids alone; soups and liquid meal replacements help people lose weight. Most research suggests that it is only the sugars consumed in drinks that bypass physiological regulatory controls.[16]

Studies sponsored by the American Beverage Association (ABA) invariably question the validity of this science. Perhaps because the members of the scientific advisory committee providing recommendations for the 2010 Dietary Guidelines did not consider the effects of industry sponsorship when evaluating the existing research, they reported the evidence on liquid calories as conflicted and in need of further investigation.[17] Maybe so, but the idea seems reasonable that liquid calories are absorbed more quickly than is good for health.

FRUCTOSE: METABOLIZED LIKE ALCOHOL

The sweeteners in sodas, usually HFCS but sometimes sucrose (table sugar), are both about half glucose and half fructose. HFCS contains more fructose than sucrose, but how much more and whether the extra amount makes any biological difference is a matter of ongoing debate. At the moment, I see the research as showing little difference in the health effects of HFCS and sucrose, even though HFCS has somewhat more fructose and the body metabolizes glucose and fructose in different ways. Glucose is an immediate source of energy for the brain and other body functions. Excess glucose is deposited as glycogen (a storage form of carbohydrate) and then, if sufficiently in excess of energy needs, as body fat.

Fructose, in contrast, is almost entirely metabolized in the liver. Many studies indicate an association between added fructose—not the fructose that occurs naturally in fruits—with metabolic problems.[18] But fructose is rarely added to foods on its own. More typically, it is added in combination with glucose as part of sucrose or HFCS. Fructose-containing sugars of any kind cause the cells of the body to resist the action of insulin. This hormone usually allows body cells to take up glucose from the blood. When cells are unable to respond to insulin and instead resist its action, levels of blood glucose increase—a symptom of diabetes. When fructose is consumed in excessive amounts, it is converted to fat in the liver and causes a rise in levels of blood triglycerides.

Blood glucose and triglycerides are two components of what is called the "metabolic syndrome," a condition well established to raise the risk of heart disease and type 2 diabetes, and discussed further in Chapter 5. According to Dr. Lustig, the rise in these risk factors makes the effects of excessive fructose similar to those of excessive alcohol intake. Fructose, he says, causes nonalcoholic fatty liver disease, a debilitating condition similar to that caused by alcohol. He characterizes excessive fructose as an epidemic—toxic, poisonous, addictive, and just as bad as alcohol but without the buzz.[19]

He does have a way with words. Indeed, as I fondly tell him, he does hyperbole better than anyone else I know. I say this because I view the jury as still out on the liver effects of sugars. A study conducted in Finland, for example, found just the opposite—a higher intake of fructose to be associated with a reduced risk of fatty liver disease, at least in older adults. A systematic review and analysis concluded that the existing studies are insufficient to distinguish the effects of any sugar on liver health from those of excess calories.[20] These particular studies were funded by independent agencies, but they agree with a study and review supported in part by the soda industry that also attribute the deposition of liver fat to excess calories.[21] I'd like to see further independently funded research studies to clarify the health effects of fructose, consumed separately and in combination with glucose.

Dr. Lustig's concerns about fatty liver and other health effects focus on *added* fructose in diets. He is not worried about the fructose in fruit or even in an occasional soda or piece of candy. Indeed, he says, small amounts of fructose appear to improve insulin sensitivity. It's the higher doses that cause problems. How much higher? The 50 grams of daily sugars he views as compatible with good health include about 25 grams of fructose, but twice that much reaches the threshold for toxicity. In between is a no-man's-land that depends on the rest of the diet and lifestyle.

But consider what these amounts mean. It only takes one 16-ounce Coke or Pepsi to reach 50 grams of sugars and 25 grams of fructose. That one drink takes care of the sugar allowance for an entire day. Two such drinks bring fructose to the threshold of toxicity. Extreme as this may seem, other researchers view Lustig's cutoff points as too generous. As I explain in Chapter 5, their studies conclude that just one 12-ounce soda a day—the daily amount available to every American of any age—increases the risk of coronary heart disease, type 2 diabetes, or stroke. They also find high sugar intakes to be associated with an overall increase in the risk of death—but *only* when those sugars are consumed in beverages.[22]

How to make sense of this? While waiting for researchers to clarify health issues related to fructose versus glucose, it makes sense to consume fewer sugars of any kind, especially in liquid form. This advice makes even more sense in light of current attempts to decide whether sugars and the foods that contain them induce symptoms of addiction.

ARE SUGARS—AND SODAS—ADDICTIVE?

Coca-Cola has been cocaine-free for more than a century, but could the sugars and caffeine in colas be similarly addictive? In research conducted using animals and people, sugars and caffeine independently induce symptoms of dependence and withdrawal. Both substances encourage habitual daily use. Although they could have a greater effect in combination, researchers find it difficult to say whether sugars and caffeine, singly or together, are addictive in the usual sense—inducing cravings, an inability to stop the cravings, misery when the craved substance is unavailable, and willingness to engage in risky behavior to obtain it. Practically everyone likes the taste of sugars, some more than others, and foods high in sugars have been shown to activate reward systems in the brain.[23] But whether pleasure, liking, desire, and reward constitute addiction remains a hotly debated question.

Studies aim to discover whether the feelings that some people develop when they eat sugar or consume sodas meet the criteria for true addiction. If the effects of sugars on the brain are similar to those of psychoactive drugs, it would be easier to explain why people overeat and gain weight. Some observations suggest that sugars could be addictive. Sweetness is well established to reinforce the desire to eat. We want to eat what we like. Researchers have induced laboratory animals to prefer sugar to cocaine under some conditions. They also observe neurochemical changes typical of addictive behavior among people who consume sugars frequently. Although some researchers interpret these kinds of observations as evidence for sugar addiction, others do not.[24]

Addiction researchers are especially interested in sodas because they contain another potentially addictive substance, caffeine, as well as sugars. The caffeine in sodas is low—less than 40 milligrams in a 12-ounce serving—but that may be enough to stimulate dependence, especially in combination with sugars. Although manufacturers say they add caffeine as a flavor enhancer, experiments prove otherwise. People cannot detect a taste difference between sugar-sweetened cola drinks with and without caffeine. The caffeine is there for a different purpose; it makes people enjoy drinking the product even more than does sugar on its own. At least one study found that the addition of even small amounts of caffeine to sugary drinks makes people drink more of them.[25]

Moderate amounts of caffeine stimulate the central nervous system and make people feel more alert, energetic, and cheery, although high doses induce anxiety and shakiness and interfere with sleep. Even though caffeine has stronger effects in children, some researchers consider the effects of moderate amounts on young children to be relatively innocuous. But addiction researchers believe that even small amounts of caffeine can induce symptoms of dependence in susceptible individuals. Some even view caffeine as a psychoactive drug.[26]

It is difficult to know how seriously to accept such views. Caffeine attracts researchers who want to find something wrong with it. Endless studies over the years have suggested that caffeine raises risks for heart disease, heartburn, cancer, infertility, fetal growth retardation, spontaneous abortion, breast lumps, osteoporosis, ulcers, and any number of other health problems. These are a lot of problems to blame on one substance, and it is not surprising that the observed effects tend to be small, inconsistent, and less than thoroughly convincing.

In 2012, however, several young people died after consuming large amounts of heavily caffeinated, sugar-sweetened energy drinks, 5-Hour Energy and Monster Energy. While investigators were trying to decide whether the products or something else caused the deaths, the FDA released a long list of reported health problems associated with such drinks. The agency reminded everyone that when it said caffeine was GRAS (generally recognized as safe) in the 1950s, it intended that designation to apply only to cola drinks like Coke and Pepsi. Once manufacturers began adding higher amounts of caffeine to beverages as well as putting caffeine into foods such as Cracker Jack, jelly beans, gummy bears, brownies, mints, maple syrup, and chewing gum, the FDA would have to reconsider the safety of such practices.[27]

The question of addiction is important to resolve. If sugars and sodas are addictive, advocates would be legally justified in insisting that they not be marketed to children. But whether these foods are addictive or not, people love the taste of sweetness, and the more the better, up to what the food industry calls the "bliss point"—the taste perceived as optimal by participants in sensory tests. Food and beverage manufacturers discovered long ago that putting as much sugar as they could into their products was an easy way to promote sales, and they market sweetness aggressively.[28]

But sugars alone do not determine how sodas taste. The bubbles, color, and recognizable brand names also are reasons why so many people like sodas.[29] In 1984, when Coca-Cola's blind taste tests demonstrated conclusively that participants preferred sweeter drinks, the company made a massive marketing blunder. In line with the test results, the company introduced a sweeter New Coke, but consumers immediately rejected it. Brands trump taste. Brands influence taste perception more than the taste itself. When it comes to sodas, customers buy the brand.

Sodas and Health

4

Dietary Advice

Sugars and Sugary Drinks

Health authorities have long been troubled by the large amounts of sugars and sugary drinks in American diets. As early as 1942, the Council on Food and Nutrition of the American Medical Association viewed wartime sugar rationing as a boon for health. Eating less sugar would force people to eat healthier foods and improve nutrient intake. The council noted a 20 percent increase in soft drink consumption since 1939, and urged physicians to tell patients not to consume sugar or carbonated beverages between meals. Far ahead of its time, the council recommended changes to the food environment to make it easier for the public to choose healthier foods and drinks. It suggested limits on soft drink advertising, on sales of candy and soft drinks near schools, and on indiscriminate use of soft drinks by the military—this at a time when per capita production of soft drinks was a mere three 6.5-ounce bottles per week.[1]

Then as now, health authorities were concerned about the effects of sugars on the nutritional quality of daily diets. Because sugar calories are "empty," eating large amounts—or drinking large volumes of sodas—could displace nutritious foods in the diet and lead to inadequate intake of essential vitamins and minerals. Research continues to support that idea. A review of studies examining intake of fourteen vitamins and minerals found drinking soda to be linked to reduced intake of all of them. Researchers say that the more calories consumed from sodas, the more unlikely it is that diets can provide nutrients at recommended levels.[2]

But nutrient deficiencies are no longer the main concern about soda intake. During the twentieth century, the most prevalent diseases related to diet shifted from those caused by inadequate food intake to those caused by too much food. Health authorities have continued to complain about excessive sugar, but now because it promotes weight gain and raises risks for chronic diseases—type 2 diabetes, heart disease, and the like.

By the mid-1970s, evidence on the role of diet in chronic disease induced the Senate Select Committee on Nutrition and Human Needs, chaired by George McGovern (D-S.D.), to hold hearings on "diet and killer diseases," a phrase guaranteed to get the attention of companies making foods high in sugar, salt, and fat. By then, soft drinks already accounted for 23 percent of sugar usage and were the largest single source of added sugars in American diets. The hearings led to development of a report entitled *Dietary Goals for the United States*, published in February 1977 (Figure 4.1). The report elicited so much protest over its "eat less" recommendations that the committee was forced to tone it down. Nevertheless, the revised goals, which appeared in December 1977, called for a startling 45 percent reduction in intake to bring sugars down to 10 percent or less of calories. How? "In reviewing ways of cutting the consumption of refined and processed sugars, the most obvious item for general reduction is soft drinks. Total elimination of soft drinks from the diet, for many people, would bring at least half the recommended reduction of consumption of such sugars."[3]

In part to head off the controversy generated by the Dietary Goals, the USDA and the Department of Health and Human Services (HHS) joined together to produce what they hoped would be less provocative advice. They released the first Dietary Guidelines for Americans in 1980, and have issued them at five-year intervals ever since. All editions have advised reductions in sugar. The 1980 guideline said to "avoid too much sugar." So did the guidelines in 1985 and, with minor modifications, those in 1990 and 1995 (Table 4.1). The explanations for the sugar guidelines sometimes—but not always—have included recommendations to reduce soda intake.

From 1980 to 2010, no doubt under pressure from food companies, the advice of federal agencies about sugars grew increasingly complex and convoluted. As shown in the table, the straightforward "avoid..." became "choose and prepare..." or "reduce the intake of..." Although most editions of the guidelines recognized the large contribution of drinks to sugar intake, they evaded clear, forceful statements about the need to reduce or eliminate them. By 2010, sugars had disappeared as a separate guideline and were folded in with "solid fats"—butter, animal fats, and the like—under the

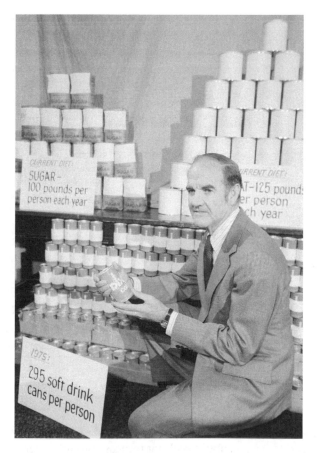

FIGURE 4.1 U.S. senator George McGovern (D-S.D.) displays the amount of sugars and sodas consumed by the average American in 1975. The photo is from a press conference in January 1977 announcing the release of the first edition of the *Dietary Goals for the United States*. AP photo used with permission.

obfuscating abbreviation "SoFAS," standing for the combination of solid fats and added sugars.

The ninety-five-page brochure that explains the 2010 guidelines states that no more than 5 to 15 percent of calories should come from SoFAS. It is difficult to know what the federal agencies intended this to mean in practice. Charts in the brochure specify a daily allowance of 258 calories from SoFAS on a 2,000-calorie diet. Fats provide more than twice the calories of sugars (9 per gram as compared to 4), so even a minimal intake of animal fat would take up much of the allowance. One tablespoon of butter, for example, is 100 calories, leaving only 158 calories for sugars and additional

TABLE 4.1 Evolution of dietary guidelines about sugar and soft drinks, 1980 to 2010

YEAR	SUGAR GUIDELINE	ADVICE ABOUT SOFT DRINKS
1980	Avoid too much sugar	"Eat less of foods containing these sugars, such as candy, soft drinks…"
1985	Avoid too much sugar	"Use less of all sugars…Examples include soft drinks…"
1990	Use sugars only in moderation	No specific mention.
1995	Choose a diet moderate in sugars	No specific mention.
2000	Choose beverages and foods to moderate your intake of sugars	"Intake of a lot of foods high in added sugars, like soft drinks, is of concern…Limit your use of these beverages…"
2005	Choose and prepare foods and beverages with little added sugars or caloric sweeteners	Notes that soft drinks contribute 33 percent of added sugars to U.S. diets.
2010	Reduce the intake of calories from solid fats and added sugars (SoFAS)	Notes that sodas, energy drinks, sports drinks, and juice drinks together contribute 46 percent of added sugars. Advises: "Drink few or no regular sodas."
2015 (advisory)	Decrease dietary intake from added sugars	Reduce consumption of sugar-sweetened beverages

SOURCE: USDA and HHS. Dietary Guidelines for Americans, 1980 to 2010. The 2015 advice comes from the scientific report of the Dietary Guidelines Advisory Committee.

solid fats. Unless the diet contains no animal fats at all, the 2010 guidelines imply that added sugars should account for less than 10 percent of calories.[4]

To achieve this reduction, the USDA says to "reduce intake of added sugars" and to "drink few or no regular sodas"—but not until pages 45 and 67, respectively. Could sugar and soda industry lobbying have anything to do with the minimization of attention to sugars and sodas in federal dietary guidelines? I cannot imagine how federal agencies could have come up with a term as unhelpful as SoFAS, and lobbying is the only explanation that makes sense. At the very least, lobbying induces the agencies to avoid issuing guidelines that suggest eating less of specific food products.

Fortunately, the scientific committee reviewing the research for the 2015 guidelines dropped SoFAS and instead simply said, "To decrease dietary intake from added sugars, the U.S. population should reduce consumption of sugar-sweetened beverages." The committee also urged the development and implementation of policies and programs to limit such drinks.[5] Its report is just advisory, however, and whether the agencies adopted this advice in the new guidelines would not be known until their release at the end of 2015.

USDA'S FOOD GUIDES

Ostensibly, dietary guidelines are intended for use by government policy makers and health professionals as the basis for developing nutrition education programs and for setting standards for federal food assistance programs. Although they invariably generate widespread press attention, they are not meant to be seen or used by the general public. Instead, for public education the USDA prepares food guides—pyramids and plates—derived from the dietary guidelines. Since the early 1900s, the USDA has produced food guides for public education about healthful food choices. These first mentioned the need to reduce sugar intake in 1979 but did not emphasize that need until 1992, when the agency released the first Food Guide Pyramid. This put little symbols at the very top—the "eat less" sector—to indicate added sugars from soft drinks and other sources. Its advice: "Choose fewer foods that are high in sugars—candy, sweet desserts, and soft drinks."[6] The 2005 revision of the pyramid dropped that statement and merely listed sodas as an example of foods that could be consumed as part of daily "discretionary" calories. These changes reflected the more conservative, industry-friendly policies of the administration of President George W. Bush, which extended to matters as detailed as dietary advice for children as well as adults.

For children, the USDA developed a special food guide in 1999. Its pyramid for kids ages 2 to 6 displayed soda pop prominently in the "eat less" tip.[7] But when the USDA released a new pyramid for children in 2005, the design eliminated all traces of "eat less" messages. Like the 2005 pyramid for adults, it emphasized physical activity. Figure 4.2 compares the 1999 and 2005 food guides for children.

In 2011, however, the USDA exhibited some courage. It issued an entirely new food guide, MyPlate, along with "selected messages to help consumers focus on key behaviors." These included some surprisingly direct advice: "Drink water instead of sugary drinks." Parents, said the USDA, should limit sugary beverages. It said: "Sip smarter: Soda and other sweet drinks contain a lot of sugar and are high in calories. Offer water, 100% juice, or fat-free milk when kids are thirsty."[8]

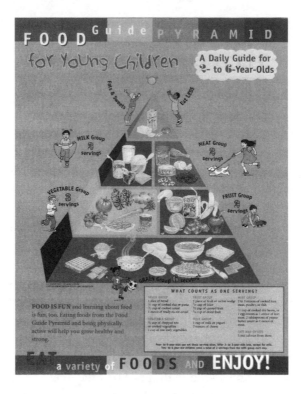

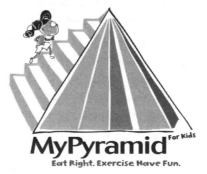

FIGURE 4.2 The USDA's Clinton-era 1999 food guide for children (top panel) and the George W. Bush–era 2005 MyPyramid for Preschoolers (bottom panel). The earlier version placed sodas among the "eat less" fats and sweets group. The later one did not. Like the 2005 pyramid for adults, the 2005 pyramid for children diverted attention from the need to make healthier food choices and instead emphasized physical activity.

A DIGRESSION: "OTHER SWEET DRINKS"

Although this book is mainly concerned with carbonated cola sodas made by the Coca-Cola and PepsiCo companies, this is a good place to stop and consider the vast array of other sugary drinks available in the marketplace, many of which these companies also produce. In Table 4.2, I categorize the universe of sugar-sweetened beverages, and list some of the other substances typically added to them. Overall, these drinks contribute an astonishing amount of sugar to American diets, all of it in liquid form. The 2010 Dietary Guidelines brochure provided the percentages. It said 35.7 percent of total sugars derived from the combination of sodas, energy drinks, and sports drinks; 10.5 percent from juice drinks (excluding 100 percent juices); and 3.5 percent from teas. Together, these added up to 49.7 percent of total sugars consumed. To this percentage must be added the smaller contributions of sweetened coffees, waters, and milk drinks. It is fair to say that drinks with added sugars contributed half the total amount of sugars in American diets in 2010, and apparently still do.[9]

Table 4.2 lists these drinks in two broad categories—sodas, which are always carbonated, and non-sodas, which may or may not be carbonated. What most distinguishes non-soda sugary drinks from sodas is how they are marketed. Producers of non-sodas invariably promote the drinks as healthier no matter how much sugar they contain. Although some of these drinks do contain less sugar than sodas, others have as much or more. Marketers tend to disguise the amounts by using healthier-sounding euphemisms for sugars such as honey, juice from concentrate, pure natural cane juice, or blue agave nectar. Along with sugars, some drinks also add erythritol, a relatively indigestible—and, therefore, calorie-free—sugar alcohol.

TABLE 4.2 Sugar-sweetened beverages: categories

DRINKS WITH ADDED SUGARS	OTHER ADDED INGREDIENTS
Sodas, carbonated	
Sodas, soft drinks, pop, soda pop	Flavors: colas, fruit, ginger, others
Non-sodas, sometimes carbonated	
Energy drinks	Caffeine, some nutrients, other stimulants
Sports drinks	Electrolytes, some vitamins
Fruit drinks, punches, ades	Fruit juice (usually much less than 100%)
Teas, coffees	Flavors
Waters	Flavors, nutrients
Milks	Flavors: chocolate, strawberry, others

The juice drinks are marketed to appear as though they are juices, although many contain very little real juice (the percentage must be stated on the label). But no matter how much sugar or how little juice they contain, these drinks are advertised as "natural" or "organic," terms that convey the aura of health. I know many health-conscious people who would never dream of drinking a Coke or Pepsi but think Snapple—a soft drink in which sugar is the second ingredient after water—is a healthier alternative. Healthier, you are supposed to believe and quite likely do, means sports and energy drinks and anything with juice in it.[10] If you share such beliefs, you had best take a close look at the labels and ingredient list of any beverage you buy.

You may have noted the omission of fruit juices from this table. Although 100 percent juices have just as much sugar as soda, the sugar is not *added*; it occurs naturally in the fruit. The sugar in juices is accompanied by all of the vitamins, minerals, and other nutrients in the original fruit, except for those lost when the fiber is squeezed out. Despite their sweetness, fruit juices are relatively minor sources of sugars in U.S. diets, mainly because most people do not drink them in large volumes.

Nevertheless, although whole fruits are better nutritionally, 100 percent fruit juices are a much better option than any other sugary drink as long as the amounts remain small. How small? Because juices as well as other sugar-sweetened drinks promote obesity and tooth decay, the American Academy of Pediatrics advises parents not to give any fruit juice to infants under 6 months. For children up to age 6, it advises no more than 4 to 6 ounces a day. For older children, it suggests a limit of 12 ounces a day. Parents, the academy says, should never permit children to sip on juice throughout the day or at bedtime. Instead, children should be offered whole fruits, water, or low-fat milk.[11] This is good advice for adults as well.

THE CONTROVERSIAL "PERCENT OF CALORIES" SUGAR RECOMMENDATION

Cutting down on sugars, sodas, and other sugary drinks is good advice, but no reasonable person suggests eliminating them entirely. I certainly don't. I love sweet tastes. But how much sugar is it reasonable to consume? At least since the 1977 Dietary Goals, health officials have consistently recommended an upper limit of 10 percent of calories from added sugars. In 1992, the USDA's Food Guide Pyramid suggested 6, 12, and 18 teaspoons of sugars for daily diets of 1,600, 2,200, and 2,800 calories, respectively. This worked out to 7, 10, and 13 percent of calorie intake, respectively, for an average of 10 percent. By that time, health officials in several European countries had recommended much the same.[12]

In 2002, despite this apparent international consensus, the Institute of Medicine (IOM) issued new Dietary Reference Intakes—standards of nutrient intake for the population—with a surprisingly high allowance for sugars. The IOM said that people could safely consume sugars up to 25 percent of daily calories. The institute based this percentage on studies comparing the effects of high and low sugar consumption on the intake of nutrients—not the effects of sugars on weight gain or chronic diseases. The studies, mostly done on people who were not overweight, showed little or no effect of sugars on nutrient adequacy except at the very highest levels of intake. A later review found that calorie intake—not sugar intake—is the prime predictor of nutrient adequacy; if calories are adequate, nutrient intake is likely to be adequate except at the extreme high end of sugar consumption.[13]

In setting the 25 percent sugar cutoff point, the IOM was interested only in the effects of sugars on intake of vitamins and minerals. The IOM did not consider the effects of high sugar intake on calorie intake, body weight, or diseases for which obesity is a risk factor. Even so, it intended 25 percent as an upper limit of safety. It most definitely did not intend to recommend consuming 25 percent of calories from sugars or even to agree that 25 percent was an acceptable level of sugar intake.

Consider the difference between 10 percent and 25 percent of calories from added sugars. If you consume about 2,000 calories a day, 10 percent means 200 calories, or 50 grams of added sugars—about the amount in one 16-ounce soda. The higher percentage is 2.5 times that amount. The sugar and soft drink industries enormously prefer 25 percent over 10 percent, and they invoke the IOM report every chance they get.

The most famous example of industry objections to the 10 percent sugar limit involved the Geneva-based World Health Organization (WHO). In the early 2000s, the WHO began developing a global strategy to reduce obesity and related chronic diseases. In 2003, this agency issued a background report advising its member nations to reduce consumption of added sugars to the usual 10 percent or less of daily calories. Despite the long history of that recommendation, national and international sugar and soft drink trade associations objected vehemently. American sugar lobbying groups enlisted senators from sugar-growing states to demand withdrawal of U.S. funding from WHO. Sugar lobbyists wrote position papers arguing against the guideline and invoking the IOM's 25 percent "recommendation." They induced government lawyers to forward these documents to Geneva. The WHO's final report on the global strategy said to "limit the intake of free [added] sugars" but dropped the 10 percent target.[14] Under these circumstances, U.S. dietary guidelines in the mid-2000s could hardly be expected to say anything stronger.

Since then, the role of sugars and soft drinks in obesity has become a much larger issue, not only in the United States but internationally. In March 2014, the WHO tried again. It issued draft proposals for intake of free sugars based largely on two research reports it had commissioned. Sugars, the WHO advised, should make up less than 10 percent of total calories per day—and less than 5 percent would be even better. Its final report in January 2015 confirmed these recommendations.[15]

The WHO reports pointed out that the risk of obesity was more than 50 percent higher among groups with the highest soda consumption as compared to those with the lowest. WHO based the "5 percent would be even better" recommendation on its commissioned report on sugars and tooth decay. This found sugar intake to be closely associated with tooth decay, "with good but not overwhelming evidence indicating that tooth decay is lower when the intake of added sugars is less than 10 percent of calories." Other investigators said even 5 percent is too high and that to prevent dental caries sugars should account for no more than 3 percent of daily calories.[16] I will have much more to say about sugars, sodas, and tooth decay in Chapter 6.

WHO is not the only agency to recommend that added sugars make up less than 10 percent of calories. Because intake of sugars and sodas is associated with metabolic abnormalities, adverse health conditions, shortfalls of essential nutrients, greater energy intake, and higher body weight, the American Heart Association (AHA) recommends that women consume no more than 100 calories per day from added sugars (25 grams), and men no more than 150 calories per day (38 grams). These come to 5 percent and 7.5 percent, respectively, of a 2,000-calorie daily diet. Following the AHA's recommendation allows for no more than one 8-ounce soda a day for women and one 12-ounce soda for men in a day—and those sodas contain all the sugar allowed for an entire day. The Canadian Heart and Stroke Foundation says much the same: no more than 10 percent of calories from added sugars and ideally less than 5 percent.[17] By these standards, the 10 percent sugar recommendation is generous. It is also likely to be somewhat more realistic.

In 2012, the IOM's Weight of the Nation study tackled environmental factors that promote obesity. Among its strategies to improve the environment of food choice was this: "Adopt policies and implement practices to reduce overconsumption of sugar-sweetened beverages." To do so, the report suggested banning soft drinks in schools, taxing the drinks, encouraging health care providers to counsel patients on the health risks of sodas, and developing social marketing campaigns to reduce intake. Other policy analysts agree, and call for national dietary guidelines to make clear that sugary drinks should be consumed infrequently.[18]

It should be evident from this account that health officials are deeply concerned about soda intake, mainly because of the sugar content but also because of the growing body of research linking soda consumption to obesity, type 2 diabetes, and other chronic conditions. The next chapter examines those linkages.

5

The Health Issues

Obesity, Diabetes, and More

Research studies—many and varied—link sodas to poor diets. People who typically drink sodas tend to make other unhealthful diet and lifestyle choices. Nevertheless, studies often link one or another ingredient in sodas, mostly sugars, to a broad array of chronic health conditions, most notably obesity, type 2 diabetes, and coronary artery disease, but also stroke, dental disease, bone disease, gout, asthma, cancers, rheumatoid arthritis, behavioral problems, and even psychological disorders and premature aging, not to mention addiction. The Center for Science in the Public Interest summarizes these associations as "Toxi-Cola" (Figure 5.1).

These constitute an unusually broad array of conditions to attribute to sugary beverages, and it is not surprising that the evidence is far more compelling for some of the links than others. The association of sodas with these conditions, as I explain below, does not necessarily imply that sodas are their cause.

In this chapter and Chapter 6, I review this evidence. But first, let's pause to consider the scientific challenges involved in demonstrating that sodas cause such illnesses independent of other dietary, behavioral, environmental, or genetic influences. Even the most avid consumers of sodas eat many other foods every day, and researchers must take special care to distinguish the effects of a single beverage from those of the diet as a whole, let alone the effects of the sugars in sodas from the calories they provide. Sodas could simply be the tip of the iceberg—a marker of unhealthful lifestyle practices or poor quality diets.

By this time, many dozens of studies have attempted to single out the health effects of sodas from those of other possible causes. These studies vary

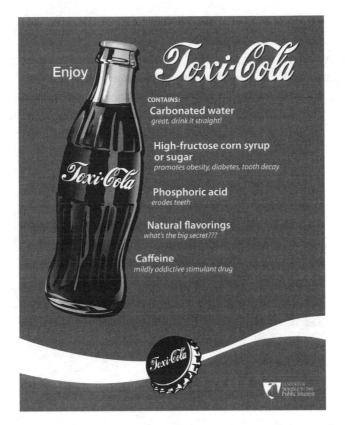

FIGURE 5.1 The Center for Science in the Public Interest's Toxi-Cola poster. This venerable consumer advocacy group argues that because soda ingredients cause so many health problems, the drinks ought to be labeled as toxic. Courtesy of Michael Jacobson.

in experimental design, methods of analysis, results, and interpretation. To make sense of them, other researchers have conducted meta-analyses, systematic reviews using defined criteria for deciding in advance which studies to examine and how to evaluate their methods and results. Meta-analyses also vary—in the definition of sodas, in the number and types of studies chosen for analysis, and in how the results of these studies are interpreted.

To further complicate an already complicated picture, the soda industry sponsors its own research studies, a topic I take up in detail in Chapter 19. For now, I'll just mention that practically all studies reporting adverse effects of sodas on health were funded by grants from government agencies or private foundations. In sharp contrast, studies finding no such association were almost invariably paid for by soda companies or their trade associa-tion.[1] This distinction is so blatant that you can safely assume that almost any study concluding that sodas or their sugars have no adverse health effects was paid for in some way by a soda industry group.

With this caveat in mind, most independently funded studies arrive at the same conclusion: habitual soda consumption is not good for health. They find soda drinking to be strongly associated with higher calorie in-takes, poor-quality diets, and overweight and obesity in children and adults, as well as with conditions for which obesity raises risks, among them type 2 diabetes and heart disease.

GUILT BY ASSOCIATION

One more caveat: the meaning of "associated." As epidemiologists endlessly repeat, association means correlation; it does not necessarily mean causa-tion. The most obvious association of sodas to health is their increased pro-duction in parallel with the prevalence of obesity, as I show in Figure 5.2.

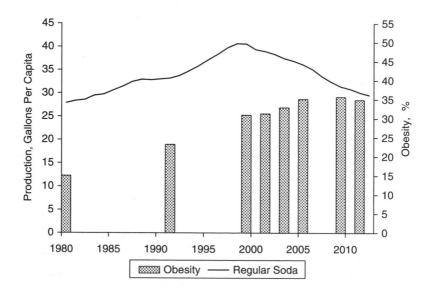

FIGURE 5.2 Guilt by association: trends in production of regular (sugar-sweetened) sodas and in the prevalence of obesity, United States, 1980 to 2012. Sources: Beverage Marketing Corporation, *Carbonated Soft Drinks in the U.S.*, 2013: Exhibits 1.2 and 3.20, and the Centers for Disease Control and Prevention.

Because sodas provide a third of the sugars in American diets, this figure should and does look just like the one presented earlier for sugars (Figure 3.3).

From 1980 to 2000, production—and, therefore, consumption—of regular sodas rose from 27 gallons per capita per year to more than 40. Since then, soda production has declined. Also from 1980 to 2000, the overall prevalence of obesity in the United States doubled from less than 15 percent to about 30 percent. Although the prevalence of obesity has continued to increase, it increased more slowly from about 2000 on, and since 2005 seems to be leveling off. Another association: the prevalence of obesity among specific population groups more or less parallels their patterns of soda consumption. Both soda consumption and obesity are highest among African and Hispanic Americans, followed by whites and Asians. None of these associations proves that sodas *cause* obesity. Similar associations can be observed with intake of sugars, as we saw in Chapter 3, but also with fast food and larger portion sizes.[2] To confirm that sodas contribute to causation, researchers have produced other evidence that links sodas to multiple health problems, as we will now see.

MORE CALORIES

As mentioned earlier, researchers report the diets of habitual soda drinkers to be of poorer nutritional quality than those of people who seldom or never drink sodas. Most also find that soda drinkers consume more calories. Despite these findings, the scientific advisory committee to the 2010 Dietary Guidelines came to a cautious conclusion. It found the evidence linking sodas to higher calorie intakes to be "limited," meaning suggestive of a link but not definitive. More recent evidence continues to support the idea that soda drinkers do not compensate for soda calories by reducing intake of calories from other sources. A survey of New York City residents, for example, observed that soda drinkers consume nearly 600 more calories a day from all sources than people who abstain from sodas. If nothing else, soda drinkers tend to eat more snacks.[3]

CHILDHOOD OBESITY

Studies of childhood obesity provide the most compelling evidence linking sodas to poor health. Children who habitually drink sodas take in more calories, eat worse diets, and weigh more than those who do not. The ever-cautious 2010 Dietary Guidelines Advisory Committee judged this evidence as "strong" (translation: as good as such evidence gets) and sufficient to conclude that "consumption of sugar-sweetened beverages in childhood should be discouraged."[4] Many studies point to this conclusion. Here is a quick summary of their findings.

- Most, but not all, studies of the effects of sugar-sweetened beverages on children's health associate soda intake with higher calorie intakes and body weight.[5]
- The more sodas children consume, the higher their risk of obesity.[6]
- The addition of even one soda a day to a child's diet increases the chance of overweight.[7]
- Even children under the age of five put on more weight if they drink sodas.[8]
- Sodas do not induce satiety in young children.[9]
- Children and adolescents who reduce soda consumption gain less weight or reduce their level of overweight. The benefits are more pronounced among overweight children.[10]

In 2014, the Obesity Society judged evidence that sugary drinks cause obesity as "suggestive, but not definitive," although more compelling for children than for adults. Children, the society said, should minimize intake of these drinks. Independently funded systematic reviews of such studies also conclude that the evidence is compelling enough to justify public health campaigns to reduce children's soda intake. In contrast, a review funded by Coca-Cola denies that sodas have anything to do with childhood obesity and instead concludes that its cause is lack of physical activity.[11] As I explain in later chapters, switching the focus to physical activity is a frequent response of the soda industry to charges that its products might be harmful to health.

ADULT OBESITY

Because the diets and lifestyles of adults are more complicated than those of children, the effects of soft drinks on their health are more difficult to interpret. The 2010 Dietary Guidelines Advisory Committee viewed the evidence linking sodas to higher calorie intake in adults as "limited" and the evidence linking sodas to increased body weight as "moderate," meaning that some evidence exists but it could be a lot stronger. Many of the studies it reviewed showed only a small effect of sodas on weight gain, or suggested that soda drinking only affects some people, or found that only high levels of soda intake are linked to obesity.[12] But the previously cited New York City study identified a clear correlation between increased soda consumption and the prevalence of obesity among residents.

Because most studies of sodas and obesity tend to produce similar results, meta-analyses of those studies do too. They conclude that habitual consumption of sodas is associated with increases in calorie intake and body weight, and that replacing sugary drinks with water and low-calorie beverages helps maintain healthier weights. These correlations are seen among populations in poor countries as well as rich ones. For adults too, researchers conclude that the link to obesity is strong enough to justify campaigns to reduce soda intake.[13] Such campaigns are especially needed, they say, because obesity is such a prominent risk factor for type 2 diabetes, coronary heart disease, and other leading causes of chronic illness and death.

METABOLIC SYNDROME

These obesity-related conditions have a potential cause in common—soda-induced "metabolic syndrome." This is the name given to a collection of measurable risk factors: above-normal sugar and triglycerides in blood, a thick waist, and lower-than-normal HDL (high-density lipoprotein—the "good" cholesterol). The more of these risk factors displayed, the greater the chance of developing chronic diseases such as type 2 diabetes and coronary heart disease. Habitual soda consumption is associated with these conditions, undoubtedly because of the sugars. When the intake of sugars exceeds the body's need for energy and its storage capacity, the sugars are converted to fat in the liver, circulate as triglycerides in blood, raise blood levels of the "bad" LDL (low-density lipoprotein) cholesterol, reduce blood levels of HDL cholesterol, and are deposited as body fat. It doesn't help that sodas deliver sugars in liquid form. Substituting water for sugary drinks helps to reduce markers of the metabolic syndrome.[14]

TYPE 2 DIABETES

Obesity unquestionably raises the risk for type 2 diabetes (formerly known as adult-onset diabetes) in children and adults. The prevalence of this form of diabetes has increased in parallel with the rising prevalence of obesity. This is happening worldwide. Type 2 diabetes has become an international public health crisis. The disease is personally debilitating; even mild cases are expensive to treat and lifelong. Over time, uncontrolled diabetes damages the circulatory system and can lead to kidney failure, blindness, gangrene, and foot amputations, among other dreadful consequences. These effects are especially disheartening because type 2 diabetes is almost entirely preventable. Most people who have it are overweight or obese. Preventing type 2 diabetes means avoiding weight gain, and weight loss can eliminate most of its symptoms.[15]

If sodas cause an increase in calorie intake and the risk of obesity, then it makes sense that they also increase the risk of type 2 diabetes. Excessive intake of sugars—in amounts over and above the body's ability to metabolize them quickly—changes hormonal balance, causes cells to resist the action of insulin, raises blood sugar levels, and leads to metabolic syndrome.

Do sugars and sodas increase diabetes risk independent of obesity? Evidence suggests that they could. The prevalence of type 2 diabetes has increased in parallel with obesity, but also with the increased availability of total sugars, high-fructose corn syrup (HFCS), and sodas in the food supply. One international study suggests that the addition of 150 calories per capita per day from all sugars, including HFCS, to a country's food supply increases its diabetes prevalence by 1.1 percent. This amount is the equivalent of only one can of soda. Studies show that American adults who increase their intake of sugary drinks are more likely to gain weight and to develop type 2 diabetes than those who do not. A European study of 350,000 people in eight countries found that for every 12-ounce sugary drink added to a person's daily intake, the risk of diabetes increased by 22 percent.[16] Taken together, these studies indicate that levels of daily consumption of sugars and, therefore, sugary drinks could be enough to explain the prevalence of type-2 diabetes in a country, regardless of its obesity prevalence.

This kind of research explains why the American Beverage Association (ABA) feels obliged to issue a statement addressing a "common myth: that drinking sugar-sweetened beverages *causes* Type 2 diabetes. The truth is, type 2 diabetes is caused by genetics and lifestyle factors.... [The solution] starts with proper nutrition education and being physically active. Simply put? Balance what you eat and drink with what you do." The ABA statement does not mention that drinking less soda might be the quickest way to achieve this kind of balance.[17]

HEART DISEASE AND STROKE

Routine consumption of sugary drinks is associated with a higher risk of coronary heart disease and strokes. Sugars raise blood pressure and blood fats independently of their effects on body weight, so sodas would also be expected to do so. Habitual intake of one 12-ounce soda a day, some researchers say, increases the risk of high blood pressure by at least 6 percent. Other researchers report that consumption of just one 8-ounce soda a day increases the risk of stroke, and 16 ounces a day increases the risk by 22 percent. As noted earlier, the American Heart Association used such findings to recommend that women consume no more than 100 calories a day from added sugars and men no more than 150—the equivalent of 8 or 12 ounces of soda.[18] For women, 100 calories is 5 percent of the total for the day, half the 10 percent typically recommended, and only a quarter of average intake. Even the most diligently health-conscious person will find so low a level of sugar intake difficult to achieve. If you eat a reasonably healthy diet and do not overeat calories, do you really need to restrict added sugars to under 10 percent of calories? I do not think current evidence permits a clear answer to that question, but overall, everyone would be better off eating less sugar.

CANCERS

It is troubling to think that sugary drinks might raise the risk of cancer, but sugars and sodas have both been linked to an increased risk of pancreatic cancer and to the estrogen-dependent form of endometrial cancer. In response to publication of these studies, Coca-Cola funded its own meta-analysis of studies of soft drinks and cancer. Its study judged the scientific quality of the previous research to be poor and concluded that sodas have no association with cancer risk.[19] Settling this question requires further research from independent investigators.

When it comes to diet sodas, the Internet is full of sites arguing that artificial sweeteners cause cancer. As I explained in Chapter 1, consumer concerns induced Coca-Cola and PepsiCo to remove or promise to remove the potential carcinogen 4-methylimidazole (4-MeI) from the caramel coloring agents in diet sodas. Although the FDA and other public and private health authorities maintain that the chemicals in diet sodas are safe at current levels of intake, concerns remain. Studies using experimental animals suggest that very high doses of some chemical sweeteners could increase cancer risk, but research on humans has yet to confirm these findings. The American Cancer Society, the American Institute for Cancer Research, and the National Cancer Institute say they have no evidence that artificial sweeteners increase the risk of cancer—or any other health problem—in humans.[20] Whether or not they cause cancer, I'm not a user of artificial sweeteners and I don't buy products containing them. I do not like their bitter aftertaste, and much prefer sugar (in moderation, of course).

PREMATURE DEATH

Obesity, type 2 diabetes, heart disease, and stroke—and the risk factors for these conditions, sugars among them—have been shown to increase overall mortality. In mice, even low levels of sugar intake have been associated with reduced survival.[21] In humans, researchers have shown soda consumption to be similarly linked. Sugar intake is associated with an increased risk of mortality from all causes—but only when consumed in beverages.[22] One group of investigators examined the relationship of soda consumption to deaths from all causes by linking data from 114 international dietary surveys to mortality statistics from the World Health Organization. On this basis, they estimated that sugar-sweetened beverages are responsible for 184,000 obesity-related deaths a year. Of these deaths, they attributed 132,000 to diabetes, 45,000 to cardiovascular disease, and 4,600 to cancer. The data show that mortality related to sugary drink consumption is lowest in Japan, where soda drinking and obesity are low, but is highest in Mexico, where soda drinking and obesity set world records.[23]

OTHER HEALTH EFFECTS

As I said earlier, researchers link frequent soda consumption with many health conditions beyond the ones just discussed. With the exception of tooth decay, to which I devote Chapter 6, the evidence associating the other conditions to soda consumption is still largely preliminary—somewhat suggestive but by no means definitive.

With respect to osteoporosis, for example, it is theoretically possible that the phosphoric acid in sodas might leach calcium from bones and weaken them. Feeding sodas to rats reduces levels of blood calcium. Researchers associate frequent soda consumption with low blood calcium in children and with bone fractures, particularly in girls. Older women who habitually drink colas are more likely to have low bone mineral density than those who do not.[24] This may seem like sufficient evidence, but the studies do not clearly indicate whether the effects are due to sodas specifically or to generally poor diets lacking in bone minerals.

Similarly, researchers link frequent soda consumption to kidney stones, asthma, gout, rheumatoid arthritis, and depression in adults, and to behavior problems in young children. Even considering the combined effects of sugars and caffeine, I find it hard to believe that any one food could be linked to so many health problems, unless sodas are an indicator of poor health habits in general and poor diets in particular. One study, for example, observed a correlation between consumption of sugary drinks and earlier menarche, independent of body weight. Associations like these require confirmation from further research.[25]

In seeking a unifying explanation, researchers have looked into the effects of sodas on cell aging. The body's cells can only divide a finite number of times. Each time they divide, the ends of their chromosomes—special sequences of DNA called telomeres—become a bit shorter, making telomere length a potential marker of aging. In 2014, researchers reported that the telomeres in the cells of habitual drinkers of regular carbonated sodas—but not diet sodas, noncarbonated sugary drinks, or fruit juices—were shorter than those of people who did not consume such drinks. This suggested that sodas might make cells age faster, leading to headlines such as this one from *Time* magazine: "Soda May Age You as Much as Smoking." Maybe, but I consider this finding highly preliminary, especially because other scientists have criticized the study's methods and are concerned that some of its authors may have a commercial interest in selling tests for telomere length.[26]

Let's agree that more research is needed to clarify the effects of sodas on conditions other than obesity, type 2 diabetes, and heart disease. But surely we can agree that the evidence linking sodas to these conditions alone is more than sufficient to recommend limits on consumption. To summarize:[27]

- Sodas contribute one-third of total daily sugar intake.
- Soda sugars promote increased calorie intake.
- Sodas decrease the body's ability to compensate for excess calories.
- Sodas increase the risk of obesity and of metabolic risk factors for type 2 diabetes, heart disease, and stroke.

- Reducing intake of sodas and their sugars reduces metabolic abnormalities and disease risks.

THE SODA INDUSTRY'S SPIN ON THE SCIENCE

By this time, you must have noted that when I talk about studies linking sodas to health problems, I mention who pays for them. Given how hard it is to obtain unambiguous results from nutrition studies, it is understandable why the soda industry would want to fund its own research and make sure it is designed and conducted by trusted investigators. In Chapter 19, I talk about the almost entirely predictable results of soda industry sponsorship. But the soda industry is also diligent in casting doubt on science that might suggest that its products cause harm. The cartoon in Figure 5.3 comments on this point.

In 2012, for example, the *New England Journal of Medicine* published several studies suggesting that soda consumption raised the risk of obesity. In response, the ABA issued a lengthy rebuttal. It said [*with my translations*]:[28]

- Obesity is caused by an imbalance between calories consumed from all foods and beverages and those burned through physical activity. [*Never mind what you eat or drink; physical activity is what matters.*]

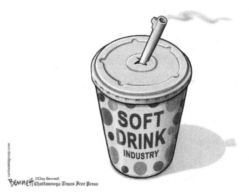

FIGURE 5.3 A cartoonist's take on the soft drink industry. Clay Bennett's substitution of a gun for a straw in this soda pop container not only suggests that soft drinks are killing people but also comments on how aggressively the industry defends its products against charges that they might do so. Used with the permission of Clay Bennett, the Washington Post Writers Group, and the Cartoonist Group. All rights reserved.

- Sugar-sweetened beverages only contribute 7 percent of the calories in the average American's diet. [*This is such a small percentage that you can ignore it, even though sodas contribute a third of daily sugar intake.*]
- These studies do not—and cannot—establish causation, nor do they present clinically meaningful findings. Focusing on total diet and physical activity is most likely to have a real and lasting effect. [*Pay no attention to the sugars and empty calories in sodas.*]
- The limitations of these studies include measurement errors in the intake of sugar-sweetened beverages; self-reported height and weight; the potential for confounding or unknown factors; the lack of evaluation of the proportion of the total energy intake derived from sugar-sweetened beverages; and study cohorts restricted to persons of European ancestry. [*Ignore the research, even though it is voluminous, consistent, and compelling.*]

WHAT IS AT STAKE?

Sodas may not be the only cause of obesity and obesity-related health problems, but they are clearly important contributors. Soda companies know this. In 2014, as it has for a decade, Coca-Cola listed obesity in its annual report to the Securities and Exchange Commission as the leading threat to its potential profitability:

> Consumers, public health officials and government officials are highly concerned about the public health consequences of obesity, particularly among young people. In addition, some researchers, health advocates and dietary guidelines are suggesting that consumption of sugar-sweetened beverages, including those sweetened with HFCS or other nutritive sweeteners, is a primary cause of increased obesity rates and are encouraging consumers to reduce or eliminate consumption of such products. Increasing public concern about obesity; possible new or increased taxes on sugar-sweetened beverages by government entities to reduce consumption or to raise revenue; additional governmental regulations concerning the marketing, labeling, packaging or sale of our sugar-sweetened beverages; and negative publicity resulting from actual or threatened

legal actions against us or other companies in our industry relating to the marketing, labeling or sale of sugar-sweetened beverages may reduce demand for or increase the cost of our sugar-sweetened beverages, which could adversely affect our profitability.[29]

Like cigarette companies, soda companies have a vested interest in selling more of their products, regardless of health consequences. Even if soda company executives would like to promote public heath, their business objectives must invariably take precedence over health objectives. The health consequences of these business objectives constitute the most compelling reason for advocating reduced soda consumption, as illustrated in Chapter 6 and throughout this book.

6

Advocacy

Soda-Free Teeth

In considering how sodas affect health, it is easy to forget about dental caries—the medical term for tooth decay or cavities. Although caries affects practically everyone and is the single most common chronic disease in children and adults worldwide, most of us rarely think of it as a public health crisis. The Centers for Disease Control and Prevention (CDC), for example, conducts separate surveys of the prevalence of decayed, missing, or filled teeth (DMFT) but does not include tooth decay on its list of chronic diseases. Until recently, the World Health Organization (WHO) hardly mentioned caries as a preventable chronic disease. WHO's 2010 resolution on the marketing of junk foods and sodas to children emphasized the need to reduce risks for obesity and type 2 diabetes but said nothing about tooth decay. Although oral health is monitored by groups who track the global burden of disease, tooth decay appears almost as an afterthought in many of their reports.[1]

This omission is unfortunate. Decayed teeth can be life-threatening when infections spread from the mouth to other vital organs. Studies link tooth decay and gum infections to heart disease, for example. More commonly, tooth decay can make life miserable, especially for young children. Deciduous or baby teeth remain in children's mouths from the time they are about 6 months old until age 11 or 12. Decay of these teeth is painful and disfiguring, makes eating difficult, and can lead to nutrient deficiencies, stunting, and wasting even among children in families able to provide sufficient food. Young children with untreated tooth decay are especially vulnerable to stunting and wasting and to the resulting poor cognitive development, school performance, and overall health.[2]

The omission is especially unfortunate because tooth decay is almost entirely preventable: by brushing teeth after meals, drinking fluoridated water, and applying topical fluoride to teeth. Seeing a dentist regularly and having teeth cleaned professionally also helps. Even so, the best way to prevent tooth decay is to eliminate its underlying cause: the sugars in foods and drinks.

In the United States, nearly half of all children under the age of 12 show signs of decay in their primary teeth, and more than 90 percent of adults have permanent teeth that are decayed, missing, or filled. This percentage increases in direct proportion to annual sugar consumption, even when the water is fluoridated. The more sugars consumed, the higher the DFMT percentage. The only world populations displaying low rates of tooth decay are those in extreme poverty who have yet to be exposed to sweets and sodas. Researchers view the introduction of sugary foods and drinks into such populations as a public health hazard of massive proportions. Specifically to prevent tooth decay in adults and children, health authorities say that sugar intake should be restricted to 2 to 3 percent of daily calories, with 5 percent of calories a pragmatic goal.[3] Let me remind you that for someone on a diet of 2,000 calories a day, 5 percent of calories is reached by the amount of sugar in just one 8-ounce soda. I have no trouble understanding why tooth decay is so widely ignored outside the dental community. Sugars are hard to avoid. Most Americans would find limiting sugars to 5 percent of calories impossibly restrictive. Cavities may be common, may hurt, and may be expensive to fix, but once fixed the problem is solved. Because medical specialization assigns obesity to doctors but tooth decay to dentists, it is easy to forget that tooth decay is a health problem and not just a matter of cosmetics. And like many modern health problems, tooth decay is the result of a combination of factors—diet, but also genetics, inadequate oral hygiene, and lack of access to fluoridated water.

But obesity and tooth decay share one factor in common—sodas. Sodas, as this chapter explains, are a *major* contributing factor to tooth decay. Preventing tooth decay is another urgent reason to advocate for reduced soda consumption.

SUGARS, SODAS, AND TOOTH DECAY

Observers have suspected that sugary foods cause tooth decay since the time of Aristotle (384–322 BCE). Ahead of his time on this and many other health issues, Aristotle asked: "Why do figs, which are soft and sweet, destroy the teeth? Do they, owing to their stickiness, penetrate into the gums, and, because they are soft, insinuate themselves into the 30 spaces between the teeth, and, being hot, quickly cause decay?"[4]

I am not sure about the "hot" part, but by the 1950s modern investigators considered the evidence for the role of sugars in tooth decay to be "overwhelming," and by the late 1970s they labeled it "inescapable." The evidence includes animal tests and epidemiologic associations, as well as controlled human studies. Even more compelling, the mechanism of causation has a well-established biological basis. Certain species of bacteria in the mouth are able to use sugars to form sticky polymers that adhere to teeth and provide a platform for the attachment of even more bacteria. As a byproduct of their metabolism, these bacteria secrete acids that dissolve tooth enamel. Although questions still remain about the relative caries-forming capacity of different kinds of sugars, the amounts needed to cause decay, and the modifying effects of fluoride and tooth-brushing, dental scientists generally agree that exposing teeth to any form of sugar promotes caries development. They also agree that the more frequent the exposure to sugars, the higher the number of decayed, missing, and filled teeth—called the "DMFT score" in adults and the "dmft score" in children.[5]

Any form of sugar means any sugar, solid or liquid. Sodas are not sticky, but bathing the teeth in sugar water promotes bacterial growth and the metabolism of sugars to acids. The risk of tooth decay increases with the frequency of exposure to sugar and its duration, which is another reason sipping sugary drinks over time is not a good idea. But sodas have one other decay-promoting characteristic: they are highly acidic (pH 2.6)—as acidic as vinegar.[6] The acids in sodas dissolve tooth enamel, as generations of junior high school students have gleefully demonstrated by dropping baby teeth into glasses of Coca-Cola. Although any acid will dissolve teeth, sodas also contain sugars. The sugar-plus-acid combination is doubly bad for teeth, and frequent, prolonged consumption makes the combined effects even worse.

By now, a great many studies confirm that sugary drinks not only contribute to tooth decay but are a *principal* cause. The more such drinks consumed, the worse the dental problems. Studies find exceptionally high levels of tooth decay and dental erosion among Olympic athletes, for example, problems attributed to their frequent consumption of sports drinks.[7]

But international studies identify sodas as the single most important cause of dental erosion in children—greater than any other dietary factor, including milk, juice, and sports drinks, or, in adults, illicit drugs—even when mitigated by fluoride. The caries-producing effects of soda consumption are most pronounced among children in developing countries, where dental

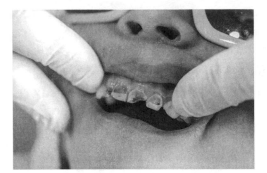

FIGURE 6.1 The teeth of a young child from Ecuador with severe dental erosion caused by frequent consumption of sugar-sweetened beverages and foods. Dental problems this acute cause pain and impair the ability to chew foods properly, leading to malnutrition, learning disabilities, and poor school performance. Photo: Sean Jones. Used with permission of Dr. Karen Sokal-Gutierrez.

care and fluoridated water are expensive or unavailable and where the marketing of soft drinks is particularly intense. The relationship of sodas to tooth decay is so clear that dental researchers can predict the extent of dental caries in young children by the amount of soda they consume. Dentists say they "can spot frequent pop drinkers easily by looking at their teeth" and that "sweetened soda is to teeth as cigarettes are to lungs."[8]

None of this would be much of a problem if dental decay were limited to tiny points that could be easily fixed. But in young children especially, frequent and prolonged exposure of teeth to soft drinks leads to erosion—the dissolving away of large portions of tooth enamel. This happens more frequently to children who have weaker enamel as a result of poor nutritional status. Figure 6.1 shows what severe dental erosion looks like. Soda-induced dental erosion is a modern example of what used to be called baby bottle tooth decay, a problem still seen in infants put to bed sucking on formula, juices, or other sugary drinks. A more recent manifestation in the United States is "Mountain Dew mouth," seen in many low-income areas but particularly in parts of rural Appalachia, where adequate dental care is almost nonexistent.[9]

PUBLIC HEALTH RECOMMENDATIONS

Because soft drinks so clearly cause tooth decay and dental erosion even when oral hygiene, fluoride, and other dietary factors are accounted for, the

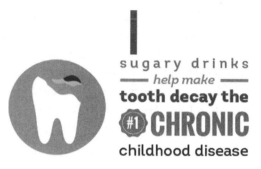

FIGURE 6.2 Section of a "Sugar Bites" infographic emphasizing the role of sugary drinks in tooth decay. The infographic was produced by First 5 Contra Costa and Healthy and Active Before 5, two organizations in Contra Costa County, California, as part of a Social Marketing Campaign to prevent childhood obesity: "Juice drinks, soda, flavored milk and sports drinks can destroy teeth, cause obesity, and lead to type II diabetes."

American Dental Association recommends total avoidance of sugary drinks, especially between meals. Since the early 2000s, the WHO has called for limits on sugar intake expressly to prevent dental disease. The WHO advises two preventive measures: consume no more than 10 percent of total calories from added sugars, and do not consume sugary foods and drinks more than four times per day. To support these recommendations, the WHO also advises environmental interventions: ban soft drink vending machines, and discourage the sale of sweets and unhealthy foods inside or near school premises and at sports events. In 2014, the WHO cited dental disease as the leading reason for limiting sugar calories to no more than 5 percent of daily intake. By now, the evidence linking sodas to tooth decay is so strong that some researchers think sodas should carry warning labels.[10] Indeed, some health departments have initiated campaigns such as the one illustrated in Figure 6.2.

THE SODA INDUSTRY'S RESPONSE

The American Beverage Association insists that sodas are only a minor factor in development of tooth decay or erosion.

> While some critics say beverages are a unique factor in causing tooth decay, the facts state otherwise.... Several factors contribute to the formation of dental cavities, including the types of food consumed, the length of time foods are retained in the mouth and a

person's level of oral hygiene and access to professional dental care. Science tells us that individual susceptibility to both dental cavities and tooth erosion varies depending on a person's behavior, lifestyle, diet and genetic make-up.... The good news is the number of cavities among children has declined significantly in America for the past several decades.... We should all do our part to enhance oral health by brushing and flossing our teeth and making regular visits to the dentist.[11]

The prevalence of tooth decay has indeed declined among U.S. children, but only in those older than 5 years; caries rates are going up among children ages 2 to 5. During the 1990s, DMFT scores in adults fell among all age groups, but they are still quite high, increase with age, and are much higher in low-income groups.[12]

But casting doubt on the science is only one of the soda industry's strategies for dealing with its tooth decay problem. To encourage dentists to emphasize professional care, sealants, and better oral hygiene rather than urging less soda consumption, the Coca-Cola Foundation in 2003 donated a million dollars to the charitable arm of the American Academy of Pediatric Dentistry. The gift was intended to promote education and research; Coke agreed to distribute the academy's educational messages and materials. The academy's 2012 policy statement on diet and dental health notes that soft drinks are associated with tooth decay and obesity, but it says nothing about avoiding sodas. Instead, it euphemistically notes the importance of "educating the public about the association between frequent consumption of carbohydrates and caries." Appalled, the Center for Science in the Public Interest said Coke was paying for "innocence by association."[13] If nothing else, such gifts buy silence.

SUCCESSFUL ADVOCACY: THE CHILDREN'S ORAL HEALTH AND NUTRITION PROJECT

The origin of the international Children's Oral Health and Nutrition Project can be traced to the experience of Karen Sokal-Gutierrez as a U.S. Peace Corps volunteer in Ecuador in the late 1970s. Then, as shown in the faded photograph in Figure 6.3, children may have had other health problems, but their teeth and smiles were beautiful. Not coincidentally, they had little access to sodas and other sugary foods.

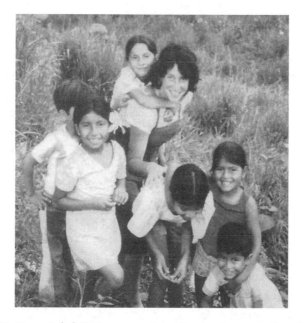

FIGURE 6.3 Dr. Karen Sokal-Gutierrez as a Peace Corps volunteer in Ecuador in the late 1970s. The children, who had little or no exposure to sodas and sugary snacks, had beautiful teeth and lovely smiles. Photo courtesy of Dr. Karen Sokal-Gutierrez.

Twenty years later, and by then a medical doctor, she revisited the country and was shocked to see that many children had rotted and eroded teeth. Heavily advertised sodas and other commercial sweetened products had taken over local markets and replaced traditional foods.

Today Dr. Sokal-Gutierrez is a professor of public health at the University of California, Berkeley, where she directs the Children's Oral Health and Nutrition Project.[14] Its aim is to reduce tooth decay and prevent malnutrition among children from birth through age 6 in developing countries. One of its most important goals is to reduce children's consumption of soda. The project involves four actions that together cost about $5 per child per year:

- Educating parents, children, health workers, and teachers about nutrition and oral health
- Providing toothbrushes and toothpaste to all family members
- Applying fluoride varnish to children's teeth three times per year
- Providing yearly dental exams for children and referrals to dental treatment

Dr. Sokal-Gutierrez began the project in El Salvador and eventually reached about two thousand children and their families. Over the course of six years, from 2004 to 2010, she and her colleagues in that country were able to promote and observe significant reductions in soda consumption. They could link reduced soda drinking to deep reductions in tooth decay, mouth pain, and childhood malnutrition, and could demonstrate that the children who fared best were those involved in the project from birth. She was able to extend the project to Honduras in 2009, Ecuador and Nepal in 2010, Vietnam in 2011, and India in 2012. Other developing countries also want to adopt this intervention. Reducing soda intake continues to be a critical factor in the success of these projects. They prove that advocacy to reduce soda intake pays off in healthier teeth and healthier children.

ADVOCATE: SODA-FREE TEETH

If you would like to get involved in efforts to reduce kids' soda intake as a means of protecting their teeth, here are some suggestions for how to engage in the debate about this issue and to take action in your own community.

Understand the Issue

- Tooth decay is a major public health problem, especially among children.
- Tooth decay and dental erosion cause pain and can lead to deficient nutrient intake and poor overall health.
- Frequent consumption of sugary foods and drinks is a well-established cause of tooth decay.
- Sodas are a particular cause of tooth decay because of their combination of sugars and acids.
- Reducing soda intake is a well-established preventive measure.

Engage in the Debate

When it comes to sodas and tooth decay, industry arguments are not difficult to counter. The evidence that links sodas to dental caries is strong, consistent, and based firmly in biology. Table 6.1 summarizes some of the soda industry's arguments and ways advocates can respond to them.

TABLE 6.1 Topic for debate: do sodas cause dental caries?

THE SODA INDUSTRY SAYS	ADVOCATES SAY
Many factors other than diet influence tooth decay.	Yes they do, but research consistently identifies sodas as a major cause.
Tooth decay can be prevented by appropriate oral hygiene.	Yes it can, but brushing must be frequent to compensate for soda exposure, and not everyone can afford toothpaste and brushes.
Tooth decay can be prevented by topical fluoride treatment and fluoridating water supplies.	Yes it can, but these treatments do not fully compensate for frequent soda exposure. They are also expensive and not everyone has access to them.
It's up to parents to prevent their children from consuming sugary foods and drinks.	It's up to soda companies to stop marketing to children, especially in places where children are not necessarily under parental supervision.
Tooth decay is declining in many places where soda intake is increasing, as a result of better oral hygiene, fluoride sealants, and dental care.	Tooth decay is increasing in many places where sodas are marketed aggressively and preventive methods are unavailable or expensive.

Take Action

To advocate for healthier teeth and healthier children in your community, you can:

- Include dental decay as a reason for advocating soda reduction.
- Demand removal of sugary drinks from schools and around schools.
- Monitor what kids drink; encourage healthier alternatives.
- Demand restrictions on marketing sodas to children.
- Develop or support policies to make safe drinking water widely available at no cost.
- Develop or support campaigns to educate parents and children about the effects of sodas on teeth. State, national, and international dental associations often sponsor campaigns using slogans such as "Drinks destroy teeth" and "Sip all day, get decay."[15]

The Soda Industry and
How It Works

7

Meet Big Soda

An Overview

It is now time to introduce the soft drink industry and its major players: Coca-Cola, PepsiCo, and Dr Pepper Snapple—collectively, Big Soda. The industry as a whole, however, is a massive enterprise involving thousands of companies and hundreds of thousands of people engaged in manufacturing beverage syrups or concentrates; in bottling, canning, preparing, or distributing finished products; and in selling soda cans, bottles, or fountain drinks to consumers everywhere in the world. Soda companies produce and sell the equivalent of nearly two *trillion* 12-ounce servings of fountain or packaged beverages every year.[1]

In doing so, the companies engaged in this industry perform one or more of four distinct tasks: producing syrup, bottling or canning the drinks, distributing the syrup or drinks, or selling the drinks, bottles, or cans. Table 7.1 summarizes the supply chain for carbonated sodas.

Nearly 4,900 companies throughout the world are engaged in producing syrups or bottling sodas, and 1,350 of them are in the United States. Until recently, these companies could be divided neatly into two categories: those making syrup and flavor concentrates for packaged sodas or fountain drinks, and those engaged in bottling or canning the finished products. Coca-Cola, for example, was largely a syrup producer; it left the bottling almost entirely to franchise companies located everywhere sodas are sold. In 2009, however, PepsiCo bought out its North American bottlers, and Coca-Cola did the same the following year. In other regions, some bottlers continue to be separate companies. But producing the syrup controls the

TABLE 7.1 The supply chain for carbonated sodas

COMPANY'S PURPOSE	CONTRIBUTION TO SODA PRODUCTION AND SALES
Syrup producer	• Receives, weighs, and blends flavoring ingredients and sweeteners • Manufactures and packages concentrates, beverage bases, and syrups
Bottler	• Blends syrup with carbonated water • Bottles or cans the products • Seals the containers • Packages and boxes the sodas for shipping
Distributor	Transports bottles, cans, and syrups to: • Supermarkets, retailers • Food service operations, public and institutional • Convenience stores, gas stations • Vending machines
Retailer	Fountain drinks • Blends syrup with carbonated water • Serves with ice Bottles and cans • Receives, stocks, sells

enterprise; every company further down the supply chain depends on getting syrup from the manufacturer.

Most finished soft drinks are sold directly to retailers. Nearly half of all U.S. sales are to supermarket chains and retailers such as Walmart and Target. The next-largest distribution channel is food service, which accounts for one-fifth of sales. McDonald's, for example, is such an important customer that Coca-Cola has a special division for it. Then come convenience stores, drugstores, gas stations, and other such outlets, which collectively account for more than 10 percent of sales. Vending machines bring another 10 percent.

Even this brief description demonstrates that the soda business involves many companies with a vested interest in its success. The stakeholders in the soda business include the soda companies themselves, of course, but also those that supply sugar and other raw ingredients, make syrup, produce carbon dioxide, fabricate the cans and bottles, can and bottle the products, make dispensers and vending machines, deliver ingredients, and supply and service the factories, dispensers, and vending machines. Sodas help support the restaurants, convenience stores, grocery stores, sports facilities, and movie theaters that sell drinks to customers, as well as the advertising agencies employed to market the products and the media venues in which advertisements appear. In later chapters, I will explain how a seemingly infinite number of individuals, nonprofit organizations, educational institutions, health and environmental groups, and business associations benefit from soda company philanthropy, partnerships, and marketing. Because all of these entities depend on sodas for their livelihoods or function, they constitute an unusually wide-ranging support system for Big Soda. Indeed, one of Coca-Cola's guiding rules is to ensure that everyone who touches its products along the way to the consumer should make money doing so. This is a business strategy guaranteed to ensure deep and lasting devotion.[2]

THE GLOBAL SOFT DRINK INDUSTRY

Although the two largest producers—and now bottlers—of sodas are American companies, this industry is decidedly global. In 2012, worldwide sales of all kinds of beverages (including bottled water) generated revenues variably estimated at from $200 billion to $800 billion, depending on the range of beverage products included in the analysis.[3]

To see where international sales of sugar-sweetened beverages fit into this broad context, Table 7.2 lists the percent of total revenue generated by various categories of drinks.

Except for bottled water and diet cola, everything else on this list comes with added sugars. Together, sugary drinks account for 65 percent of worldwide sales of all beverages. According to one of the research firms tracking such things, the world's three largest soft drink companies—Coca-Cola,

TABLE 7.2 Percent of global revenue generated by categories of beverages, 2012

BEVERAGE CATEGORY	PERCENT OF TOTAL REVENUE
Carbonated cola	38
Bottled water	19
Carbonated diet cola	16
Other carbonated sodas	9
Lemonade	8
Sports drinks	6
Energy drinks	4

SOURCE: *Global Soft Drink & Bottled Water Manufacturing*, IBISworld, January 2013.

TABLE 7.3 Global market share, revenues, and profits from sales of soft drinks, Big Soda, 2012

COMPANY	MARKET SHARE, PERCENT	REVENUE, $ BILLION	PROFIT, $ BILLION	PROFIT
Coca-Cola	25	48	11	23%
PepsiCo	18	34	5	15%
Coca-Cola FEMSA	6	11	2	18%
Average for the 3 companies	49	93	18	19%

SOURCE: *Global Soft Drink & Bottled Water Manufacturing*, IBISWorld, January 2013.

PepsiCo, and Coca-Cola FEMSA (the Latin American partner)—generated $93 billion in sales in 2012, as shown in Table 7.3. This industry is famously profitable. These three companies averaged profits of 19 percent that year, but profits are now declining somewhat along with soda sales.

The international soft drink industry, according to business analysts, is moderately consolidated, mature (in the business sense), and highly globalized. Despite the dominance of Coca-Cola and PepsiCo, the remaining half of the global market is shared among countless small brands and private labels sold through supermarket chains such as Walmart in the United States and Sainsbury in the United Kingdom, or, in developing countries, in niche markets catering to local tastes. Consolidation is expected to increase as larger companies buy up the more successful smaller ones.

Reflecting the maturity of this industry, the number of companies involved in the business has been declining for years, and further declines are expected. Whereas sales of bottled waters, sports drinks, and energy drinks are increasing in industrialized countries, sales of sodas are falling. To compensate for this loss, soda companies are increasingly marketing to developing world economies. Although the United States, Canada, and Mexico together produce more than one-third of the world's soft drinks, and European countries produce almost another third, the remaining third is shared among a great many other countries in which opportunities for sales expansion seem unlimited.

The United States may be the largest market for soft drinks, but other leading markets—notably those of China, Brazil, and Mexico—are middle-income countries. The soda industry expects future growth to derive from sales in those three countries as well as in India, Asia, and throughout Africa. In Chapter 9, I present a more detailed discussion of international soda marketing, but for now let's return to how Big Soda operates in the United States.

THE U.S. SODA INDUSTRY

In the United States, many of the companies engaged in beverage manufacturing belong to the industry trade group, the American Beverage Association (ABA). This association's role, among others, is to promote the value of
its member companies to the U.S. economy. The soda industry, it says, "has
a direct economic impact of $141.22 billion, provides more than 233,000
jobs, and helps to support hundreds of thousands more that depend, in
part, on beverage sales for their livelihoods."[4] Moreover, says the ABA, the
companies and their employees pay more than $14 billion in state taxes and
nearly $23 billion in federal business and income taxes, and contribute hun-
dreds of millions of dollars to charitable causes. Although the ABA does not
say so directly, its point is that any public health campaign to reduce soda
intake will cost jobs and harm the economy. You may recall that cigarette
companies set the standard for use of such arguments. But in promoting the
value of their industries to the economy, neither considers the economic or
personal costs of the diseases their products may cause.

Like the cigarette industry, the U.S. soda industry is dominated by a
very few companies, in this case Coca-Cola, PepsiCo, and Dr Pepper Snapple. Table 7.4 lists the leading producers of carbonated soft drinks, in rank
order. In 2014, Coca-Cola led the market with a 42.3 percent share that includes both diet and regular (sugar-sweetened) beverages, but Coke's U.S.
sales represent just 20 percent of the company's global sales. Pepsi comes
next, followed by Dr Pepper Snapple, which also markets 7UP in the United
States (in Europe, 7UP is marketed by PepsiCo.) Other companies hold much

TABLE 7.4 The leading U.S. companies that produce
carbonated sodas, 2014

RANK	COMPANY	PERCENT VOLUME*
1	Coca-Cola	42.3
2	PepsiCo	27.5
3	Dr Pepper Snapple	17.1
4	Cott Corporation	4.2
5	National Beverage	2.9
6	Monster Beverage	1.7
	All other	4.3

* Refers to *all* brands made by the company.

SOURCE: Adapted from *Beverage Digest*, March 26, 2015. Coca-Cola
bought a 16.7% equity stake in Monster Beverage in 2014.

TABLE 7.5 Leading specific U.S. brands of carbonated soft drinks, 2014

SALES RANK	BRAND*	MARKET SHARE, PERCENT
1	Coca-Cola	17.6
2	Pepsi-Cola	8.8
3	Diet Coke	8.5
4	Mountain Dew (PepsiCo)	6.9
5	Dr Pepper	6.8
6	Sprite (Coca-Cola)	6.0
7	Diet Pepsi	4.3
8	Fanta (Coca-Cola)	2.2

* All are sugar-sweetened except for Diet Coke and Diet Pepsi. Adapted from *Beverage Digest*, March 26, 2015.

smaller market shares. In contrast to this industry's global concentration, which is considered moderate, the U.S. soda industry is highly concentrated, and remarkably so: the three leading companies control nearly 90 percent of the market. Just the top two control nearly 70 percent. In 2014, Coca-Cola bought a 16.7 percent share of Monster Beverage in a partnership clearly designed to further expand the market share of both companies.[5]

What brands do these companies sell? Among hundreds, Table 7.5 lists the eight leading brands of carbonated soft drinks in the United States. Six of these top brands are sugar-sweetened. In 2014, Coca-Cola's sugar-sweetened brands (regular Coke, Sprite, and Fanta) together held a market share of nearly 26 percent. The two leading sugary Pepsi brands (Pepsi plus Mountain Dew) held nearly a 16 percent share. The two other brands in the top ten are Diet Mountain Dew and Coke Zero, with shares of about 2 percent each.

Nevertheless, the big news in 2014 was Pepsi-Cola's replacement of Diet Coke at the number two position. Diet Coke had held that rank since 2010, but its sales fell by 6.6 percent in the previous year—a result, according to *Beverage Digest*, of consumers' "withdrawal of enthusiasm for aspartame and other legacy diet sweeteners."[6]

This table demonstrates that concentration in the soda industry extends to specific brands. The leading brands of sugar-sweetened sodas, each manufactured by one of the three leading companies, account for almost half of all soft drink sales in the United States. Now let's take a brief look at these major players: Coke, Pepsi, Dr Pepper Snapple, and their trade group, the American Beverage Association.

Coca-Cola

In the more than one hundred years since it was founded in 1886, The Coca-Cola Company (its official abbreviation is TCCC) has become an internationally recognized symbol of business success. The company, which employs about 150,000 people, earned $11 billion in profits on revenues of $48 billion in 2012 (Table 7.3). In April 2015, a share of Coca-Cola sold for $41, but its market capitalization—the value of all its stock—was more than $178 billion. The previous year, the company rewarded its chief executive, Muhtar Kent, with $18.2 million in salary, bonuses, perquisites, stocks, and stock options. He also owned more than 260,000 shares of Coca-Cola stock, worth an additional $11 million.[7] Throughout its history, Coca-Cola has generated impressive wealth for its executives and investors.

During this history, Coca-Cola became firmly established as a ubiquitous icon of American culture. Business analysts frequently acknowledge Coca-Cola as the top-ranked global brand—not just in the category of foods or beverages, but among *all* brands. After a thirteen-year run in the leading position, the company fell to second place after Apple in 2013.[8] It is still extremely popular with the public. In mid-2015, Coca-Cola's Facebook page had more than 89 million "likes." As I discuss in later chapters, the company routinely wins the industry's highest awards for effective advertising, leadership, and social responsibility.

Shelves of books are devoted to the history of the company and its marketing practices, to biographies of its leaders, to its vast collections of memorabilia, and even to recipes that include its signature product as an ingredient. I list and describe some of these works in the bibliographic note in Appendix 3. Although these books also cover some of the company's less attractive business practices, particularly in developing countries, the sheer number of these volumes attests to the position held by this maker of flavored sugar water as a quintessentially American economic and cultural institution.

Coca-Cola is best known for its namesake brand, but it also markets 3,500 different products under 500 brand names in more than 200 countries and territories. Fanta and Fresca are some of the better known non-cola brands, but the company also owns Dasani water, Minute Maid juice, and Glacéau Vitaminwater, as well as smaller international brands such as VegitaBeta in Japan and Inca Kola in Peru. Some non-colas, such as Fanta, are sold internationally in dozens of flavors. In Macedonia, for example, you can buy Orange, Lemon, and Melon Fanta, but also Shokata (elderflower) and Bamboocha (translated, more or less, as "terrific"). I find it hard to get my head around this fact: Coca-Cola provides more than 1.8 billion servings a day of everything in its product lines. That's billions, every day. The company maintains this reach through a system that involves 250 bottlers worldwide.[9]

It is worth taking a minute to think about Coca-Cola's business model. This is a relatively small—but very rich—company founded on the manufacture of syrup. Historically, it left the more labor- and capital-intensive production of the actual sodas (and the risks that go with it) to franchise operations. The company controls sales of the syrup, but it also decides who gets the franchises, how the syrup is produced and distributed, and how the final products are packaged and advertised. It exerts this control through complete or partial ownership of the franchises. By the mid-1980s, Coca-Cola owned one-third of its bottling operations. In 2006, it consolidated the North American bottling operations into a new and distinct corporate entity, Coca-Cola Enterprises (CCE). Five years later, Coca-Cola took over CCE's entire North American business, changed that company's name to Coca-Cola Refreshments (CCR), and folded most of its U.S. and Canadian businesses into this new corporation.

Although the overseas business model keeps the bottling corporations separate, the parent Coca-Cola Company (TCCC) typically and deliberately owns no more than a 49 percent share of any franchise operation. Holding less than a majority share allows Coca-Cola to control the bottling operations in various countries without being saddled with legal or moral responsibility for anything the local bottlers do with respect to labor rights, water use, or environmental damage, issues I take up in later chapters.[10]

PepsiCo

Pepsi is the leading soft drink produced by a company increasingly focused on its snack food operations. Beverages account for just under half of all PepsiCo sales, but Pepsi is still the company's flagship product. It is also a popular company; its Facebook page in late 2014 recorded nearly 33 million "likes." In addition to Pepsi and Mountain Dew, the sports drink Gatorade, Tropicana juices, and Aquafina and other bottled waters, PepsiCo owns Frito-Lay, Lipton Tea, and Quaker Oats, among other brands. Twenty-two of its brands each bring in more than a billion dollars a year, and the entire Pepsi portfolio generated revenues of more than $65 billion in 2012, for a profit of nearly $11 billion. Like Coca-Cola, Pepsi sells its carbonated beverages in more than two hundred countries and territories. Among its brands of drinks, Manzanita Sol and Mirinda especially target Hispanic markets.[11]

In mid-2015, a share of PepsiCo cost just over $96 for a market capitalization of more than $142 billion. Coca-Cola has higher revenues, but PepsiCo is not doing badly. Its shares, like those of Coca-Cola, have doubled in value since 2009. In 2013, PepsiCo paid its chief executive, Indra Nooyi, a base salary of $1.6 million, stock awards of $7.5 million, a performance-based bonus of $4 million, $102,772 for use of the company aircraft, and $30,463 for ground transportation—more than $13 million in total.[12] By 2015, she owned nearly 722,000 shares of PepsiCo stock, valued at more than $69 million.

Pepsi is a larger company than Coca-Cola—it employs 278,000 people worldwide, 106,000 of them in the United States—but you would never know that from comparing soda revenues. In the soda universe, Pepsi is decidedly number two. Whether it tries harder is debatable, but its competition with Coca-Cola has long been known as the "soda wars." Years ago, critics recognized the absurdity of the conflict as a form of sibling rivalry—and among twins at that: "They look the same, they taste the same, and they bubble into foam the same."[13] The latest skirmish occurred in 2014, when Pepsi displaced Diet Coke as the second-highest-selling soft drink in America.

Dr Pepper Snapple

This company, much smaller than either Coke or Pepsi, used to be a division of Cadbury Schweppes but after a series of mergers and acquisitions ended up in its present form in 2008. The company now produces more than fifty different drinks under its principal labels: Dr Pepper, 7UP, Royal Crown, A & W, and Canada Dry. But it also owns Nehi, Hawaiian Punch, and Deja Blue, among others. Its integrated syrup, concentrate, and bottling operations brought in nearly $6 billion in revenues in 2012, for a tidy profit of $1.3 billion. Fourteen percent of its sales are to Walmart, and nearly 90 percent are in the United States, with the rest mainly in Canada, Mexico, and the Caribbean. Carbonated beverages account for 80 percent of sales.

Dr Pepper holds licensing agreements with both Coca-Cola and PepsiCo to distribute its beverages in the United States and to bottle and distribute its products in other countries. Rather than attempting a hopeless competition with Coke and Pepsi over cola sales, Dr Pepper focuses on flavored soft drinks: "Without flavors, we'd be just another cola company." The company's sales in the United States have been relatively flat in recent years but are increasing elsewhere, enough to explain why its stock price continues to rise and nearly tripled in value between 2009 and 2014. Business analysts do not expect Dr Pepper to ever outsell Coke and Pepsi but think it "will likely plug along profitably, though slowly, over time."[14]

The American Beverage Association (ABA)

The ABA is the soda industry's principal trade association, public relations agent, and staunch defender. It originated in 1919 as the American Bottlers of Carbonated Beverages but changed its name to the National Soft Drink Association in 1966. Recognizing that industry growth increasingly involved sports and energy drinks and other nontraditional beverages, the group adopted the current name in 2004. The ABA represents dozens of beverage producers, bottlers, distributors, franchise companies, and support industries, but bottlers predominate, particularly those connected to Coca-Cola, PepsiCo, and Dr Pepper Snapple.

The ABA describes itself as a neutral forum for members to discuss common issues; a liaison between the industry, government, and the public; and a strong voice for the industry in legislative and regulatory matters. Its staff consists of legislative, scientific, technical, regulatory, legal, and communications experts devoted to representing the interests of member companies. The ABA lobbies aggressively on behalf of the industry and weighs in loudly, forcefully, and persistently on a broad range of issues affecting the soda marketing environment, as I point out in later chapters.[15]

SUGARY DRINK PROFITABILITY: BUSINESS STRATEGIES

In the most recent addition to my library of books about this industry, the historian Bartow Elmore describes its business model as "Coca-Cola capitalism." By this, he means that this industry outsources the making of its products and, therefore, the social, environmental, and financial risks entailed in their production. The soda industry, he says, must be understood as an extractive industry. Like other extraction industries, it draws on natural resources and transfers the cost of those resources—water and agricultural land for growing sugar and corn, for example—to taxpayers. The public pays for municipal water supplies used to make soft drinks, for the railroads and highways used to transport the drinks, for the corn subsidies that reduce the price of high-fructose corn syrup (HFCS), for cleaning up the mess made by discarded cans and plastic bottles, and for the health care of soda drinkers who become ill.[16]

This business model explains why, despite slow growth and declining sales in some markets, sugary drinks generate hefty profits. Profits are driven by marketing and by overseas sales, as I discuss in later chapters, but Big Soda companies keep costs low by outsourcing many of them. They also take advantage of the tax system to benefit their investors. In 2013, for example, the average tax rate for the soda industry was 19 percent, substantially below that of most individual taxpayers. To achieve low tax rates, soda companies move their worldwide concentrate headquarters to Singapore (Coca-Cola) or Ireland (PepsiCo). Coca-Cola's tax rate was 15 percent in 2012, while Pepsi's was 21 percent. By one analysis, Coca-Cola keeps 88 percent of its cash overseas, which amounted to more than $13.9 billion in 2013.[17]

Publicly traded corporations are required to disclose information about who invests in them. Coca-Cola's largest and most famous stockholder is Warren Buffett's Berkshire Hathaway, which owned 400 million shares valued at more than $16 billion in April 2015. The other major institutional holders of the soda Big Three are mutual funds and banks. The Vanguard Group, for example, is the second-leading investor in Coca-Cola (244.5 million shares), number one in PepsiCo (93 million), and number two in Dr Pepper Snapple (16 million). The State Street Corporation is the number three investor in Coke and number two in Pepsi. BlackRock Institutional Trust shows up as a top-ten investor in all three companies. The values of investor holdings run into the billions. If your retirement funds are invested with these companies, you—like Warren Buffett—will want soda stocks to continue to increase in value and will do and say nothing that might reduce the value of those stocks.

Again, let me point to the irony of all this. These extraordinary profits and returns come from the sale of products that cost practically nothing to manufacture. Their principal ingredient—water—comes at low cost from the tap at taxpayer expense. Their most expensive ingredient is the sugar or HFCS sweetener, but both are relatively cheap as a result of price stabilization of cane and beet sugar and subsidies for corn. In many gas stations, supermarkets, and fast-food chains, sodas are used as "loss leaders," underpriced items attracting customers into stores where sodas cost less than bottled water. Figure 7.1 presents an example.

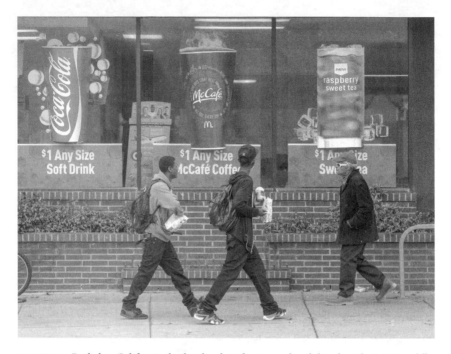

FIGURE 7.1 Berkeley, California, high school students on a lunch break at the McDonald's on University Avenue. Fountain drinks cost so little to produce that fast-food chains can offer them for a fixed, low price, no matter how large the container. This photo, taken by Gael McKeon on October 20, 2014, is part of a photo essay on Berkeley's successful soda tax initiative discussed in Chapter 27. Used with permission.

PRESSURES ON SODA INDUSTRY PROFITS: BUSINESS AND HEALTH

While the business community still ranks Coke and Pepsi among the top-ten brands in America and the companies' overall sales and profits are still highly robust, many signs indicate that sodas are in trouble. The persistent decline in soda sales since the late 1990s is only the most visible such sign, but it is the one that most disturbs investors. Activist shareholders are demanding that PepsiCo spin off its less profitable beverages and focus entirely on snack sales. Other investors, concerned that 75 percent of Coca-Cola beverages are high in sugar, want more diversification in the company's product portfolio. Soda suppliers and bottlers face increasing competition from SodaStream and other makers of home carbonation machines. Transporters and bottlers fear that Coca-Cola's Freestyle cartridge-based soda-dispensing machines could put them out of business. Others worry that Pepsi's computerized, personalized, and customized Spire dispensers could replace traditional fountains.[18]

From the soda industry's standpoint, however, the single biggest threat to its long-term profitability is obesity. For a century, Coca-Cola and PepsiCo have been accustomed to enthusiastic public support. The idea that the public might hold these companies responsible for childhood obesity, let alone accountable for it, comes as an unwelcome surprise. How obesity became a threat to soda sales and what the companies are doing to counter this threat come next.

8

Obesity

Big Soda's Response

You might think the biggest threat posed by obesity is the risk of chronic disease, but the soda industry's concern is quite different: loss of sales. If you can prevent obesity by drinking less soda, you might actually do that. The industry recognized this threat long before obesity became the prominent public health concern that it is today. When the Senate Select Committee on Nutrition and Human Needs wrote the Dietary Goals in 1977, the soda industry needed to respond to the "drink less soda" recommendation. But industry officials suspected that an overt attack on the goals might create an "untenable, anti-soda backlash."[1] Instead, soda companies used less confrontational tactics. They recruited sympathetic scientists to attack the Dietary Goals as unjustified, and arranged for the industry trade association, then called the National Soft-Drink Association, to do the talking for them. The association framed its rebuttal in ways sure to resonate with the public:

- Sodas bring pleasure and have a place in balanced diets.
- Personal choice is a fundamental freedom of American citizenship.
- Parents know how to decide what their children eat and drink.

The soda industry's position, then and now, is that obesity is strictly a matter of individual and parental responsibility (see Figure 8.1).

Throughout this book, I maintain that it is much easier for individuals to make responsible personal choices in a healthier food environment backed up by supportive public policies.[2] In this chapter, I explain how the

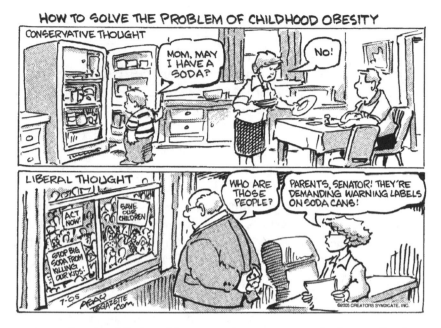

FIGURE 8.1 A cartoonist's view of the contrast between conservative (personal) and liberal (policy) views about how to prevent childhood obesity. The soda industry argues that because obesity is a matter of personal responsibility, government has no business suggesting that people would be healthier drinking less soda. Chuck Asay, Creators Syndicate. Used with permission.

industry's 1977 expressions of doubt about the role of sodas in obesity remain central to its current "playbook"—the term advocates use to describe the standard talking points used by the tobacco industry and now any industry selling a product that is not good for health. Although the soda industry's basic arguments remain the same, it has refined the playbook over the years in response to increasingly urgent concerns about the role of sugary drinks in obesity.

Recall from Chapter 4 that from 1980 to 2000, federal dietary guidelines said little about drinking less soda. These were precisely the years in which the prevalence of obesity increased sharply among children as well as adults. In 2001, the U.S. surgeon general, then Dr. David Satcher, issued a call to action to prevent obesity, especially among schoolchildren. While not mentioning sugary drinks by name, he urged the USDA to mandate healthy beverages in schools during meals and sports events and to enforce standards prohibiting foods of minimal nutritional value from school meals and vending machines. All foods and beverages served at schools, he said, should contribute to eating patterns consistent with the Dietary Guidelines.[3]

To investment analysts, this suggestion from the nation's top doctor was nothing short of alarming. In reports released in 2003, researchers in three international banking firms warned food and beverage companies that they must act quickly to turn the obesity crisis into a business opportunity. Soda companies got the message. In 2007, a Coca-Cola marketing executive told a reporter from *Advertising Age*, "Our Achilles heel is the discussion about obesity....It's gone from a small, manageable U.S. issue to a huge global issue. It dilutes our marketing and works against it. It's a huge, huge issue."[4]

That soda companies were aware of the way concerns about obesity might threaten profits is evident from Coca-Cola's annual reports to the U.S. Securities and Exchange Commission (SEC), which I mentioned in Chapter 5. The SEC requires corporations to disclose factors that might pose a risk to meeting growth targets. As it had in annual SEC filings since at least 2003, Coca-Cola listed obesity as its primary risk. Obesity, as the company wrote in its 2013 report, "represents a significant challenge to our industry." Its explanation echoed phrases used in 1977:

> We understand and recognize that obesity is a complex public health challenge and are committed to being a part of the solution. We recognize the uniqueness of consumers' lifestyles and dietary choices. All of our products can be part of an active, healthy lifestyle that includes a sensible and balanced diet, proper hydration and regular physical activity. However, when it comes to weight management, all calories count, whatever food or beverage they come from, including calories from our beverages.[5]

BIG SODA'S PUBLIC RELATIONS PLAYBOOK

Since the 1970s, the soda industry has remained firmly "on message" and its playbook themes are familiar and predictable.[6] Its messages, methods, and actions aim to achieve three goals: avoid public criticism, head off government regulation, and protect sales. I am awestruck by how well soda companies manage these tasks. Their strategies are astonishingly comprehensive. No community group is too inconsequential to receive a grant from the Coke or Pepsi corporate foundations. No city contemplating a soda tax is too small or too poor to be the target of a massive and lavishly funded counteroffensive.

No issue that might affect marketing is too trivial to be ignored by industry lobbyists.

To public health advocates familiar with the actions of tobacco companies, the response of soda companies to obesity seems all too familiar. Soda is not tobacco, of course, and the problems it causes depend on how much is consumed and how often. But the soda industry's playbook—the script it follows—is a carbon copy of the one used by cigarette companies to deflect attention from the hazards of smoking. Figure 8.2 illustrates this point.

As Professors Kelly Brownell and Kenneth Warner wrote in the *Milbank Quarterly* in 2009, the cigarette industry's playbook invariably

emphasized personal responsibility, paying scientists who delivered research that instilled doubt, criticizing the "junk" science that found harms associated with smoking, making self-regulatory

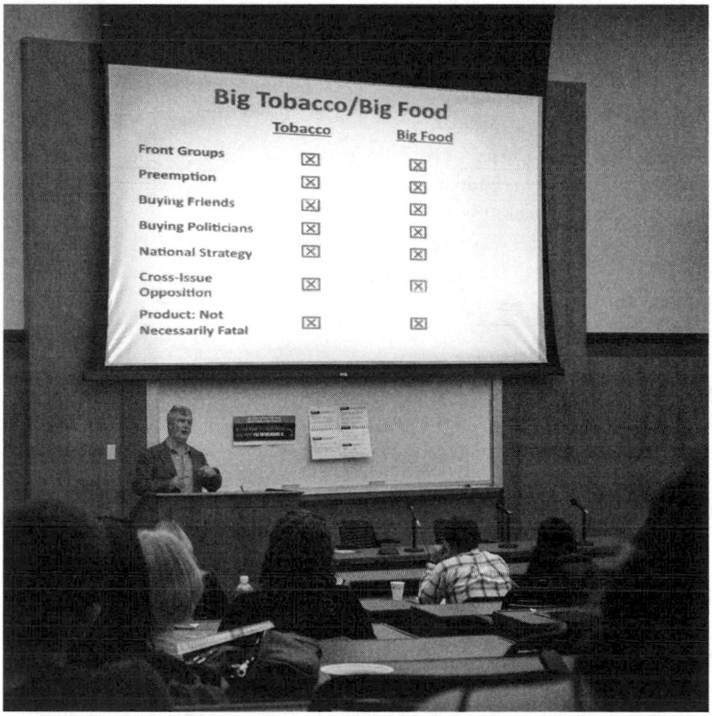

FIGURE 8.2 Big Tobacco and Big Food use similar political strategies. In October 2014, just before the ultimately successful vote for a soda tax in Berkeley, California (Chapter 27), Mark Pertschuk, a longtime advocate for anti-smoking policies and grassroots approaches to social change, pointed out the parallels. Photo by Gael McKeon. Used with permission.

pledges, lobbying with massive resources to stifle government action, introducing "safer" products, and simultaneously manipulating and denying both the addictive nature of their products and their marketing to children...Because obesity is now a major global problem, the world cannot afford a repeat of the tobacco history, in which industry talks about the moral high ground but does not occupy it.[7]

In Table 8.1, I summarize the strategies used by soda companies to counter the threat of obesity to sales and profits. For convenience, I divide the industry's methods into four categories. The first, covered in this chapter, deals with the efforts of soda companies to position themselves and their industry as deeply committed to health and wellness. The second, discussed in Chapters 9 to 16, demonstrates how soda companies market

TABLE 8.1 The soda industry's four-part playbook in reaction to obesity: summary

1. Emphasize devotion to health and wellness (this chapter)
   - Reframe the issues
   - Divert attention to physical activity
   - Introduce and promote "better for you" products
   - Self-regulate marketing to children
   - Create coalitions to promote the reframed messages
2. Sell to everyone, everywhere (Chapters 9–16)
   - Put millions into advertising and marketing
   - Use celebrities and sports heroes
   - Market to children
   - Market to minorities
   - Market to developing countries
3. Build allies: create conflicts of interest among potential critics (Chapters 17–22)
   - Engage in philanthropy: provide funds for students, athletes, playgrounds, city parks
   - Form partnerships and alliances with health professional groups, minority groups, anti-hunger groups
   - Sponsor nutrition research, athletic and sports activities
   - Engage in and emphasize corporate social responsibility
4. Play hardball: protect corporate interests (Chapters 23–27)
   - Attack the science as "junk"
   - Attack the critics as "nannies"
   - Form advocacy groups posing as "grassroots" (but really "astroturf")
   - Fund campaigns and legal challenges to soda taxes, soda caps, labeling of genetically modified foods (GMOs)
   - Fund public relations firms posing as public interest groups
   - Lobby state and federal officials
   - Contribute to election campaigns

their products in every imaginable way, in every place imaginable, and to every imaginable person. In the third category, I explain how the soda industry uses "softball" tactics—those that appear open and friendly—to build allies and neutralize potential critics (Chapters 17 to 22). While engaged in these softer approaches, soda companies simultaneously employ the more aggressive "hardball" tactics covered in Chapters 23 to 27. But for now, let's look at how soda companies attempt to appear as part of the solution to obesity, rather than its cause. As Coca-Cola says in its 2013 filing with the SEC, "We understand and recognize that obesity is a complex public health challenge and are committed to being a part of the solution."

EMPHASIZE DEVOTION TO HEALTH AND WELLNESS

Soda industry rhetoric in response to concerns about obesity is best seen in statements from its trade association, now called the American Beverage Association (ABA). The ABA deals with the obesity issue head on: "The headlines are hard to ignore. America needs to lose weight." The association

> is concerned about the obesity issue in America and is proudly doing its part to help improve health and wellness...All of our industry's beverages can be enjoyed as part of a balanced lifestyle.... While beverages and food play a role in determining good health, so do other important factors. In fact, it is generally accepted that obesity involves three main factors: genetics, diet and exercise. We know that obesity is a serious and complex problem that is best addressed by living a balanced lifestyle—consuming a variety of foods and beverages in moderation and getting plenty of exercise. Quite simply, overweight and obesity are a result of an imbalance between calories consumed and calories burned.[8]

In sum, the ABA's statement translates to mean that obesity is about anything other than "drink less soda."

Reframe the Issues

On a website devoted to clearing up its version of myths about sodas, the ABA says, "FACT: Obesity is a complex condition, that can't be boiled down to one specific product or ingredient. Many health organizations, including the Mayo Clinic, have found multiple risk factors, including genetics, age, stress, and even lack of sleep."[9] Such statements aim to deflect attention from the health effects of sodas by emphasizing anything other than sugars and calories. Its update of the 1977 framing devices looks like this [*with my comments added*]:

- Sodas can be part of healthful diets. [*Yes, but only in small amounts.*]
- Other foods and beverages also contribute calories. [*They do, but sodas contribute one-third of the sugar consumed in the United States and with other sugary drinks contribute half. Their calories are empty, and they are well established to promote poor health.*]
- Genetics is the key determinant of obesity. [*Genetics has not changed since 1980.*]
- Physical activity is more important. [*Activity is important, but it takes considerable effort to balance excessive calorie intake.*]

Divert Attention to Physical Activity

I call the idea that obesity is about physical activity, not what you eat, the "physical activity diversion." In 2013, to pick just one instance, Coca-Cola placed a full-page ad in the *New York Times* (May 8): "At Coca-Cola, we believe active lifestyles lead to happier lives. That's why we are committed to creating awareness around choice and movement, to help people make the most informed decisions for themselves and their families." The soda industry aimed its 2014 "Mixify" campaign at teenagers: "Balance what you eat and drink with what you do. That's how you Mixify."

Don't get me wrong. I greatly favor physical activity for its substantial physiological, social, psychological, and health benefits, but, as I discuss in Chapter 17, it is much easier to overeat than it is to work off excess calories. That is why Coca-Cola's 2013 video showing how effortless it is to burn off the 140 "happy calories" from a 12-ounce soft drink—75 seconds of laughing out loud, for example—elicited dismay if not outrage. Coca-Cola marketers meant this approach to be amusing, but the commercial message was so far from the reality of calorie balance that several countries banned it.[10]

Introduce and Promote "Better for You" Products

Business analysts view both Coca-Cola and PepsiCo as drivers of today's burgeoning health-and-wellness market—referred to in the trade by the abbreviation *HW*. Both companies, they say, are taking initiatives to promote their HW profiles by expanding sales of existing HW products (e.g., Diet Coke and Diet Pepsi), developing new HW products (Coke Zero, Pepsi Max), and acquiring smaller companies that make HW carbonated drinks, HW juice, HW functional drinks, HW bottled water, and HW ready-to-drink teas. Better-for-you products, they say, make good business sense.[11] Yes, but they make the best health sense when unsweetened.

Coca-Cola's anti-obesity efforts. In May 2013, Coca-Cola used playbook rhetoric to announce a new initiative, "Coming Together:" "Beating obesity will take all of us.... [A]s the world's leading beverage company, we can play an important role by creating awareness around choice, helping consumers make the most informed decisions for themselves and their families, and by inspiring people everywhere to find the fun in movement."[12] In that spirit, the company said, it would commit to the following actions in every country in which it does business:

- Offer low- or no-calorie beverage options
- Provide transparent nutrition information, featuring calories on the front of all packages
- Help get people moving by supporting physical activity programs
- Market responsibly, including no advertising to children under 12

In 2013, the Coca-Cola webpage prominently displayed this message: "Help us fight obesity." A click on that statement sent readers to an infographic explaining the company's global commitments, and a dedicated website (www.comingtogether.com). A jazzy Coca-Cola cartoon video advertisement linked physical activity to happiness: if you are happy, you are moving; if you are moving, you are happy—and Coke makes you happy too. Another Coca-Cola video, "Coming Together," explained that 180 of Coke's 650 beverage products were low in calories, and that the company had reduced the number of calories per serving in its overall beverage profile by 22 percent. To public health advocates, these promises and claims were so far from the reality of Coca-Cola marketing practices that the Center for

Science in the Public Interest issued its own satirical version of the video with commentary, "Coming Together, Translated."[13]

Business analysts also were dubious. In a case study of Coca-Cola's communication strategies to deal with the obesity problem, they noted:

> Coca-Cola's major challenge is finding a balance between supporting anti-obesity efforts and selling products many claim contribute to the very issue Coca-Cola is taking efforts to eliminate.... [M]any perceive the company's anti-obesity efforts as disingenuous attempts at damage control to keep sales up. Continuing to engage in discussions about scientific studies and Coca-Cola product nutrition will be essential in ensuring Coca-Cola is perceived as transparent and genuinely concerned in consumers' wellbeing, rather than simply concerned with profit.... By acknowledging the obesity issue and spending millions of dollars on anti-obesity efforts, Coca-Cola is demonstrating corporate social responsibility—if not in its products, then at least in its community involvement.... The challenge is for Coca-Cola to find a way to be taken seriously as a player in anti-obesity efforts while simultaneously increasing sales and offering consumers the products they love.[14]

Advocates most definitely do perceive the company's anti-obesity efforts as disingenuous and view profit as the determining motive for all of its actions. If companies fail to put profits first, they get into trouble, as PepsiCo's HW efforts demonstrated.

PepsiCo's ill-fated attempt to promote wellness. Although PepsiCo's 2013 SEC filing mentioned obesity only within the context of "health concerns (whether or not valid) about our products," the company's CEO, Indra Nooyi, discussed obesity in her 2012 annual report: "Intensifying consumer and government focus on health and wellness is changing the relative growth trajectory of our categories and products. Consumers are clearly changing their habits, preferences and consumption patterns."[15] Pepsi, she suggested, was responding to these changes in beverage preferences by making healthier products.

Revealingly, Pepsi groups its products into three categories: "Fun for You" (e.g., Pepsi, Mountain Dew, and other sugar-sweetened beverages), "Better for You" (Pepsi NEXT), and "Good for You" (Aquafina, Gatorade). Pepsi's 2012 annual report said: "Importantly, we offer low- or zero-calorie

and smaller-portioned options, such as 8 ounce cans, for almost every drink
we make. To further help our customers manage calories...we launched
Pepsi NEXT, a game-changer in the cola category." Pepsi NEXT, in the
"Better for You" category, is a reduced-sugar version that contains 35 calories in 7.5 ounces. But is Gatorade really "good for you"? It still has half the
sugar of Pepsi along with a few added electrolyte minerals.

PepsiCo tends to be more cautious than Coca-Cola when talking about
obesity, perhaps because it got burned so badly when it did. In 2008, Pepsi attempted to position itself as a wellness company. *Fortune* magazine celebrated
this initiative with an admiring cover profile of the beautifully dressed Indra
Nooyi: "The Pepsi Challenge: Can This Snack and Soda Giant Go Healthy?"
Pepsi, *Fortune* noted, "was so early getting beyond soda pop and into the
healthier, faster-growing noncarbonated beverages (bottled water, sports
drinks, and teas) that it commands half the U.S. market...Not that PepsiCo is
anywhere near becoming purely a health-food company, mind you....But its
acquisitions and product reformulations...indicate the strategic shift is more
than show."[16] The cover quoted Nooyi: "If all you want is to get double-digit
earnings growth and nothing else, than I'm the wrong person."

An equally admiring *New Yorker* profile in 2011 had Nooyi insisting
that taste was not a sufficient rationale for making products. Pepsi, she said,
must also "aspire to higher values than the day-to-day business of making
soft drinks and snacks." Her long-term strategy: expand the nutrition portfolio and increase the products in the "Good for You" category.[17]

It took just a year, however, for the business press to begin writing
scathing stories about the failure of this strategy: Diet Coke had recently
replaced Pepsi as the number two best-selling soft drink. The stories were
accompanied by photographs of Nooyi that were noticeably unattractive.
Indeed, the comparison to earlier photographs was so striking that I could
predict how well PepsiCo's stock was doing by how the press portrayed her.
Investors charged that Pepsi's health-and-wellness strategy amounted to
public relations, not business reality, and insisted that the company refocus
attention on its core product, full-sugar Pepsi. Nooyi assured critics that she
had always been a fan of regular Pepsi: "I'm the only person who drinks
blue-can Pepsi on this floor....I drink blue-can Pepsi exclusively."[18] The articles quoting her did not say how much Pepsi she drank, or how often.

By 2013, Pepsi's renewed marketing investment in its sugary beverages
had paid off. Earnings were up; calls for Nooyi's resignation were down. She
again looked stunning in press photographs. Nooyi, investment analysts

pointed out, "had taken a great deal of criticism for focusing on healthy products that took attention away from Pepsi's older brands. The goals she laid out last year were a direct response to that, and she's earned some breathing room. Provided, of course, that Pepsi continues at this clip."[19]

For soda companies, this experience was an object lesson. You can promote health as much as you like, if and only if sales continue to grow by percentages that satisfy investors.

Self-Regulate Marketing to Children

As an example of how unrealistic it is to expect soda companies to address obesity voluntarily, consider self-regulation by industry of advertising to children. Under pressure from health advocates, the soda industry has pledged to restrict such marketing. Food and beverage companies promised to stop marketing in schools, to only market beverages that meet nutrition standards, and to adhere to self-established standards for use of licensed cartoon and other characters. They also say they will not market to children under age 12 anywhere. As the ABA explains, the soda industry wants to help educate children, provide them with nutritious beverage options, and give students a range of lower-calorie, smaller-portion beverage options.[20] I talk about the extent to which soda companies actually meet these pledges in later chapters, but here I explain why soda industry self-regulation is not effective and unlikely to become effective.

Soda companies participated in development of the marketing guidelines developed by the Children's Food and Beverage Advertising Initiative (CFBAI), a project of the Council of Better Business Bureaus. CFBAI guidelines are voluntary and place some restrictions on advertising sodas to children under age 12. Coke and Pepsi were among the companies that agreed, among other things, to use at least half their child-directed advertising for promoting messages that encourage good nutrition or healthy lifestyles. From the start, child health advocates questioned the sincerity of the guidelines. Would food companies simply shift their marketing to venues not covered by the guidelines? Would anyone monitor progress to hold companies accountable for meeting their pledges?

Advocates had reason to be skeptical. Soda companies were using multiple methods to reach children with "drink soda" messages. If anything, the companies were *increasing* their marketing to children. As reported by the Yale Rudd Center in 2011:

Even though children and teens should rarely, if ever, consume the sugary drinks and energy drinks analyzed in this report, beverage companies continue to market them aggressively in virtually every medium where young people spend their time: TV, radio, websites, social media, smartphones, local retailers, and community events.... Regular soda brands, including Coca-Cola, Dr Pepper, Pepsi, Mountain Dew, 7Up, and Sprite were consistently among the brands seen or heard most often by children and teens.[21]

In its 2014 update of this report, the Rudd Center found that companies had spent $866 million the previous year to advertise unhealthy drinks in all media, more than four times the amount they had spent to advertise 100 percent juice and water. The report also observed that preschoolers were exposed to 39 percent more television ads for PepsiCo sugary drinks than in 2010, and children ages 6 to 11 were seeing 25 percent more. The increases were even more pronounced among Hispanic children.[22] If soda companies are self-regulating marketing to children, they are not succeeding very well.

Create Coalitions to Promote the Reframed Messages

Soda companies were founding members of the Healthy Weight Commitment Foundation, a "CEO-led coalition of over 230 organizations working together to help families and schools reduce obesity—especially childhood obesity—by 2015." This group emerged in response to First Lady Michelle Obama's Let's Move! campaign to reduce childhood obesity within a generation. She is its honorary chair. The foundation made two notable commitments. The first was to develop a "Together Counts" campaign to promote the advantages of family meals and physical activity. The second was to reduce production by 1.5 trillion calories annually by the end of 2015 by developing new reduced-calorie products and introducing smaller portion sizes. In 2013, the foundation announced that it had already achieved this goal, three years ahead of schedule.[23] This sounds like a laudable accomplishment, but if my calculations are correct, it amounts to an average reduction of less than 15 calories per person per day, an amount hardly measurable on an individual basis.

Coca-Cola says it is proud to be a founding member of this organization: "Partnerships like this reinforce that when we all work together we can create a greater impact to help reduce obesity, especially childhood obesity, in society." They could, but this partnership says and does nothing about adhering to nutrition standards for marketing to children. What the partnership does do is to keep Coca-Cola brands in the public eye, stave off regulation, and, by some accounts, improve the company's bottom line. Lower-calorie food and beverage products were said to have driven 82 percent of Coca-Cola's sales growth in the United States during the five-year period ending in 2012.[24]

CAN SODA COMPANIES HELP SOLVE THE OBESITY PROBLEM?

Like all publicly traded corporations, soda companies are obliged to focus primarily on sales and growth targets. Even if they might like to, they cannot focus on health unless doing so promotes consistent corporate growth. For the soda industry, the proposed solutions to obesity cause irreconcilable conflicts. This book has more to say about industry "healthwashing" in Chapter 17. But now let's turn to the soda industry's second strategy for achieving corporate growth targets—selling to everyone, everywhere.

9

Marketing Sugary Drinks

Seven Basic Principles

In a rational world, selling soft drinks ought to be a tough challenge. People do not need sodas for health, welfare, or safety. Soda marketing must, therefore, create demand for the products, build brand loyalty, and above all establish a social environment in which drinking sodas anytime, anywhere, often, and in large amounts is considered not only desirable but entirely normal. The best explanation I can find for the popularity of these drinks comes from, of all people, the pop artist Andy Warhol: "A Coke is a Coke and no amount of money can get you a better Coke than the one the bum on the corner is drinking. All the Cokes are the same and all the Cokes are good."[1] You and I can argue about how "good"—or how democratic—sodas might be, but Warhol was not referring to their health effects. He was talking about their marketing.

Marketing sodas as icons has a long history. Coca-Cola first advertised its bottled drinks in newspapers in 1902. Within just a few years the company was advertising widely in magazines and distributing enormous numbers of signs and novelty items marked with its logo—today's highly prized collectibles.[2] In response, sales grew.

The Great Depression of the 1930s forced nearly two thousand bottlers out of business, and soda sales fell by half. The industry had to come up with new marketing strategies. One was to introduce larger sizes but keep the price about the same. The original sodas came in 6.5-ounce bottles. In 1939, Pepsi broke that tradition and introduced a 12-ounce bottle with its now classic jingle:[3]

> Pepsi-Cola hits the spot,
> Twelve full ounces, that's a lot.
> Twice as much for a nickel, too,
> Pepsi-Cola is the drink for you.

By the 1920s, the principal elements of Coca-Cola's advertising were well established. Marketing emphasized pleasure and sociability: "the pause that refreshes." Advertisements depicted active, attractive, happy people enjoying the drink, often in nostalgic settings. One micromanaging executive in the 1930s issued precise rules: the name Coca-Cola was never to be split into two lines; paintings or color photographs must show brunettes rather than blondes; young women should always be depicted as wholesome, not sophisticated.[4] Soda marketers modified these principles over time, but not by much. Today, Coke and Pepsi commercials still feature lively, attractive, and thin young people—although now of diverse ethnicities—having a wonderful time drinking sodas.

Did soda executives ever have second thoughts about the effects of their products on health? Once obesity became a recognizable problem, at least one did. In 2012, Todd Putman, a marketing executive for Coca-Cola from 1997 to 2000, confessed regrets in a speech to food and public health advocates: "It took me 10 years to figure out that I have a large karmic debt to pay for the number of Cokes I sold across this country." The company, he said, cared about only one thing: "share of stomach." "He was astonished," he later told *New York Times* reporter Michael Moss, "by the ferociousness with which the company pursued customers…the marketing division's efforts boiled down to one question: 'How can we drive more ounces into more bodies more often?'"[5] The soda industry did just that by following marketing principles that I am summarizing by grouping them into seven categories.

THE FIRST PRINCIPLE OF SODA MARKETING: ADVERTISE

In the mid-1980s, Roger Enrico, then president and CEO of PepsiCo, explained how soda marketing works:

> Americans don't drink fifty gallons of soft drinks apiece each year because they have to.…[Y]ou choose soft drinks…because companies like Pepsi and people like me spend a great deal of time and energy

to encourage you. We do this with print advertising. With coupons in newspapers. With signs at stadiums and billboards on highways. With eye-catching displays in supermarkets and convenience stores. With catchy jingles in radio ads. And we do it with television commercials.[6]

Soda makers sink fortunes into doing these things. For the year 2013, the trade magazine *Advertising Age* reported that Coca-Cola spent $3.3 billion to market its products worldwide and Pepsi spent $2.4 billion. Such amounts, astronomical as they are, are small percentages of Coke's $47 billion and Pepsi's $66 billion in sales revenues that year. The magazine also provides information about companies' U.S. advertising expenditures for specific products, as shown in Table 9.1. In 2014, when global Coke sales fell by 1 percent—the first decline since 1999—the company's CEO, Muhtar Kent, assured reporters that Coca-Cola planned to take firm action. The company would increase its annual marketing budget to "north of $4 billion." To put this amount in context: in 2014, Coca-Cola's "north of $4 billion" advertising budget equaled or exceeded the gross domestic product of twenty-seven countries in the world.[7]

From these few examples, you can assume that any nationally advertised soft drink brand is backed by at least $20 million or so in marketing, and more for the more popular brands. Such staggering amounts—$169 million to advertise Gatorade, for example—apply only to marketing expenses funneled through U.S. advertising agencies. They do not apply to international marketing. They also do not include the additional amounts spent on

TABLE 9.1 Advertising expenditures for specific sugary drink brands, United States, 2013

SOFT DRINK BRAND	U.S. ADVERTISING EXPENDITURES, $ MILLIONS
Coca-Cola Company	
Coca-Cola	202.2
Glacéau Vitaminwater	22.9
Powerade	18.6
PepsiCo	
Pepsi	225.0
Gatorade	169.0
Mountain Dew	50.4

SOURCE: *Advertising Age*, June 22, 2014.

websites, trade shows, supermarket product placements, or behind-the-scenes lobbying, litigation, partnerships, research support, or philanthropy. On average, the Big Soda companies spend about 5 cents just to advertise every gallon of Coke, Pepsi, or Dr Pepper.[8] This may not sound like much, but it adds up quickly when gallons run into the billions annually (Figure 2.2).

Advertising Age also tracks where the marketing takes place—the media channels. Television continues to be the leading venue for soda advertising, with cable and Spanish-language TV attracting more dollars each year. Advertising in newspapers is rare except for major announcements or defensive statements, as illustrated in later chapters. The companies still advertise in magazines, but not nearly as much as they used to. They also still advertise on billboards. And they continue to produce signs with brand logos for grocery stores, gas stations, fast-food restaurants, sports arenas, scoreboards, vending machines, schools, and any other place where they can be seen. A study in Philadelphia, for example, found that two-thirds of the city's retailers displayed advertisements for sugary beverages. Its authors also observed impressive stacks of beverage packs near the entrances of 30 percent of retail stores and more than 40 percent of convenience stores, gas stations, and takeout restaurants. Coca-Cola works with retailers on how best to use such displays and considers them a critically important sales strategy, as illustrated in Figure 9.1.[9]

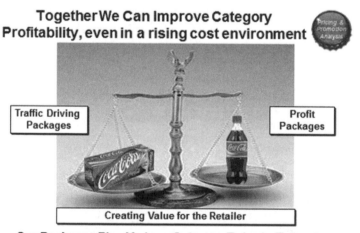

FIGURE 9.1 How Coca-Cola generates profits for retailers. The illustration is from a Coca-Cola slide presentation to the Food Marketing Institute in May 2007, explaining how to obtain the highest profits from soda sales.

TABLE 9.2 U.S. advertising expenditures for all products, Coca-Cola and PepsiCo, by media channel, 2012*

VENUE	COCA-COLA, $ MILLIONS	PEPSICO $ MILLIONS
Television		
Network TV	127	249
Cable TV	81	324
Spanish-language TV	21	29
Magazines	34	125
Network & local radio	9	25
Outdoors	27	24
Internet	9	29

* Dollars rounded off.

SOURCE: *Advertising Age*, June 22, 2013.

By far the fastest-growing venue for soda advertising is the Internet, with its display ads, banners, and pop-ups. The companies also have their own websites, of course, in multiple versions even within the United States, and in multilingual versions for the countries in which they operate. Table 9.2 summarizes Coke and Pepsi's total advertising expenditures for all of their products combined, by media channel.

THE SECOND PRINCIPLE: BE STRATEGIC

The marketing philosophy used by soda companies is summarized succinctly by Mark Pendergrast in his peerless history of the Coca-Cola Company (see Appendix 3). Pendergrast distills thirty-five business lessons from this history, among them some philosophical approaches to successful marketing:

- Believe in your product.
- Develop a mystique (hence the secret formula).
- Advertise an image, not a product.
- Appeal to universal human desires.

Coca-Cola's use of this last approach is particularly effective. To cite just one example: Coca-Cola's Ramadan campaign in 2014, "#OpenUp, pays tribute to the holy month by spreading happiness and encouraging people to open up to each other, rekindle lost connections and mend unresolved tensions." The videos show stories of how families bond together over drinks of Coca-Cola.[10]

THE THIRD PRINCIPLE: BE UBIQUITOUS

Pendergrast offers another lesson: "Make your product widely available." At least since the 1920s, Coca-Cola's explicit goal has been to ensure that its products are always "within arm's reach of desire." Beverage makers sell products to grocery stores and convenience stores, gas stations, drugstores, business supply stores, sports stadiums, concession stands, movie theaters, airports, casinos, restaurants, museums, schools, hospitals, prisons, and everywhere it can install a vending machine. Marketing methods vary at each of these locations and often include promotional spending. Table 9.3 summarizes the primary sales channels for soda marketing. Most soda cans and bottles are sold in supermarkets, mass retailers such as Walmart, and convenience stores, in that order. As drug and convenience stores increasingly stock grocery items, they too can be expected to increase promotion of bottled and canned drinks.[11]

THE FOURTH PRINCIPLE: MARKET SODAS BY EVERY MEANS POSSIBLE

I still have trouble grasping the comprehensiveness of soda companies' sales strategies. Coke and Pepsi each have a century's worth of marketing experience. From that experience, Pendergrast distills the lessons "Market your product wisely," "Involve your customers," and "Understand that there

TABLE 9.3 The major soda sales channels, 2012

SALES CHANNEL	MARKET SHARE, PERCENT
Off-Premise	
Supermarkets	27.6
Mass retailers	11.5
Convenience stores	9.8
Drugstores	2.1
All other	12.0
On-Premise	
Food service	24.2
Vending machines	10.7
All other	2.1

SOURCE: Adapted from Beverage Marketing Corporation, *Carbonated Soft Drinks in the U.S.*, 2013, Table 8.1.

is no saturation point." These adages mean that if companies use innovative methods, especially those that engage consumers, there should be no limit to the amount of soda they can sell. In Table 9.4, I give a few selected examples of soda industry marketing methods consistent with Pendergrast's advice.

Later chapters cover many additional examples, but I will just mention one more here: Coca-Cola's sponsorship in 2015 of one of London's premier tourist attractions, the enormous Ferris wheel known as the London Eye. The Eye used to shine blue at night, but it now shines Coca-Cola red, causing at least one critic to complain that while most cities were introducing anti-obesity initiatives, London had instead chosen "to hand over the single biggest advertising hoarding in the city to one of the principal drivers of an epidemic that threatens to engulf us and overwhelm the NHS [National Health Service]."[12]

TABLE 9.4 Examples of marketing methods used by soda companies to reach a broad range of customers, build brand loyalty, and create a positive brand image

Collectibles	Coke and Pepsi sell memorabilia in stores and via websites: cups, trays, calendars, toys, photographs, clothing, and pet supplies. Dozens of books—field guides, price guides, encyclopedias—describe these items.
Vending machines	Coke "happiness" machines dispense gifts while photographing surprised recipients and creating viral videos (U.S.). Coke machines dispense "sharing cans" that can be twisted in half (Singapore). Coke machines require people in India and Pakistan to cooperate to obtain soda.
Personalized cans	Coke replaces its standard branding with 150 popular names, supported by media campaigns in the U.K., Israel, and now other countries. Machines produce personalized names on-site.
Social media	Coke and Pepsi host multiple websites. In 2012, Coke redesigned its main site in magazine format, Coca-Cola Journey, "a multimillion dollar effort over multiyears." Pepsi hosts a corporate site, a global site, and a site devoted to beverage facts. Both companies use Facebook, Twitter, and other media. Both companies use contests and prizes to generate followers and "likes."
Military employment	Coke pledges 800 job and career opportunities for veterans.
Market research	Coke opens Shopper Experience Innovation Center for testing marketing strategies in simulated displays; employs facial recognition software to track responses.
Marketing training	Coke Solutions offers programs, suggestions and tools for increasing soda sales in supermarkets, convenience stores, and restaurants.

THE FIFTH PRINCIPLE: USE MUSIC AND SPORTS CELEBRITIES

Celebrities help sell products, especially to young people. Pendergrast lists two more rules: "Use celebrity endorsements wisely—but sparingly" and "When you do use celebrities, use some local celebs." Celebrities are effective in reaching fans, but they are especially effective in reaching target groups: the young and hip, teenagers, minorities, or even residents of specific parts of the country. Pepsi's $50 million deal with the pop star Beyoncé and its arrangements with controversial hip-hop artists are examples (see Chapter 14). In 2013, Pepsi targeted customers in the neglected American heartland, the "flyover states," for national ad campaigns featuring country music singer Jason Aldean. As one commentator pointed out, the targeted areas are among those with the highest rates of obesity in the country: "Of course this is purely about market share, but in [a] time where soda makers are being routinely blamed for much of our nation's expanding seat-size, the sophisticated targeting of regions where obesity rates have already reached alarming rates is notable. That can't be good news for those in frontline states like Missouri, Oklahoma, Texas or Michigan."[13]

Sports celebrities perform two marketing functions: they influence fans, and they shift the focus to physical activity. Their endorsements imply that obesity is about what you do, not what you eat or drink. In 2012, Coca-Cola signed the professional basketball player LeBron James to a $16 million, six-year endorsement deal, and Pepsi signed Robinson Cano, then a baseball player with the New York Yankees, and basketball player Kobe Bryant. Both Coca-Cola and PepsiCo invest heavily in sponsorship of international sports teams, as discussed in Chapter 18. Public health advocates note how frequently young people are exposed to advertising by professional athletes, who are almost always promoting energy-dense, nutrient-poor foods and beverages. Countries worldwide, they suggest, should implement policies restricting such advertising.[14]

From the standpoint of the soda industry, celebrity marketing is not only useful but essential. In a speech at a conference titled "Masters of Marketing," Joseph Tripodi, the chief marketing officer of Coca-Cola explained, "In our business you have to be constantly recruiting younger people into your franchise.... Otherwise you won't have a business long term.... Finding new ways to engage consumers presents a particular opportunity for Coca-Cola and other companies as well. . . . It's really important for us as a big global brand to lead culture, not just follow it."[15]

THE SIXTH PRINCIPLE: KEEP PRICES LOW

Pendergrast lists three other rules for soda producers:

- Sell a cheaply produced item.
- Ensure that everyone who touches your product before it reaches the consumer makes substantial amounts of money.
- Make your product affordable to everyone.

Sodas are famously profitable. Consumers buy bottled and canned drinks at about double their cost to the retailer, and fountain sodas make higher profits than anything else in the fast-food industry. Low soda prices are an incentive to buy, and higher prices discourage soda purchases—the rationale for the soda tax initiatives discussed in later chapters. Soda companies can offer products at low prices because the cost of the basic ingredients is so low. The water comes from municipal supplies, the cost of carbonation is trivial, and the most expensive ingredient is sugar or high-fructose corn syrup (HFCS). Bottles and cans add to the cost of production, which explains why Coca-Cola is so interested in promoting do-it-yourself Freestyle cartridges. These were in twenty thousand locations by 2014. Cost reduction also explains why Pepsi is pushing its do-it-yourself, thousand-choice Spire beverage machines.[16]

Cans and Bottles

In 2012, the Beverage Marketing Corporation said that the wholesale, nondiscounted price of a 24-unit case of 12-ounce cans or bottles was $11.12, or 46 cents each.[17] Based on my observations of the impossibly complex cost options at retail stores, this price seems implausibly high. Otherwise, soda companies would have to be selling cans and bottles at deep discounts, as I show in Table 9.5.

This bewildering array of price options is only for 12-ounce sizes. The prices of other sizes are equally bewildering. It is also bewilderingly difficult to obtain this information. Many stores do not keep shelf labels up to date

TABLE 9.5 Comparison shopping: the retail cost of 12-ounce bottles or cans of Coke or Pepsi, August 2013

SALES VENUE	PACKAGE	COCA-COLA RETAIL PRICE	COCA-COLA PRICE PER 12-OUNCE UNIT	PEPSI RETAIL PRICE,	PEPSI PRICE PER 12-OUNCE UNIT
Drugstore	12-pack, cans	$6.99	58¢	—	—
Gas station	24-pack, cans	$7.99	33¢	$7.99	33¢
Walmart	6-pack, cans	$2.12	35¢	$1.88	31¢
	8-pack, bottles	$4.38	55¢	$3.98	50¢
	12-pack, cans	$4.98	42¢	$4.98	42¢
	24-pack, cans	$7.98	33¢	$7.98	33¢
	24-pack, bottles	$10.98	46¢		
Wegmans	4-pack, bottles	—	—	$3.29	82¢
	6-pack, bottles	5 for $11.00	37¢	—	—
	8-pack, bottles	$4.49	56¢	$3.99	50¢
	12-pack, cans	3 for $12.99	36¢	3 for $10.98	31¢
	24-pack, cans	—	—	$7.99	33¢

or do not bother to mark the prices on stacks of soda packs. Without going to the checkout counter, I was only able to find retail prices in Walmart with the help of two friendly Pepsi employees who were stocking the section. Even so, some conclusions should be evident from this table:

- Some stores carry Coke or Pepsi, but not both, and must have a deal with a company.
- Sodas are more expensive in bottles than in cans.
- Coke is usually as expensive as or more expensive than Pepsi. (Price wars?)
- Sodas in drugstores are more expensive than those in gas stations or Walmart.
- Prices decrease with increasing number of units (but exceptions are frequent).
- Many packages are priced well below the theoretical 46-cent wholesale cost.
- Comparative shopping is extremely difficult.

On this last point, you need a calculator and a store that is diligent about keeping up with shelf labels to figure out the best buy. Do they make the

comparisons so difficult on purpose? And what about Walmart? The low
price of its six-packs of cans could be because that particular item was a loss
leader to entice people into the store, but Walmart's massive buying power
is also a consideration. Its sales volume allows it to force the lowest possible
prices from its suppliers. The much smaller supermarket chain Wegmans
must have a similar arrangement. The low-priced Coke six-pack in Wegmans
was on special that day, but I would have had to buy five of them to get that
price. Beyond occasions when stores offer loss leaders, I have a hard time
believing that any store loses money on sodas given the vast amount of
supermarket floor and shelf space they occupy.[18]

Mexican Coca-Cola

Although I did not list it in the table, I must mention one other 12-ounce
Coca-Cola: "hecho in Mexico." In 2013, I began seeing Mexican Coke sold in
U.S. drugstores, liquor stores, and bodegas, always at premium prices—an
impressive $1.69 at a Wegmans and an even more impressive $2.99 at a drugstore, for just one 12-ounce bottle. They get away with this because Mexican
Coke comes with an aura of hipster appeal. It is imported and, ostensibly,
made with sugar (sucrose) rather than HFCS. I use "ostensibly" because
Mexican Coca-Cola has been made with varying proportions of HFCS for
some time now, but you cannot tell this from the labels. Imported products
are supposed to carry FDA-authorized Nutrition Facts labels, but some of
the bottles I've seen do not. A bottle of Mexican Coke from a Brooklyn

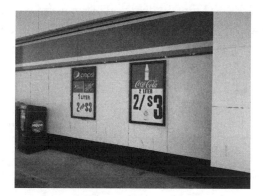

FIGURE 9.2 Soda signs, New Hampshire gas station, 2012. This station offered two
2-liter bottles—4 liters—of Coca-Cola for $3 in late 2012, but sold 2 liters of Diet Pepsi
or Mountain Dew for the same price. Photo by author.

bodega came with an ersatz, pasted-on label that listed ingredients as "Carbonated Water, Hig [*sic*] Fructose, Corn Syrup, and/Or Sugar." You decide if it is worth the much higher price.

Table 9.5 says nothing about vending machines. This is because vending machines have dispensed 20-ounce—not 12-ounce—drinks since the late 1990s. Larger bottles generally cost less per ounce, and their low cost is widely advertised. I photographed the sign shown in Figure 9.2 in a New Hampshire gas station late in 2012. It advertised four liters of Coke for $3.00, but two liters of diet Pepsi or Mountain Dew for the same price. This place, unusual in my experience, sold Coke at half the price of Pepsi.

Fountain Drinks

If you can believe it, the basic cost of fountain drinks is even more complicated to compute. In 2012, according to the Beverage Marketing Corporation, the average wholesale cost of a 5-gallon container of syrup was $35.47. Let's take a breath and work through the math. Mixed with carbonated water at ratio of 5 to 1, the syrup makes 30 gallons of soda. This means 3,840 ounces. The soda gets poured into cups filled at least one-third with ice, so a 12-ounce cup contains only about 8 ounces of the original mix. If you are still with me, the 5 gallons of syrup could end up filling 480 12-ounce cups at a wholesale cost of 7.3 cents each. To this cost must be added that of the carbonation, ice, cup, straw, and cover, as well as overhead. These bring the cost up to 12 cents or so, the penny-per-ounce figure I quoted in an earlier chapter.[19] Consider this: fountain drink sellers make money as long as they charge more than 1 cent per ounce. To see how this works out for fountain drinks at a New York City McDonald's in August 2013, take a look at Table 9.6.

TABLE 9.6 Retail cost of sodas at McDonald's, Manhattan, 2013

SIZE	OUNCES	COST TO McDONALD'S	COST TO CUSTOMER	PROFIT PER DRINK*
Small	16	16¢	$1.39	$1.23
Medium	21	21¢	$1.89	$1.68
Large	32	32¢	$2.29	$1.97

* Cost to customer less cost to McDonald's.

TABLE 9.7 Retail cost of sodas, movie theaters, Manhattan, 2013

SIZE	OUNCES	COST TO THEATER	COST TO CUSTOMER	PROFIT*
Film Forum				
Small	12	12¢	$3.00	$2.88
Medium	16	16¢	$3.50	$3.33
Large	24	24¢	$4.25	$4.01
Regal Multiplex				
Small	30	30¢	$4.75	$4.45
Medium	44	44¢	$5.25	$4.81
Large	51	51¢	$5.75	$5.24

* Cost to customer less cost to theaters.

These figures, approximate as they are, make it clear why fast-food places can offer drinks of any size for a dollar and still make money (see Figure 7.1). They also explain why retailers train employees to promote supersize servings. To make this point even more forcefully, take a look at soda prices in one upscale and one mass-market movie theater in lower Manhattan (Table 9.7). Movie theaters derive as much as 40 percent of their income from concession stands, and the markup on sodas easily explains why.

The Film Forum shows foreign, independent, and classic movies. Its sodas are all Cokes served in elegantly designed cups, remarkable for their comparatively small sizes. The Film Forum "large" is fully 6 ounces smaller than the "small" at the Regal Theater, where soda cups are typical of sizes at any other multiplex. For fountain drinks, the larger the cup, the higher the profit. This is why movie theater owners oppose menu label laws requiring them to display calories. If customers knew the calories in soft drinks, they might be warned off the larger sizes.

Federal Sugar Price Policies

It is not possible to talk about soda prices without saying something about the major reason their prices are so low: federal subsidies and price supports. These, to say the least, are also convoluted. The government subsidizes corn farmers, thereby reducing the price of HFCS. But it also subsidizes the production of ethanol from corn, which depletes corn stores and inflates HFCS prices. Even so, HFCS is less expensive than

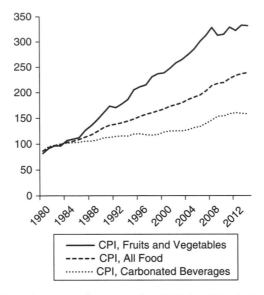

FIGURE 9.3 Trends in the Consumer Price Index (CPI) for all foods, fruits and vegetables, and sodas, 1980 to 2013. The soda CPI increased more slowly than that for all foods, but much more slowly than the CPI for fruits and vegetables. These values from the U.S. Bureau of Labor Statistics represent the yearly (twelve-month) average CPI for urban consumers, adjusted for inflation, compared to a baseline in the early 1980s.

sucrose, but the gap has narrowed in recent years. And then there are the government's arcane sugar policies: quotas on domestic beet sugar, but tariffs on imported cane and beet sugar. Although both policies maintain the cost of sugar at a level higher than world market prices, sugar is still not very expensive.[20] Relative to the rise in the Consumer Price Index (CPI) for fruits, vegetables, and many other foods since 1980, the CPI for sodas has also risen, but much more slowly (Figure 9.3). Low prices, please recall, encourage consumption.

THE SEVENTH PRINCIPLE: SELL TO EVERYONE

In the next several chapters, I describe how soda companies aim their marketing efforts to target children, minorities, and populations of developing countries. Here, I want to briefly mention soda companies' attempts to engage and influence the lesbian, gay, bisexual, and transgender (LGBT) community. Coca-Cola, for example, supports groups such as the Point Foundation, which raises funds for LGBT student scholarships. Soda industry donations to this community sometimes pay off handsomely. During the 2014 election campaign to tax sodas in San Francisco (see Chapter 27), the American Beverage Association (ABA) contributed $45,000 to the Harvey Milk LGBT Democratic Club. The money was well spent. The club publicly opposed the tax and endorsed the ABA's anti-tax ("No on E") television advertisements—in English and Spanish.[21]

The industry's relationships with this community, however, do not always go so smoothly. In 2013, soon after the Russian government passed a law banning pro-LGBT statements in public or private, the U.S. advocacy group Queer Nation organized a protest against Coca-Cola's sponsorship of the Winter Olympic Games in Sochi (Figure 9.4).[22]

The Sochi protesters created a parody of a Coca-Cola commercial showing LGBT demonstrators forcibly carried off by Russian police. In response, Coca-Cola created the "It's Beautiful" ad, in which people throughout the world, among them a gay Jewish couple, sing "America the Beautiful" in a variety of foreign languages. This may have pleased the gay community, but the ad, shown during the 2014 Super Bowl, caused a furor among conservative Americans distressed that the lyrics were in languages other than English.[23]

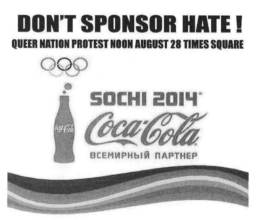

FIGURE 9.4 Queer Nation poster announcing a demonstration in New York City to protest Coca-Cola's sponsorship of the Olympic Games in Russia, 2014. This LGBT advocacy group was objecting to the company's support of the Games in a country whose leadership had just enacted an anti-LGBT law.

Then Coca-Cola further offended the LGBT community by editing out a gay marriage scene from one of its international commercials. This video featured, among other happy or amusing occasions, a wedding between two young men. Although the ad was aired in several countries, Coke's marketers deleted that scene from the version shown in predominantly Catholic Ireland and instead substituted a clip with an interracial couple. Gay marriage is not legal in Ireland, Coke explained.[24] But by 2015, it was.

Coca-Cola points out that it has been named one of the ten most-diverse companies for twelve consecutive years, has been honored by the Human Rights Campaign as the best place to work for eight straight years, and has won numerous other awards for its diversity efforts. PepsiCo scored 100 percent in the 2014 Corporate Equality Index, earning a designation as one of the "Best Places to Work for LGBT Equality," perhaps because of its titanium-level ($80,000) donation to the fifteenth annual Out & Equal Workplace Summit.[25] These gifts may support sexual diversity but, as the Harvey Milk LGBT Democratic Club episode illustrates, they also promote the soda industry's agenda.

Targeting Children

10

Starting Early

Marketing to Infants, Children, and Teens

In the summer of 2013, First Lady Michelle Obama addressed the annual conference of the National Council of La Raza, a meeting sponsored in part by Coca-Cola and PepsiCo. Both companies had long supported Hispanic organizations, a topic I discuss further in Chapter 14. Mrs. Obama called on participants to reclaim the health of their children:

> And that starts by using our power as consumers to hold companies responsible for the food they make and how they market it to our kids. In 2008 alone, companies spent well over half a billion dollars on food, beverage and restaurant ads in Latino media markets—many of them for unhealthy products. And those of us with kids who have seen our kids begging and pleading for something they saw on TV, we know just how persuasive these ads can be. So we all know that the food industry has some serious work to do when it comes to how they market food to our kids.[1]

This was not the first time the First Lady had expressed concern about the effects of food marketing on children's diets and health. Soon after launching Let's Move! in 2010, she admonished the Grocery Manufacturers Association "to entirely rethink the products that you're offering, the information that you provide about these products, and how you market those products to our children...This isn't about finding creative ways to market products as healthy."[2]

In such remarks, the First Lady did not refer to sodas. Her campaign's most notable contribution to the soda debate was the statement accompanying the 2011 release of the USDA's MyPlate food guide: "Drink water instead of sugary drinks." But she had plenty of reason to be concerned about the effects of food and beverage marketing on children. Promoting foods and drinks to adults may be fair game. After all, adults are supposed to be able to distinguish sales pitches from other kinds of information. We can argue about how well most of us can make this distinction, but there is no question that young children cannot, leaving them especially vulnerable to advertising messages. Research demonstrates without question that marketing induces children to prefer advertised products, pester their parents to buy them, and eat or drink advertised products. It is especially effective with low-income and minority children. Since most such marketing is for sodas and junk foods, it stands in direct competition with the goals of public health.[3]

Marketing also targets parents effectively. In the 1990s, for example, soda companies licensed their brands to be placed on infant feeding bottles such as those illustrated in Figure 10.1. A study demonstrated that parents who bought these bottles were four times more likely to fill them with soda than those who used regular bottles. Complaints from nutrition advocates and unfavorable publicity forced the manufacturer to stop making them. Another example: children fed identical foods packaged with either McDonald's labels or unbranded labels say that they greatly prefer the McDonald's foods.[4] And recall from Chapter 1 that children who insist they prefer Coke or Pepsi over a store brand of soda cannot tell the difference in blind taste tests.

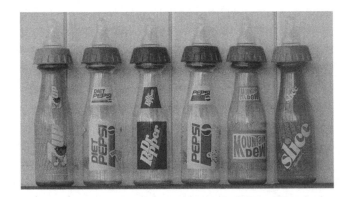

FIGURE 10.1 Soda logos on infant feeding bottles produced by the Munchkin Bottling Company, Los Angeles, California, mid-1990s. When researchers found the bottles to be four times more likely to be filled with soda than bottles without soda company logos, protests from child health advocates convinced Munchkin to stop making them. Photo courtesy of Dr. Kelly Brownell.

TELEVISION: THE QUICKEST AND MOST EFFECTIVE ROUTE TO REACHING KIDS

In 2005, the Institute of Medicine (IOM) issued a report, *Marketing to Children and Youth: Threat or Opportunity*. Among its other contributions, this report summarized research on the effects of televised food and beverage commercials on children. Food advertising, the IOM found, induces children to recognize and prefer brands, to pester parents to buy advertised brands, and to believe they are *supposed* to be choosing branded foods. TV commercials strongly influence children's desire for food products, their requests for marketed products, and their overall diets. Children, the IOM said, are the primary focus of many marketing initiatives, most of which focus on foods of poor nutritional quality. The IOM's tough conclusion: food marketing undermines parental authority, poses a direct threat to the health of America's children, and should be curtailed.

Despite this report, soda commercials on television continue to be rampant. Prior to industry pledges to stop marketing to children under age 12, about 10 percent of commercials on kids' Saturday morning television programs were for sugary drinks of one kind or another. Then, children viewed most soda commercials on television programs aimed at adults. They still do. Not all children drink soda and not all watch television, but children who are soda drinkers are more likely to be television watchers. Soda drinking is so closely linked to watching television that its consumption can be predicted by formula: the probability that children will consume sodas up to three times per week rises by 50 percent for every hour a day they watch television, and by 60 percent if they are watching commercials.[5]

To put this finding another way: for every one hundred soda commercials watched on television, a child's soda consumption increases by 10 percent. Furthermore, soda-drinking children who watch television are more likely to be obese, and not just because the activity is sedentary. Watching commercials for sodas is independently associated with obesity as well as with drinking sodas.[6]

By 2011, the American Academy of Pediatrics judged such evidence so compelling that it called for a ban on junk-food advertising during children's television hours. The academy urged pediatricians to ask two questions about media use at every office visit: How much time do children spend in front of a screen each day? Is a TV set or Internet connection in the child's bedroom? Pediatricians want parents to understand that the first line of defense against obesity-promoting marketing is to reduce TV hours and keep media out of kids' rooms.[7]

DIGITAL MEDIA: THE NEW MARKETING FRONTIER

The 2005 IOM report focused on television advertising, largely because most marketing to children then took place on television. It still does. But soda marketers increasingly use digital media to reach children and expose them to food and beverage advertisements on popular websites. Most (but by no means all) digital marketing is aimed at teenagers—"fishing where the fish are," as marketers like to put it. The aim of digital marketing is to engage media-savvy teens through personalized, targeted messages that encourage them to feel part of a peer community centered on the brand. Soda companies use Facebook, Twitter, YouTube, games, and phone apps to reach teenagers, track their use of these media, and use the tracking information as the basis for refining the marketing methods.[8]

Digital marketing is more difficult for kids to recognize as advertising, particularly because it is interactive and delivered online or through mobile devices. It aims to get kids to share commercial messages with their friends without noticing that they have just become part of the marketing process. In 2013, investigators from the Centers for Disease Control and Prevention, alarmed that teenagers with high media exposure were more likely to drink sodas and less likely to drink water or milk, urged limits on exposure to electronic media. Such limits, they said, should be part of efforts to reduce soda intake among adolescents.[9]

SODA MARKETING TO KIDS: THE FINANCIAL INVESTMENT

In 2008, the Federal Trade Commission (FTC) attempted to find out how much money food and beverage companies were spending on marketing to children. This was a challenge. Companies consider spending data to be proprietary, and the FTC had to resort to using "compulsory process orders" (translation: subpoenas) to obtain the information from forty-four leading food and beverage companies. Adding up the data that it managed to extract from these companies, the FTC concluded that they spent $1.6 billion in total to market foods and beverages to children and adolescents. Of that amount, more than half—$870 million—was spent on marketing to children under age 12.[10]

Soda company spending accounted for 30 percent of this amount—the largest single category. But in contrast to the practices of most other food companies, soda companies only buy television commercials that target teenagers. The companies have pledged not to market directly to children under the age of 12. The word *directly*, however, leaves much room for interpretation. But before we get to that interpretation, let's finish up the question of how much money is involved.

In 2012, the FTC published a follow-up report, this time based on subpoenas to forty-eight companies. Collectively, these reported spending $1.79 billion on kids' television marketing, again with half of it aimed at children under age 12, and again with no soda industry contributions to that half. Soda companies reported spending less on television advertising to children than they did in the past—a drop from $492 million in 2006 to $395 million in 2011—presumably reflecting the withdrawal of ads from programs aimed at young children. Yes, soda companies reduced expenditures for television commercials, but they are now spending more on digital marketing.[11]

Food companies have every incentive to spend fortunes on marketing to children. It works. And in the absence of advocacy to curtail such marketing, they have no disincentive. As I explain in Chapter 11, U.S. attempts to regulate marketing to children run up against claims of First Amendment protection. Furthermore, the government considers marketing expenses of any kind to be legitimate business expenses and fully deductible from annual corporate income taxes. It is one of the great ironies of federal health policy that tax policies reward soda companies—and alcohol, cigarette, and junk-food companies—with tax write-offs for advertising to children as well as to adults.[12]

HOW MUCH SODA ADVERTISING DO CHILDREN SEE?

In 2010, the Rudd Center for Food Policy and Obesity surveyed the extent of television advertisements, product placements, and Internet marketing for sugary drinks aimed specifically at children. It identified the leading advertiser to children, accounting for 26.6 percent of the exposure, as Kraft Foods, the maker of Capri Sun and Kool-Aid drinks. Coca-Cola came next, at 24.8 percent; PepsiCo was fourth, at 13.7 percent (for all of its sugar-sweetened drinks); and Dr Pepper Snapple was fifth, at 10.2 percent. Innovation

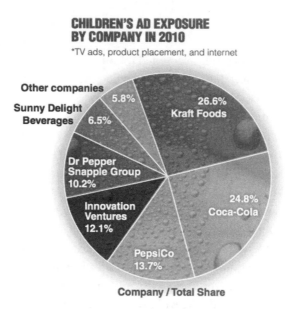

CHILDREN'S AD EXPOSURE BY COMPANY IN 2010

*TV ads, product placement, and internet

Other companies 5.8%

Sunny Delight Beverages 6.5%

Dr Pepper Snapple Group 10.2%

Innovation Ventures 12.1%

PepsiCo 13.7%

Kraft Foods 26.6%

Coca-Cola 24.8%

Company / Total Share

FIGURE 10.2 Share of money spent on marketing sugary drinks to kids, by company. Marketing by Coca-Cola, PepsiCo, and Dr Pepper Snapple for all sweetened drinks (not just sodas) accounted for nearly half of children's exposure to advertising in this category. From *Sugary Drink Facts, 2011*, courtesy of the Rudd Center for Food Policy and Obesity.

Ventures, at 12.1 percent, sells an energy drink. This distribution is shown in Figure 10.2. Together, advertising by the big three soda companies accounts for nearly 49 percent—half—of the total commercials for sugary drinks to which kids are exposed.

DO SODA COMPANIES MARKET TO CHILDREN UNDER AGE 12?

In speaking of the "karmic debt" he owed for collaborating on Coke's marketing to children, former Coca-Cola marketing executive Todd Putman noted that the company had a long-standing policy not to *directly* market to children younger than age 12 (my emphasis). But "magically, when they would turn 12, we'd suddenly attack them like a bunch of wolves.... I would say 90 percent of all soft drink marketing is targeted at 12- to 24-year-olds.... It was how we spent all of our time."[13]

I have no idea how widely Putman's views might be shared by other soda company executives, but *New York Times* reporter Michael Moss names one other in his book *Salt, Sugar, Fat*. Moss describes how Putman's former boss, Jeffrey Dunn, also acknowledged a "karma debt" and the need to do penance for his years at Coca-Cola. Dunn said he had achieved "peace of mind...by simply not thinking about what he sold."

I suspect that cynicism has long been an integral part of the job descriptions of soda company executives. In 1975, the political reporter Robert Scheer wrote a piece for *Esquire* about Pepsi's international marketing adventures based on interviews with, among others, Donald Kendall, the company's CEO from 1971 to 1986. "Most of the executives I talked to," Scheer wrote, "including Kendall, said that they had required their own children to drink milk and not spoil their appetites before dinner on Pepsi, while at the same time they were out in the world conning kids who didn't get milk to hustle up their quarters for a cola."[14]

Translation: "Directly"

I emphasized "directly" in Putman's statement because the word deserves scrutiny. In marketing terms, *direct* means television, radio, print, and Internet commercials paid for through advertising agencies. Since companies know how much they pay to advertising agencies, direct advertising is measurable. But soda companies use many other forms of marketing that are not managed by advertising agencies. These include trade shows and product placements in supermarkets, but also forms that might particularly appeal to children: toys and games, product placements on television programs, movie tie-ins, cross-promotion licenses, athletic sponsorships, celebrity endorsements, T-shirts and other giveaways, and digital media such as Facebook, Twitter, and apps of one kind or another. Do soda companies use such methods? They do, but the amount of money spent on them is not easily tracked.

Translation: "Not Below 12"

The meaning of "not below age 12" also deserves scrutiny. As early as the 1930s, Coca-Cola deliberately excluded children under the age of 12 from advertisements. But even then, the company produced vast numbers of items attractive to young children—toys and school materials, for example. As I discuss in Chapter 11, both the Coke and Pepsi websites list "responsible marketing" policies that preclude direct marketing to children under age 12. These policies state that the companies do not buy advertising on programs for which more than 35 percent of the viewers are children under age 12. This pledge covers paid advertising on television, on radio, and in print and, as Coca-Cola puts it, "where data is available, Internet and mobile phones."

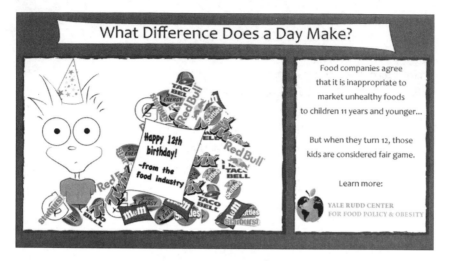

FIGURE 10.3 Food industry promises not to market to children screech to a stop on their twelfth birthdays. This illustration by Patrick Mustain comments on the absurdity of age cutoff points for marketing to children. Courtesy of the Rudd Center for Food Policy and Obesity, formerly at Yale University and since 2015 at the University of Connecticut.

Beyond the ambiguities associated with "direct" and "where data is available," the age and audience limits also leave lots of wiggle room. It makes no sense to think that one day after their twelfth birthdays children will be watching different programs than they did the day before. The Rudd Center illustrates this point in Figure 10.3. The "35 percent" rule also raises questions. The only television programs aimed primarily at children are cartoons and those on kids' TV channels. It is a sign of progress that soda companies no longer buy commercials during those programs. But many television programs aimed at adults, families, and older children are watched by younger children, and even very young children watch as many televised food advertisements as do older children. In 2014, the Rudd Center reported that food and beverage advertising to children under age 12 had increased by 8 percent on television since 2007.[15]

Putman's comments suggest that he believes Coca-Cola adheres to its promises not to market directly to children under age 12. I am willing to grant that neither Coke nor Pepsi buys media ads aimed specifically at preteens. But it seems obvious that the lines blur between advertising aimed at children older or younger than age 12, and between direct and indirect marketing. It is not difficult to observe such blurring in soda commercials. A 2013 Coca-Cola

Canada video, for example, depicts Canadian soccer stars working with teams of clearly thrilled kids, many of whom appear to be junior high age—over 12, but barely. This particular "Open Happiness" commercial appears to be aimed at younger children interested in sports and sports celebrities. So are some of the Coke and Pepsi commercials shown during other television programs watched by older children or families. These commercials may well meet the letter of the "not to under 12" pledge, but not its spirit. To illustrate the tenuousness of such arbitrary boundaries, see the marketing examples listed in Table 10.1. Would some or all of this marketing appeal to children under age 12?[16] You decide.

TABLE 10.1 Coca-Cola and Pepsi marketing activities likely to appeal to children: selected examples, 2012–2014

MEDIUM	ACTIVITY
Toys	Coca-Cola and PepsiCo license logos to hundreds of toys and games: toy cars and trucks, puzzles, plush toys, playing cards, Barbie dolls, Monopoly sets, savings banks, games, dollhouse miniatures, action figures (some with movie tie-ins), lunch boxes, comic books, and more. In 2014, Coca-Cola offers patterns for Halloween costumes to dress 7.5-ounce cans.
Boy bands	Pepsi advertisement features One Direction.
Mobile phones	Coca-Cola's all-digital marketing campaign, "Explore the world of AHH," features online phone apps and games, offers prizes for website ideas.
Websites	Coca-Cola's partnership with the World Wildlife Fund, "Arctic Home," features baby polar bears. Pepsi's "Live for Now" campaign targets global teenagers with music and entertainment, digital innovation, events, and interactive partnerships.
Fast food menu	Coca-Cola's promotion partnership with McDonald's offers "child" fountain drink.
Dispensing machines	Coca-Cola illustrates dispensing and vending machines with characters from Dr. Seuss books.
Community events	Coca-Cola sponsors "Kids Night" at Sioux Falls raceway, featuring race car rides, prizes. Coke sponsors "all-you-can-eat (and drink)" ice cream safari, annual benefit for Sacramento Zoo with entertainment and face painting for kids; it supports the Boston Museum of Science and runs ads on delivery trucks showing parents and children at the museum.
Sports events	Coca-Cola sponsors tennis clinic for teenagers in Atlanta.
Television	Coca-Cola sponsors *American Idol*, widely watched by families (discontinued in 2015).
Share-a Coke campaign	Coca-Cola issues cans and bottles with personal names as well as "Mama," "Papa," and "Grandma."

Some of the methods listed in Table 10.1 exist in a gray area not always recognizable as marketing. Pepsi's "Live for Now" and Coke's "World of AHH" campaigns obviously aim to engage teenagers. The "Share-a-Coke" campaign appeals to people of any age who like to see their names in print, and might encourage young children to ask for their own Cokes or those labeled "Mama" or "Papa." But Coca-Cola's sponsorship of community or sports events can appear as generous philanthropy, not advertising. When a tennis champion wears a Coca-Cola T-shirt or an *American Idol* judge drinks a Coke, they appear to be having fun, not marketing sugary drinks. Coca-Cola admitted its true motives when it withdrew its sponsorship of the audience-losing *American Idol* late in 2014, saying that it needed to pursue other ways to "connect with teens and leverage music as a passion point." Many child health advocates believe that these methods, while ostensibly aimed at teens or adults, encourage children younger than 12 to want Coke or Pepsi. If nothing else, soda companies have created a marketing environment in which ads for these drinks are so ubiquitous that they appear as normal, socially acceptable, and generally unnoticed features in the landscape surrounding American childhood.[17]

11

Advocacy

Stopping Soda Marketing to Kids

For more than forty years, advocates have attempted—without success—to induce the federal government to set limits on the marketing of sodas and other junk foods to children. Throughout this history, the soda and other food industries systematically and effectively opposed these attempts, even going so far as to defeat efforts to set *voluntary* nutrition standards for products that could be marketed to children. These industries much prefer self-regulation, not least to demonstrate that government intervention is unnecessary. As advocates have repeatedly demonstrated, although voluntary self-regulation may reduce the visible, quantifiable marketing to children directly paid for through advertising agencies, it freely permits food and beverage companies to promote their products "under the radar" through other means.[1] Regulations, advocates insist, are *essential* to protect children from the harm caused by food marketing.

Let's begin this account in 1970 when a group called Action for Children's Television, concerned that television commercials were having too great an influence on children's food preferences, petitioned the Federal Communications Commission (FCC) to ban advertising during children's programming. The FCC denied the petition. Without advertising, it said, children's television programs could not exist. This decision meant that business needs would take precedence over children's health. Even so, the advertising, food, and beverage industries could see that calls for restrictions on television advertising were sure to continue. To head off any chance that Congress might intervene, they created the Children's Advertising Review Unit (CARU) to develop an industry-wide program for self-regulation.

Since then, CARU has repeatedly issued guidelines for marketing self-regulation. These are voluntary, and advocates have no trouble finding examples of evasions and violations (see, for example, the items listed in Table 10.1).[2]

The Federal Trade Commission (FTC), the agency responsible for regulating advertising, entered the fray in 1978. In an act of what in today's political climate seems like either hubris or political naiveté, the FTC embarked on what the agency later viewed as a "well-intentioned, but ill-fated regulatory venture," known then and now as "KidVid," slang for "kids' video." The FTC's tough proposals were to ban television advertising to children under age 8, and also to ban advertising of sugary foods, including sodas, to children of any age. The response of the food, beverage, advertising, and television industries was, to understate the matter, vehement. Industry lobbyists induced Congress to hold hearings that ended up subjecting the FTC to merciless ridicule. Congress enacted a bill—the ironically named FTC Improvement Act of 1980—to remove the agency's authority to regulate unfair advertising to children. For the next three decades, the thoroughly traumatized FTC refused to even consider limits on food marketing to children. As one former director of the FTC explained in 2004, "Although the idea of banning certain kinds of advertisements may offer a superficial appeal . . . it is neither a workable nor an efficacious solution to the health problem of childhood obesity. The Federal Trade Commission has traveled down this road before. It is not a journey that anyone at the Commission cares to repeat."[3]

To advocates, KidVid taught harsh lessons. Federal agencies, no matter how well-meaning, would not be able to stand up to industry lobbying of a Congress more concerned about the health of corporations than that of children. Advocates had to recognize the overwhelming political power of industries that profited from marketing food and drinks to children and the willingness of such industries to go to any lengths to protect their marketing "rights." It would be unrealistic of advocates to expect such industries to act on behalf of kids' health if profits were at stake.[4]

But during those next three decades, childhood obesity emerged as a health issue of increasing public concern. In 2005, the Institute of Medicine (IOM) produced its landmark report on food marketing to children, demonstrating clear effects on children's food preferences, demands, eating habits, and body weight. On this basis, the IOM called on the FTC to revisit the idea of limits. Indeed, it issued an "or else" warning: either food companies must voluntarily self-regulate their marketing practices within two years or

Congress should enact legislation. The American Academy of Pediatrics also called for regulations on food marketing to kids.[5] Neither, however, had anywhere near the power to induce Congress to act.

But the FTC did respond. It urged CARU to take more forceful, if voluntary, actions against inappropriate marketing, and to develop nutrition standards, also voluntary, for foods that could be advertised to children. As discussed in Chapter 10, the FTC conducted a review of the extent of televised food advertising to children, required food companies to disclose how much money they were spending on children's food advertising, and did a follow-up study two years later. These studies demonstrated that self-regulation had led to some useful changes in direct paid advertising, but the indirect, "under the radar" methods of marketing to children had proliferated. Early in 2009, these findings led Congress, under the new administration of President Barack Obama, to authorize the FTC to create and lead a federal Interagency Working Group (IWG) to develop voluntary nutrition standards for food marketing to children.[6] Because the sequence of these events can be difficult to follow, Table 11.1 summarizes them.

TABLE 11.1 Time line of events in the history of unsuccessful attempts to regulate food marketing to children in the United States, 1970 to 2014

YEAR	EVENT
1970	Action for Children's Television petitions Federal Communications Commission (FCC) to ban advertising during children's programs. FCC denies petition on grounds that such programs depend on advertising for their existence.
1974	Better Business Bureau and advertising industry establish the Children's Advertising Review Unit (CARU) to promote and self-regulate responsible children's advertising.
1978	Federal Trade Commission (FTC) proposes bans on TV advertising to children under age 8 and on commercials for sugary foods to children of any age. Stakeholder industries protest, vigorously.
1980	Congress passes FTC Improvement Act; removes FTC authority to regulate food advertising to children; stops further advocacy efforts for twenty-five years.
2005	Institute of Medicine (IOM) publishes *Marketing to Children and Youth: Threat or Opportunity*; says companies must implement voluntary regulation within two years or Congress should regulate.
2006	American Academy of Pediatrics deems self-regulation ineffective; says Congress should ban junk food advertising aimed at young children. FTC urges CARU to take more forceful action on self-regulation and to develop nutrition standards. Council of Better Business Bureaus launches Children's Food and Beverage Advertising Initiative (CFBAI) to shift the mix of foods advertised to children under age 12 to healthier options, but its nutrition criteria do not apply to sodas.

(continued)

TABLE 11.1 Continued

YEAR	EVENT
2007	FTC reviews the extent of televised food advertising to children.
2008	FTC orders forty-four companies to provide data on how much they spend on marketing to children; publishes estimate of $1.6 billion; says self-regulation has gaps. International Council of Beverage Associations publishes marketing guideline for its member organizations. Coke and Pepsi commit to stop buying TV ads aimed at audiences with more than 50 percent of children under age 12.
2009	Industry report says Coke and Pepsi 96 percent in compliance with TV guidelines; 100 percent in compliance with print and Internet guidelines. Congress directs FTC to establish an Interagency Working Group (IWG) with three other federal agencies— FDA, USDA, and CDC—to set voluntary nutrition standards for food and beverage marketing to children. IWG issues preliminary standards. Industry protests ensue.
2010	White House Task Force on Childhood Obesity calls for uniform nutrition standards; says if voluntary efforts are ineffective, federal regulation should be considered. Pepsi announces "strict science-based criteria" for advertising to children under age 12. Center for Science in the Public Interest (CSPI) calls for voluntary uniform nutrition standards for food marketing to children by 2012, or else for government regulations.
2011	FTC opens IWG report to public comment. American Academy of Pediatrics issues policy statement calling for ban on junk-food advertising during children's television hours. Congress holds hearings, blocks IWG from releasing voluntary nutrition standards until it can demonstrate that benefits justify costs. Pepsi promises not to advertise to audiences of more than 35 percent children under age 12.
2012	FTC publishes follow-up report on advertising to children by forty-eight companies—$1.79 billion, half aimed at children under age 11; concludes that industry has made some progress, but could do better. Legal advocates say FTC has the authority to regulate food marketing to children; urge FTC to act more forcefully. Coke promises not to advertise to audiences of more than 35 percent children under age 12.
2013	IOM issues follow-up report; says setting limits on food marketing to children is public health priority of highest order. Coca-Cola issues policy on global self-regulation of marketing to children under age 12.
2014	Better Business Bureau's CFBAI report on compliance and progress finds soda companies to be meeting their self-regulatory commitments.

THE IWG FIASCO

When President Obama took office, advocates had every reason to be optimistic that the FTC not only would issue nutrition standards for marketing to children but also would enforce them. Shortly before the election, the *Washington Post* had asked presidential candidates about their positions on childhood obesity. To the question "Would you support national regulation of food advertising and marketing to children?" Obama replied:

The food industry overall could do substantially more to limit [children's] exposure to foods with minimal nutritional value.... [G]uidelines for advertising and marketing of foods and beverages must be finalized, and the industry should be encouraged to implement these guidelines on a voluntary basis. If voluntary adoption is not effective...these guidelines should be made mandatory and...the Federal Trade Commission should have the authority and the resources to monitor and enforce compliance.[7]

This statement echoed the "or else" admonition of the 2005 IOM committee. Soon after Obama took office, the congressionally mandated IWG, composed of representatives of four federal agencies—the FTC, FDA, USDA, and CDC—began its work. It published preliminary standards late in 2009. These standards, among others, included limits on the amounts of salt and sugar in food products that could be marketed to children up to age 17.

Even though the standards were voluntary, they scared food companies. They would preclude the marketing of the most highly profitable products—sodas, snack foods, sweetened cereals, and other foods of poor nutritional quality—even to teenagers. Uproar ensued, again revealing the extent of the food industry's investment in selling junk foods to kids. Companies and trade associations spent millions lobbying against the voluntary standards. They also created a "grassroots" organization, the Sensible Food Policy Coalition, to lobby for them. The IWG standards, they said, were an assault on First Amendment protections of commercial speech.[8]

At the time, I was not concerned about the uproar because the Obama administration still appeared to be backing the IWG report. In 2010, the White House Task Force on Childhood Obesity released a report setting the agenda for Michelle Obama's Let's Move! campaign. The task force noted that four conditions were necessary for meaningful improvement in industry self-regulation: (1) self-regulatory groups must adopt uniform nutrition standards, (2) voluntary reform must create a level playing field for industry, (3) self-regulation must apply to all forms of marketing, and (4) food companies must be presented with sufficient reasons to comply. On this last point, the report added: "The prospect of regulation or legislation has often served as a catalyst for driving meaningful reform in other industries and may do so in the context of food marketing as well."[9] This marked the third time that regulation had been invoked as a threat.

In the meantime, food companies were putting increasing effort into blocking this initiative. They induced Congress to hold hearings on the IWG guidelines in 2011. Internal staff memos revealed that the hearings were meant to be critical of the FTC. Indeed, Republican legislators complained that the guidelines reflected actions of Big Brother government, and rather than focusing on marketing, the IWG ought to be emphasizing physical activity. Faced with what seemed like overwhelming opposition, the FTC backed down. According to one account, FTC official David Vladeck "nearly wore himself out repeating that the guidelines were voluntary and had no force of law."[10] The agencies, Vladeck conceded, would abandon guidelines for children older than 11 years, would not restrict cartoons and licensed characters on food packages, and would allow marketing of the unhealthier foods at fund-raisers and sporting events.

> FTC staff has determined that, with the exception of certain in-school marketing activities, it is not necessary to encompass adolescents ages 12 to 17 within the scope of covered marketing.... In addition, the FTC staff believes that philanthropic activities, charitable events, community programs, entertainment and sporting events, and theme parks are, for the most part, directed to families or the general community and do not warrant inclusion with more specifically child-directed marketing. Moreover, it would be counterproductive to discourage food company sponsorship of these activities to the extent that many benefit children's health by promoting physical activity. Finally, the Commission staff does not contemplate recommending that food companies change the trade dress elements of their packaging or remove brand equity characters from food products that don't meet nutrition recommendations.[11]

Where was the Obama White House while all this was happening? Neither the president nor the First Lady issued statements in support of the IWG report, perhaps because the president had to stand for reelection the following year and wanted to avoid all unnecessary controversy. Rumors circulated that the White House not only had withdrawn support for the IWG report but also was pressing the FTC to back off.[12] By the end of 2011, industry lobbyists had induced Congress to insert language in an appropriations act requiring the FTC to prove in advance that the benefits of voluntary nutrition standards would exceed their cost. That action effectively killed the IWG initiative.

In 2013, the IOM issued a follow-up to its 2005 report on food marketing to children. Although health groups such as the American Academy of Pediatrics continued to press for regulations, the IOM recognized the low level of political support for restrictions on food marketing, even to children. Given the political realities, the IOM concluded that self-regulation was the only viable option. But, it said, in an almost verbatim repeat of its 2005 threat—the fourth time we have heard this—if voluntary efforts were not able to shift marketing away from unhealthy foods and beverages, "Congress should enact legislation mandating the shift on both broadcast and cable television." Limiting food and beverage marketing, the IOM insisted, is "a public health priority of the highest order."[13] Perhaps, but with a Congress unwilling to stand up for children's health, such "or else" threats are meaningless—as food companies by now are well aware.

ADVOCATE: REGULATE SODA AND JUNK FOOD MARKETING TO CHILDREN

If you are troubled by the idea that food companies can market their products to children indiscriminately and with little regard for health consequences, you can inform yourself of the issues and the rationale for regulation, join the debate, consider engaging in advocacy, and join or support organizations engaged in such advocacy.

Understand the Issue

For the food and beverage industries, marketing to children is the line drawn in the sand. They cannot risk profits by allowing such marketing to be regulated. Soda companies are willing to embrace self-regulation, perhaps because they know they can find ways around it. But the rationale for federal regulation of soda marketing to children is strongly established.

- Young people are unusually vulnerable to marketing.
- Marketing is unusually effective with children.
- Electronic marketing is not viewed by children as marketing.
- Children are especially influenced by celebrity endorsements.

- Soda marketing undermines the school environment.
- Marketing undermines parental authority over food choices.
- Soda company self-regulatory policies provide easily evaded loopholes.
- Self-regulation is demonstrably ineffective in protecting children from harm.

On this basis, federal regulation is essential and should include independently determined nutrition standards that apply to all companies, all products, and all media. Because teenagers bear the brunt of soda marketing, regulations should apply to all children up to the age of 18.

Engage in the Debate

Table 11.2 summarizes the principal arguments for and against setting clear limits on what food and drink marketers do or say to encourage children to desire, ask for, and consume their products.

TABLE 11.2 Topic for debate: the federal government should regulate food marketing to children

SODA COMPANIES SAY	ADVOCATES SAY
Self-regulation is sufficient.	Self-regulation policies do not include nutrition standards and should apply to teenagers as well as young children.
Evaluations find that soda companies fully comply with marketing policies.	Those are industry-paid evaluations. Independent investigations reveal that children are still subjected to a barrage of advertising through other channels.
The First Amendment protects our right to market to children.	The First Amendment does not permit deceptive marketing or promotion of products harmful to children.
Congress passed a law in 1980 expressly forbidding the FTC from restricting food advertising to children.	Obesity was not as prevalent a problem in 1980 as it is today; Congress needs to bring the law up to date.
Marketing to children is legal.	Marketing to children may be legal, but is not ethical; children are unable to evaluate marketing messages and are especially influenced by advertising.
Adolescents can make their own decisions.	Adolescents are exceptionally subject to peer pressure and lack impulse control.
The government should not be involved in personal food choice.	Corporations should not have the power to promote unhealthful food choices.

Take Action

Given the strong political opposition to these efforts, American advocates for children's health are limited in what they can do to achieve more responsible advertising in general, and elimination of soda and junk food marketing aimed at children in particular. While waiting for more responsible leadership in Congress, advocates can work toward intermediate, incremental goals that may lead to measurable benefits.

Hold Soda Companies Accountable for Self-Regulation

Industry self-regulation has led to some changes in marketing practices, but not nearly enough. Recent self-regulatory efforts began in 2008. In response to rising concerns about the effects of food marketing on childhood obesity and the "or else" threats of regulation, the International Council of Beverage Associations (ICBA) published guidelines on marketing to children. Companies belonging to its member associations—the American Beverage Association (ABA), for example—must promise not to pay for advertising in any media aimed at audiences in which 50 percent or more of viewers are children under the age of 12. This promise applies to advertising on TV, radio, print, Internet, phone messages, and film, including product placements.[14] These sound like impressive restrictions, but they do not apply to all of the other forms of marketing used by soda companies—toys, games, social media, and digital methods, for example.

In November 2009, Coke and Pepsi hired Accenture Media Management to evaluate their adherence to the ICBA guidelines. The Accenture study reported that the two companies paying for the study were 96 percent in compliance with the guideline on television marketing, and 100 percent in compliance on print and Internet media. By 2012, Accenture reported that, worldwide, both soda companies were 99 percent in compliance with the television guideline.[15]

Since then, both Coke and Pepsi have posted notices on their websites announcing voluntary reductions of the 50 percent kids-in-the-audience cutoff point to 35 percent, everywhere in the world. Figure 11.1 shows Coca-Cola's Global Responsible Marketing policy for eliminating direct advertising to children under age 12.

Advocacy groups tracking progress on marketing promises generally agree that soda companies are in fairly good compliance with their own stated policies—the letter of the law. But the loopholes allow other ways of

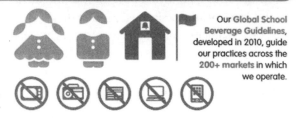

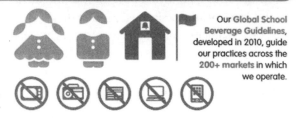

> **Market responsibly, including no advertising to children under 12 anywhere in the world**
>
> Our responsible marketing guidelines include a global industry policy to not buy advertising directly targeted at audiences that are more than 35% children under 12. This applies to TV, radio and print, and, where data is available, to the Internet and mobile phones.
>
> Our Global School Beverage Guidelines, developed in 2010, guide our practices across the 200+ markets in which we operate.
>
> **Find out more about our commitments at comingtogether.com**

FIGURE 11.1 Coca-Cola's global policy on marketing to children, 2013. The policy applies only to paid advertising specifically aimed at children under age 12. It does not apply to other forms of marketing discussed in Chapter 10, or to marketing aimed at older children or adults but still accessible to younger children.

reaching children. Food companies' reliance on self-regulation implies that they know perfectly well that their products harm children. But what can they do? No regular soda can ever meet a nutritional standard for sugars, and companies do not want to stop marketing to children if doing so reduces sales and profits.

When the advocacy group Center for Science in the Public Interest (CSPI) evaluated food companies' responsible marketing pledges in 2010, it gave both Coca-Cola and PepsiCo a dismal grade of C+—in sharp contrast to the industry-funded A+ Accenture assessment. In CSPI's view, the companies were doing a good job of adhering to their own policies, but those policies were too weak and full of loopholes to be taken seriously. Systematic reviews of the evidence have come to similar conclusions: children are still subjected to massive amounts of soda marketing, whether aimed directly at them or not. Because self-regulation is ineffective, policy action is needed.[16] But in the current political climate, such action is unlikely. Advocates must look for other ways to curb food marketing to children. They can continue to hold soda companies accountable for their promises, but also consider mounting legal challenges when opportunities arise, and look for other ways to try to deal with the problem at the local or state levels.

Use Legal Approaches
Frustrated by congressional inaction, lawyers and legal advocacy groups have begun to explore ways to use legal strategies to address childhood

obesity. They also have published interpretations of the First Amendment based on psychological research demonstrating how badly children are misled and harmed by food advertising. In their view, because the FTC regulates cigarette advertising to children, it can also regulate food advertising. On this basis, they continue to urge the FTC to use its constitutional authority to limit food marketing to children. Other legal advocates point out that the First Amendment protects free speech but does not protect *deceptive* free speech. Digital marketing in particular, they say, raises issues of deception. It violates children's privacy by disguising advertising as entertainment. It also does so by using packaging that requires children to obtain a code or provide personal information to gain access to online content, loyalty points, games, or premiums.[17]

Use Legislative Approaches

In 2013, Rep. Rosa De Lauro (D-Conn.) introduced a bill to close the loophole in the tax code that permits deductions for advertising expenses. Her bill would eliminate tax deductions for children's marketing intended to promote foods of poor nutritional quality. It also would disallow other expenses related to such marketing, including travel, gifts, promotional items, packaging, movie placements, loyalty programs, and celebrity endorsements. "Taxpayers," she said, "should not continue to subsidize a tax loophole that allows companies to deduct expenses for marketing unhealthy foods to kids."[18] By children, she meant anyone age 17 or under. Although her bill did not even get discussed, let alone pass, it brought the issue to public attention. Such bills will undoubtedly be introduced again.

Hold International Public Health Agencies Accountable

In 2010, the World Health Organization (WHO) issued recommendations on marketing to children.

> Given that the effectiveness of marketing is a function of exposure and power, the overall policy objective should be to reduce both the exposure of children to, and power of, marketing of foods high in saturated fats, *trans*-fatty acids, free sugars, or salt.... Settings where children gather should be free from all forms of marketing of foods high in saturated fats, *trans*-fatty acids, free sugars, or salt. Such settings include, but are not limited to, nurseries, schools, school grounds and pre-school centres, playgrounds, family and

child clinics and paediatric services and during any sporting and cultural activities that are held on these premises.[19]

Advocates can encourage WHO's work with member nations to implement such recommendations, monitor international compliance by issuing reports on a regular basis, and encourage WHO's donors to support such actions.

Join the Campaigns

A good place to start is with CSPI's Food Marketing Workgroup (www .foodmarketing.org), a coalition of more than two hundred organizations and experts aimed at eliminating harmful food marketing to children and other vulnerable groups. The workgroup actively identifies, investigates, and advocates changes to unhealthful marketing practices. Appendix 1 lists it and other advocacy organizations working on this issue.

12

Advocacy

Getting Sodas Out of Schools

Whereas advocates for banning soda marketing to children seem stuck with industry self-regulation, those working to remove sodas from schools have done better—although it took half a century to make real progress. From the 1960s on, advocates for children's health repeatedly petitioned the USDA to remove sodas from schools, at first to encourage schools to set higher nutrition standards and later as a measure to prevent obesity. Today, advocates joined by no less than the First Lady of the United States succeeded in banning full-sugar sodas from schools during class hours—in theory if not always in practice. But the soda industry also succeeded in protecting some of its interests. It salvaged loopholes that allow sodas to be offered at sports and other special events, and it kept vending machines in the schools. It also used its political clout to generate substantial opposition to the USDA's school nutrition standards.

As a reminder, the value of removing sodas from schools is well established. Research increasingly supports the benefits of healthier school food environments. Children in states with more restrictive school nutrition standards do not compensate by drinking more soda outside of school and are not as obese. Such benefits are even greater for low-income children.[1]

Since the 1960s, Congress has viewed sodas as "foods of minimal nutritional value" (a polite euphemism for junk foods), sold in competition with school meals. Kids who buy sodas, candies, snacks, and other "competitive" foods from à la carte lines or vending machines are less likely to participate in school meal programs run by the U.S. Department of Agriculture (USDA). The USDA, not the Department of Education, is in charge of school meals.

Unlike most other school programs, these meals are required to have separate budgets and in some schools are expected to be entirely self-supporting.[2] The USDA reimburses schools for the cost of the breakfasts and lunches based on the number of students who actually take meals produced according to its requirements. If more students take the authorized meals, the schools get more money from federal reimbursements to prepare and serve them. School districts in wealthy areas may supplement costs, but in poor districts the federal reimbursements are often the only source of school meal funding.

Competitive foods not only set a poor example to students but also undermine the financial viability of school food service operations, especially when these operations subsidize sales of sodas and snacks, which some do. This is a particularly difficult problem in low-income communities, where parents may not want to fill out government paperwork to enroll their children, and where teenagers are more heavily exposed to soda marketing.[3] The limited funding available for school meals and other discretionary purposes has encouraged many school districts to view sales of sodas and snacks as sources of badly needed revenue. This explains why advocacy to remove sodas from schools confronts opposition not only from soda companies but also from school administrators who do not want to lose that source of discretionary revenue.

HOW ADVOCATES GOT TO THIS POINT

In Table 12.1 I summarize the exceptionally complicated history of advocates' efforts to get sodas out of schools and the opposition they faced in doing so.[4] Although school meal programs in the United States have a longer history, let's start this discussion in 1946, when Congress passed the National School Lunch Act (NSLA) as "a measure of national security, to safeguard the health and well-being of the Nation's children and to encourage the domestic consumption of nutritious agricultural commodities and other food by...providing an adequate supply of food and other facilities for the establishment, maintenance, operation and expansion of nonprofit school lunch programs."[5] The NSLA specified details of what could be served and family income levels that qualified for free or reduced-price meals. In 1952, Congress passed the first of many amendments to the act, setting a decades-long pattern of nearly annual tinkering with the regulations.

TABLE 12.1 Selected events in the history of attempts to get soft drinks out of schools, 1946 to 2014

YEAR	EVENT
1946	Congress passes National School Lunch Act to promote use of surplus agricultural commodities in school meals as a means to improve the nutritional status of low-income children.
1966	Congress passes Child Nutrition Act; requires USDA to develop regulations for nutritional quality of school meals.
1970	Congress amends 1966 act to give USDA authority to control sales of competitive foods until the end of the school lunch period in or near school cafeterias during mealtimes; allows anything typically served in school meals to be sold competitively at other times and places. Effect: bans competitive foods from schools. Soda trade associations object, sue, win ruling that USDA had exceeded its authority.
1972	Congress repeals the 1970 authorization; permits sales of competitive foods during mealtimes if proceeds benefit schools or school groups; prohibits USDA from regulating competitive foods; transfers authority to state and local education boards. Effect: deregulates federal oversight of competitive foods.
1977	Congress restores USDA's regulatory authority over competitive foods but demands assurances that USDA will not ban sodas and snacks.
1978	USDA proposes rules restricting foods of minimal nutritional value—soft drinks, water ices, chewing gum, and certain candies—from the beginning of the school day until after the last lunch period; withdraws proposal in response to objections about its scope of authority.
1979	USDA re-proposes rules; PepsiCo organizes letter-writing campaign opposing USDA authority.
1980	USDA issues final rules banning vending of foods of minimal nutritional value until the end of the school lunch period. National Soft Drink Association sues to overturn "arbitrary and capricious" regulations; loses, appeals, and wins in 1983.
1983	U.S. appeals court rules that USDA cannot impose "time and place" restrictions on sales of competitive foods.
1985	USDA revises rules to prohibit sales of competitive foods of minimal nutritional value during lunch periods in cafeterias and to permit sales of sodas and other such foods at all other times and places with no restrictions on allocation of revenues. Effect: increases sales of competitive foods.
1990	Advocacy groups call for restrictions or bans on competitive foods.
1994	Sen. Patrick Leahy (D-Vt.) introduces bill to restrict or ban school sales of soft drinks and other foods of minimal nutritional value. Soda lobbyists testify against restrictions. Congress reaffirms 1985 rules. Soda companies establish exclusive "pouring rights" contracts with colleges and universities.
1995	Center for Science in the Public Interest (CSPI) petitions USDA to require competitive foods to meet nutrition standards. USDA says agency has no authority to regulate food sales outside food service areas.
1998	Soda companies offer pouring rights contracts to elementary schools as well as to junior high and high schools. CSPI publishes *Liquid Candy*; urges schools to stop selling soft drinks.

(*continued*)

TABLE 12.1 Continued

YEAR	EVENT
2000	Advocates induce at least 30 school districts to refuse to accept pouring rights contracts.
2003	Coca-Cola issues voluntary guidelines; suggests not selling sodas in elementary schools.
2004	Congress passes act requiring local school districts to develop wellness policies by 2006.
2005	American Beverage Association (ABA) announces new vending machine policy to provide lower-calorie drinks to schools. Congress directs the Centers for Disease Control and Prevention (CDC) to ask the Institute of Medicine (IOM) to recommend nutrition standards for competitive foods as well as school meals.
2006	Clinton Foundation and American Heart Association form Alliance for a Healthier Generation; forge voluntary agreement with ABA to keep vending machines in schools but remove full-sugar sodas. ABA issues school beverage guideline: no more than 66 calories per 8 ounces (100 calories per 12 ounces).
2007	IOM issues report on nutrition standards for school food; recommends that competitive foods comply with Dietary Guidelines. Soda industry agrees to support federal legislation to remove full-sugar sodas from schools.
2009	IOM issues report on nutrition standards for school meals.
2010	First Lady Michelle Obama launches Let's Move! campaign to improve school food. White House Task Force on Childhood Obesity recommends improvements in school meals. Congress passes the Healthy, Hunger-Free Kids Act; authorizes USDA to set nutrition standards for all foods sold in schools.
2011	Congress puts language in appropriations act blocking the USDA from setting volume or frequency restrictions on tomato paste and french fries in school meals.
2012	USDA releases nutrition standards for school meals based on IOM reports. Objections from industry and some school districts ensue.
2013	USDA eases off on meal standards. Releases rules for nutrition standards for competitive foods. These exclude full-sugar sodas but allow high schools to sell sodas containing no more than 40 calories per 8 ounces. Effect: full-sugar sodas cannot be sold in schools except when states allow them in "infrequent" fundraisers or outside the school day. The meaning of "infrequent" is delegated to schools.
2014	Members of Congress introduce bills to weaken or eliminate school nutrition standards. School Nutrition Association (SNA) asks Congress to delay implementation. Former SNA presidents write letter supporting the standards. USDA finds most schools to be in compliance with new standards.

By the 1960s, school officials, health authorities, and even Congress had come to recognize that sales of sodas and junk foods were competing with student participation in the meal programs. When Congress first tried to ban competitive foods from schools, soda companies objected and sued the USDA. Bans, they said, were outside the scope of the USDA's mandate and constituted an "arbitrary and capricious exercise of authority," words used to this day by soda industry lawyers. The courts agreed. This meant that the USDA's policy on competitive foods had only one restriction: sodas and snacks could not be sold in cafeterias during lunch periods. But even this limitation could be, was, and still is ignored or evaded.[6]

From the start, school meals were intended to serve two functions: to improve the nutritional status of children and to provide an outlet for surplus agricultural commodities (although cash has now replaced most of the commodities). Also from the start, the USDA's attempts to establish nutrition standards for school meals encountered strong objections from soft drink companies—often joined by principals, school boards, and state education departments reluctant to give up the income from soda sales. These groups lobbied against any proposed restriction on whether, when, or where competitive foods might be sold. The USDA tried to ban sodas, but it was forced by Congress to replace the ban with "time-and-place" restrictions. These allowed sodas to be sold, but only outside the cafeteria after the end of the last lunch period. Even so, the USDA either could not or would not enforce these rules, and schools could easily ignore them.

POURING RIGHTS CONTRACTS

While Congress fussed with time-and-place rules for competitive foods, soda companies found another way to entrench their products in schools. In the early 1990s, Coke and Pepsi began to offer large sums to colleges and universities for the exclusive right to sell their company's products on campuses. The practice continues. In 2013, PepsiCo agreed to pay the City University of New York (CUNY) $21 million over ten years for pouring rights to the university's twenty-four campuses. Pepsi celebrated this victory over Coca-Cola with advertisements for CUNY on its trucks (Figure 12.1). Also in 2013, UCLA replaced its previous soda contracts with a ten-year, $15.4 million arrangement giving Coca-Cola exclusive access to its forty-one thousand students. UCLA announced that $3 million of the proceeds would go for scholarships. It did not, however, explain how the contract might contribute to its campus-wide "social movement around health and well-being." In 2014, the University of California, Davis, dropped its long-standing agreement with Coca-Cola and signed a $10 million contract with PepsiCo; most of the money would go to support athletics. University administrators justify such contracts on the grounds that they provide needed funds for sports and academic purposes.[7]

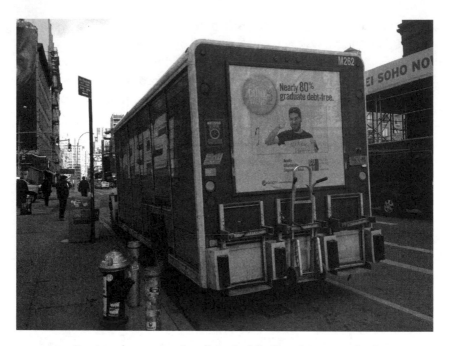

FIGURE 12.1 Pepsi truck promotes the value of a debt-free education at the City University of New York, 2013. PepsiCo had just won a $21 million pouring rights contract with the University. Photo courtesy of Daniel Bowman Simon.

These examples illustrate contracts with institutions serving college-age young adults. But in the late 1990s, in response to a decline in federal and state financing of public schools, soda companies contracted for pouring rights with high schools, middle, and even elementary schools. The contracts, often for ten years, invariably required the schools to increase the number of vending machines on their campuses—the more vending machines, the more drinks sold. The contracts may have seemed like free money, but they required the schools to pay for the sodas and other expenses. Schools had to set sales targets, meet quotas, and permit display of company logos on vending machines, cups, sportswear, brochures, and school buildings. An additional benefit to soda companies was the steady base of sales from a captive audience of children too young or too difficult to reach by conventional advertising methods. By 2005, a national survey showed that half of U.S. elementary schools and 80 percent of high schools had such contracts, mainly with Coke or Pepsi. A later survey calculated the actual size of the net profits obtained by the schools from these contracts. These were surprisingly small: less than $2 per elementary and middle school child per year, and slightly more than $4 per year per high school student.[8]

Despite such low returns—which surely could have been generated by some other means—administrators of financially strapped school districts eagerly entered into such contracts. Larger school districts auctioned pouring rights to the highest bidder, and some hired consultants to negotiate the best possible deals. Because the contracts placed school administrators in the position of encouraging students to drink more sodas, they created conflicts of interest. As the ethical issues and low financial returns became more evident, some school districts began to refuse the contracts. Today they are rare in elementary schools. In 2014, for example, the Pasco, Florida, school district gave up a ten-year, $5.7 million contract with Coca-Cola out of concern for what it might do to kids' health.[9] But pouring rights contracts still affect half of middle school children and 70 percent of high school students, and they are especially prevalent in low-income school districts.

EARLY EFFORTS TO RESTRICT SODA SALES

Because of their large, captive, impressionable audience, schools are prime locations for obesity intervention. As evidence for the links between competitive foods and obesity grew in strength, calls for bans became more urgent. Schools, parents, teachers, and food service directors in many locations wanted to create healthier food environments. But without a national policy, they had to make the changes one school at a time, with inconsistent results. Outright bans encountered vigorous objections from soda companies as well as from some parents and food service personnel. In 2013, I attended a public health conference in Boston addressed by Mayor Thomas Menino shortly before he ended his twenty-one-year term. Menino told the audience that the biggest political battle of his entire career was the one to get sodas out of the Boston public schools. He managed to do this in 2004; by 2006, Boston students were demonstrably drinking less soda.[10]

The threat of such losses induces soda companies to seek other options. In 2003, in an action that can be interpreted as a tacit admission that sodas harm kids, Coca-Cola established guidelines—voluntary, of course—for its bottlers. Bottlers were no longer to send full-sugar sodas to elementary schools. They could supply sports events and vending machines in middle and high schools, but not cafeterias. This policy, the company explained, would continue to allow educators to "raise critical resources for their schools."[11]

In 2004, Congress passed a law long sought by advocates. It required local school districts to develop wellness policies. Although the act provided no funds, it did encourage school districts to establish nutrition guidelines for school meals. It also gave advocates a mandate to push for school environments that would be free of soda contracts and vending machines. Cities began to demand the ban of sodas from schools. In 2005, legislators in forty-two states introduced two hundred bills aimed at restricting sales of competitive foods. Lawyers working with two advocacy groups, the CSPI and the Public Health Advocacy Institute, were preparing class-action lawsuits against soda companies and negotiating with Coca-Cola to withdraw *all* of its products—not just full-sugar sodas—from schools.[12]

PREEMPTING THE SODA BAN: THE CLINTON FOUNDATION'S END RUN

The American Beverage Association (ABA) responded to these threats with a new school-based policy excluding full-sugar sodas but permitting sales of those that did not exceed 66 calories per 8 ounces (an 8-ounce regular soda usually provides 100 calories). A year later, the Clinton Foundation and the American Heart Association formed the Alliance for a Healthier Generation for the express purpose of negotiating school policies with the ABA and soda companies. The alliance convinced soda companies to agree to phase out any drink with more than 66 calories per 8 ounces within five years. This policy excluded regular sodas but permitted sales of Gatorade (50 calories per 8 ounces), diet sodas, and sweetened vitamin waters. And the vending machines would remain. Former President Bill Clinton, who had brokered this deal, called soda companies "courageous" for their actions. Clinton, I must point out, had his own conflict of interest. By 2013, Coca-Cola had donated between $5 million and $10 million to his foundation.[13]

Advocates were dismayed. The alliance had betrayed their negotiations. Although they had come close to getting all sugary drinks and vending machines out of schools, the Clinton deal rescued sports drinks, sugar-sweetened waters, and the machines that sold them. In 2008, the alliance proudly announced that after just two years, companies had cut the beverage calories shipped to schools by 58 percent. A USDA study observed that 80 percent of school districts had bans or restrictions on sweetened beverages, and a study funded by the ABA concluded that school soda calories had been cut by 90 percent. Independently funded studies, however, demonstrated that sodas were still widely available, even in elementary schools.[14] The alliance deal, after all, was private, voluntary, and intended to head off the class-action lawsuit, which it succeeded in doing. As it became evident that schools were implementing the voluntary guidelines inconsistently or ignoring them, advocates again pressed for federal intervention.

ACHIEVING FEDERAL REGULATION

In 2005, Congress asked the Institute of Medicine (IOM) to develop nutrition standards for competitive foods and school meals. IOM committees issued reports on the topic from 2007 to 2009. These concluded that the nutritional content of all food in schools should align with the Dietary Guidelines. In 2010, to accomplish one of the principal goals of Michelle Obama's Let's Move! campaign, Congress passed the Healthy, Hunger-Free Kids Act. This act authorized the USDA to set nutrition standards for school meals. It issued the standards in 2012. At that point, lobbyists for the potato and pizza industries complained directly to Congress, which intervened by effectively micromanaging the USDA's rules through the appropriations process. It inserted clauses in the agricultural appropriations act forbidding the USDA to set limits on the number of times french fries could be served in a week or on the volume of tomato sauce that would allow pizza to be counted as a vegetable.[15] This lobbying outcome sent a clear signal to other food companies that if the nutrition rules did not work in their favor, they could go straight to Congress to have the rules weakened or set aside.

A year later, the USDA proposed similar rules for competitive foods. Remarkably, the soda rules turned out to be even more restrictive than those proposed by the ABA and the Alliance for a Healthier Generation.[16] They entirely ban full-sugar sodas from elementary and middle schools. High school students, however, can buy 8-ounce beverages with no more than 40 calories (60 calories in 12 ounces). This cutoff point excludes not only regular Coke and Pepsi (150 calories per 12 ounces) but also sports drinks such as Gatorade (75 calories). The 12-ounce size is the largest that can be sold, thereby eliminating the 20-ounce bottles typically sold in school vending machines. The rules also require schools to supply potable drinking water to all students at no cost. Let me be clear: to the extent that schools adhere to these standards, they represent an extraordinary victory for child health advocates.

Getting schools to follow the standards, however, is another matter. To make the rules more acceptable to school administrators, the USDA left some loopholes. The standards apply to sodas sold during the school day, but not to non-school hours, weekends, off-campus events, or school lunches brought from home, or to school birthday and other celebrations that can pile on the sugars and calories. They also do not apply to in-school fund-raisers; these are to be "infrequent," with the meaning of that word left to states to determine and enforce. Because so many decisions about school food are delegated to states, actual policies vary from outright bans on sodas to no rules at all.[17]

Despite the loopholes, advocates managed to get full-sugar sodas banned from school meals and à la carte lines, at least most of the time. And they have research on their side. Studies provide increasing evidence that soda bans lead to significant reductions in consumption. By one calculation, the ban on full-sugar sodas will cost schools no more than 74 cents per student per year. On this basis, some schools, such as those in Portland, Maine, have banned sodas entirely—no sodas of any kind on sale anywhere, not at sports events or field trips, not by parent-teacher organizations, and not even in the teachers' lounges. This, the Portland district claims, makes it part of a national trend.[18]

SODA INDUSTRY PUSHBACK

By late 2014, the USDA's nutrition standards again were under attack, this time from members of Congress opposed to government interference in personal food choice, students who complain they are not getting enough to eat, and school food service directors who insist that the rules are impossible to implement.

How much of this opposition has been organized by soda companies and their trade association is difficult to judge, but I have my suspicions. Publicly, the industry supports the new regulations. ABA president Susan Neely actually takes credit for them, as in her view they are similar to those her association initially suggested: "We just think that's highly unusual that something that the government would ultimately codify draws from a voluntary industry initiative."[19]

But in a bizarre turn of events, the School Nutrition Association (SNA), the professional association for school food service personnel and an initial supporter of Let's Move!, soon came to oppose the standards. The association derives half its income from food industry donations, and its website lists both Coke and Pepsi on the long list of corporate patrons.[20]

The SNA issued a position paper charging that students are refusing to eat the healthier meals, plate waste is increasing, and school meal revenues are falling. On this basis, the SNA induced the House to use the appropriations process to postpone the standards for a year, a move widely perceived as a first step toward overturning them. But a USDA study found that 90 percent of schools were doing just fine with the standards. When the First Lady called on advocates to oppose the House appropriations maneuver, nineteen former presidents of the SNA responded with a letter in support of the USDA's efforts.[21] Given the SNA's conflict of interest, it is understandable why it would not actively encourage its members to try to make the new standards work. But its stance isolated the SNA from health advocates, exposed its conflicted interests, and divided its membership—all collateral consequences of food industry sponsorship.

BEYOND SALES: MARKETING SODAS IN SCHOOLS

Advocates also want soda advertising out of schools, as well as soda sales. State surveys document that such advertising is extensive. In Pennsylvania, for example, soft drink advertisements pervade schools, not least on vending machines. The Maine legislature banned junk-food advertising in public schools in 2007, but when researchers followed up three years later, they found that soda advertisements continued to pervade the school landscape, unnoticed by school administrators. On average, schools displayed an average of 49 illegal posters and displayed forbidden advertising for more than 197 competitive foods, of which nearly half were products owned by Coca-Cola or PepsiCo.[22]

The National Education Policy Center's fifteenth annual report on commercialism in schools confirms these findings. It finds that food and beverage companies still display logos on vending machines; sponsor school programs, educational materials, and incentive programs; reach kids through digital media; and participate in fund-raising efforts. The report notes that even when teaching materials do not mention the sponsor's name, they reflect the sponsor's interests. They might mention, for example, that all beverages count toward hydration, or they might emphasize physical activity or state that individuals are entirely responsible for food choices. The center urges policy makers to prohibit advertising in schools.[23] But, as the Maine study indicated, prohibitions are unlikely to be effective unless schools actively enforce the rules and hold companies accountable.

Soda Company School Marketing Policies

Coca-Cola and PepsiCo both have issued policies on marketing to children in schools. Coca-Cola's says:

> As a global business, we respect and recognize the unique learning environment of schools and believe in commercial-free classrooms for children. We will make every attempt not to commercially advertise in primary schools, and we will not offer our beverages for sale in primary schools. If requested to do so by parents and caregivers or school authorities to meet hydration needs, we will endeavor to meet those requests.[24]

Ah yes, hydration. That argument is why the requirement for free, potable water in schools is so critical. PepsiCo's school marketing policy also says

TABLE 12.2 Soda company activities aimed at schools, selected examples, 2013–2014

COMPANY	ACTIONS AIMED AT ENGAGING SCHOOLS
Coca-Cola	Provided toolkit for teachers who bring classes to World of Coca-Cola in Atlanta explaining how visits can help meet state performance standards.
	My Coke Rewards for Schools (now discontinued) encouraged families to collect bottle caps with codes for points that could be redeemed for school support. The current program encourages Twitter followers to use points for sports and music events.
	Scholars Foundation offers college scholarships to high school students involved in civic engagement.
	$500,000 award to Abyssinian Development Corporation to establish a student media center in New York City's Bread & Roses Integrated Arts High School.
PepsiCo	Refresh program (now discontinued) invited school groups to compete for grants voted on by website viewers.
	Recruited Nebraska high school marching band for Super Bowl video; provided free concert in return.
	Greenville County, SC, schools awarded 25 Pepsi-Greenville Golf Tournament scholarships to 25 seniors.

that the company "commits not to engage in product advertising or mar keting communications directed to students in primary schools, except if requested by, or agreed with, the school administration for specific educational purposes. This restriction does not apply to signage at the point of sale identifying those products available for purchase."[25] These policies leave plenty of leeway for interpretation of what does and does not constitute marketing, as Table 12.2 illustrates.

Federal School Marketing Policy

Throughout the history of competitive food policies, federal regulations focused only on sales and said nothing about food or beverage marketing in schools. In 2014, the White House broke new ground. As part of Let's Move!, the White House announced new USDA policies for school wellness programs. In addition to setting goals for nutrition education and physical activity, the proposed guidelines "would ensure that foods and beverages marketed to children in schools are consistent with the recently-released [USDA] Smart Snacks in School standards. Ensuring that unhealthy food is not marketed to children is one of the First Lady's top priorities."[26]

The CSPI weighed in with strong support: "USDA's proposed updates will strengthen implementation, help parents be better informed about the policies, and provide schools with more tools and resources." The Campaign for a Commercial-Free Childhood, however, called for a ban on *all* advertising in schools: "The USDA is urging schools only to limit junk food marketing.... [This] opens the floodgates for many other types of marketing in schools, setting a dangerous precedent that goes far beyond food."[27]

But the strongest criticisms came from a group supported by food companies, the National School Board Association (NSBA), which is funded by school food service companies such as Sodexo, Aramark, and Chartwells. Its executive director, Thomas Gentzel, argued that in raising questions about food and beverage marketing in schools, the USDA had overstepped its bounds.

> As part of their curricular studies...students participating on year-book or on the school newspaper routinely engage members of the community by soliciting advertisements for restaurants and other food services to be included in their school-based publications.

The Department's proposed prohibition on food marketing would cut off an important tie to the community the public school district serves. NSBA does not believe Congress intended such a result.[28]

In mid-2015, it remained uncertain whether the marketing ban could survive such opposition.

THE ROLE OF ADVOCATES: CSPI'S NATIONAL ALLIANCE FOR NUTRITION AND ACTIVITY (NANA)

Today's school food environment may not be ideal, but it is unquestionably healthier than it was a decade ago. Much of the success in setting nutrition standards for schools, getting sodas out of schools, and putting an end to classroom-based soda marketing is due to the efforts of the CSPI and its National Alliance for Nutrition and Activity (NANA) initiative, co-founded by Margo Wootan, who has been on the CSPI's staff since 1993. In 1999, she and a committee of advocates from state health departments and health organizations got together to create this alliance.

NANA is a coalition of four hundred national, state, and local organizations devoted to health promotion and obesity prevention. Its purpose is to convince Congress and federal agencies to do more to improve the public's diet and activity patterns. NANA deserves much credit for establishing nutrition standards for school meals and setting limits on soda marketing in schools. It led efforts to induce Congress to require school wellness policies, to pass the Healthy, Hunger-Free Kids Act, and to implement the act's provisions on competitive school foods. Wootan and NANA members framed the issues, developed policy recommendations, drafted backgrounders and legislative language, identified bill sponsors, built congressional and public support, and worked with staff of the Obama administration to get the bill passed.

NANA is behind CSPI's stated policy on marketing to children in schools: companies must not be permitted to market, sell, or give away low-nutrition foods or brands anywhere on school campuses by means that include:

- Selling low-nutrition foods
- Displaying logos, brand names, spokescharacters, product names, or other product marketing anywhere
- Using educational and other incentive programs to reward schools when families buy a company's food products[29]

CSPI also partnered with the Berkeley Media Studies Group to create the Food Marketing Workgroup, another coalition—this time of organizations and academics—working to obtain a federal ban on marketing to kids in or out of school. To do this, it needed authoritative data on current marketing practices, and it successfully lobbied for a national study of food marketing in schools. Congress agreed to appropriate funds to add questions to an ongoing school health survey. The survey questions assess the use of brand and product logos on educational materials, school supplies, displays, signage, equipment, buses, or other school property, as well as companies' use of incentive and label redemption programs, in-school media, free samples and coupons, fund-raising and market research activities, and product displays and placements. The results of this survey are expected to become available in 2015 and could well form the basis of legislation.[30] Although the history of school food advocacy may appear to indicate that progress occurs at glacial speed, it also demonstrates that improvements are possible and are well worth whatever time and effort they take.

ADVOCATE: ELIMINATE SODAS FROM SCHOOLS

Understand the Issue

Sodas and other foods of minimal nutritional value should not be sold, distributed, or marketed in the school environment:

- Schools should set standards for healthy diets.
- Schools should not promote poor health.
- Sodas and other junk foods compete with participation in federally subsidized school meals.
- Children in schools with strict nutrition standards exhibit a reduced prevalence of obesity.

Engage in the Debate

The Berkeley Media Studies Group describes the debate over sodas in schools as one of conflicting "frames"—ways of explaining the issue that promote support for one position or another. It advises advocates to anticipate the frames used by opponents and to develop appropriate responses.[31] Table 12.3 presents some of these framing perspectives.

TABLE 12.3 Topic for debate: sodas and soda marketing should be banned from schools

OPPONENTS SAY	ADVOCATES SAY
Sodas are already out of schools.	Sodas can be sold at sports events and fundraisers and are still marketed in schools; lower-calorie sodas are still sold in high schools.
Banning soda sales reflects "nanny state" government; schools are making choices for which students should be responsible.	Schools have a responsibility to promote kids' health and foster learning; kids learn better when they eat more healthfully.
It's unfair to restrict kids' choices.	It's unfair to encourage kids to pay for their education by buying sodas.
Schools need the revenues from soda sales.	Studies show that profits from soda sales are quite low. Health should be placed above profit.
It's not fair if kids can't celebrate events and sports with sodas.	Healthier beverage options are available and preferable.
Soda companies do so much for our schools and schoolchildren.	Soda companies have only one goal: to sell sodas.
It's unfair to single out sodas as a problem in schools. Other foods also contribute to obesity.	Sodas provide empty calories. Kids learn better and are healthier when they consume healthier beverages.

Take Action

If you would like to get sodas out of your children's school, you can:

- Visit the school and observe the marketing and sales environment for sodas.
- Ask for a balance sheet for net revenue. Find out how much profit the school actually makes from soda sales (principals may only look at gross revenue and overlook expenses).
- Meet with the principal, teachers, and other parents to express your concerns and generate support.
- Meet with the school board to encourage policy changes.
- Write letters to local newspapers to publicize the issue and generate support.
- Join the campaigns (see Appendix 1).

13

Advocacy

Getting Kids Involved

A demonstrably effective way to counter the effects of soda marketing is to encourage children to think critically about how companies get them to recognize, want, and consume the drinks. If you have kids of your own or work with children or adolescents, you can help even the youngest understand how deliberately soda companies design strategies to reach them. As kids get older, they can take increasing responsibility for their own observations, investigations, and actions. This chapter provides suggestions for how to teach kids about sodas, soda marketing, and healthier beverage choices, and how to help kids take such actions on their own.

Talking to children about these topics is the first step. Kids catch on fast. One group of investigators, for example, conducted focus groups with children ages 8 to 17 to evaluate responses to commercials featuring sports and music celebrities. Most of the kids could recall the commercials and associate specific brands with a celebrity, especially those for Gatorade, Coke, and Pepsi. But when the kids were asked to view the commercials critically, they made these kinds of observations:

- Once Beyoncé took a sip of Pepsi, she became more alive. Instantly, she had more energy and power to dance.
- The commercial would influence my friends to buy Pepsi because they are soccer players.
- It is obvious that this ad is appealing to kids, not adults.[1]

You can teach kids to think critically about soda marketing, beginning at home, but also at other places throughout the day. To explain how to do this, I organize advocacy suggestions by place, starting with supermarkets and then moving on to homes, restaurants, neighborhoods, means of transportation, and schools. Since this entire chapter is about how to advocate, I think it's useful to begin with a quick summary of what kids need to know.

UNDERSTAND THE ISSUE

From 1977 to 1996, soda consumption increased among children. So did the frequency of consumption, the size of the average drinks, and the daily intake of soda sugars and calories. Childhood obesity went up in parallel. The good news is that since then, most kids—and some adults—have been cutting down on sugary drinks. One California study reports that consumption of sodas has fallen by about 30 percent among younger children. But the not-so-good news is that teens are drinking more soda, perhaps because so much marketing targets them, particularly those who are African American or Hispanic (Chapter 14 says more about this).[2] Some parents are still giving sodas to very young children, as shown in Table 13.1.

TABLE 13.1 Calories from sugary drinks consumed per day by boys and girls of different ages*

AGE, YEARS	AVERAGE CALORIES PER DAY	BOYS	GIRLS
2–5	69	75	63
6–11	118	128	108
12–19	225	278	175

* The calories in this table are averages; some kids consume much more.

SOURCE: BK Kit et al., "Trends in sugar-sweetened beverage consumption among youth and adults in the United States: 1999–2010," *American Journal of Clinical Nutrition* 2013;98(1):180–88.

Sugary drinks are still the third-leading source of calories in kids' diets. Only two other food categories contribute more—what the government calls "grain-based desserts" (cakes, pies, cookies, Pop-Tarts, donuts) and, if you can believe it, pizza. Kids who habitually drink sodas gain more weight and are more likely to develop obesity-associated risk factors for heart disease.[3] From these findings alone, we can safely conclude that kids' diets could use improvement. Cutting down on sodas is a good way to start.

The reasons for this are well established. Reducing soda intake means reducing intake of sugars. Sodas alone account for one-third of kids' daily sugar intake.[4] The basic facts:

- Sodas contain sugars.
- Sugars have no nutrients (their calories are "empty").
- The sugars in sodas are in liquid form and absorbed rapidly.
- Sugars in small amounts are fine. But sodas have large amounts.

With this background, kids are ready to do their own soda research. Take them on a field trip to your neighborhood supermarket and ask questions as you go along, starting with the marketing. You will, of course, need to select and tailor these questions to the age and ability of the accompanying child.

EXPLORE A SUPERMARKET

Start by looking at the entrance to the store and then walk through it. Ask:

- How many places in the store display sodas for sale? [*Be sure to look at the entryway, at the ends of aisles, and at checkout counters— prime supermarket real estate.*]
- How many feet of shelf space does the supermarket devote to sodas? Pace out the linear feet and multiply by the number of shelves. [*You're squeezing in a basic math exercise while you are at it.*]
- Why are sodas displayed in so many places? [*Marketers know that the more products customers see in supermarkets, the more they buy.*]
- Does the supermarket do anything special to make sodas appeal to kids? [*Look for cartoons, placement on lower shelves, items at the checkout counter.*]
- Do some comparative pricing. Which costs more per unit: Single bottles or multiple packs? Sodas or bottled water? [*Read these off shelf labels, if available.*]
- Why do sodas cost so little compared to water? [*Among other supporting policies, the government subsidizes corn production, which reduces the cost of high-fructose corn syrup (HFCS).*]
- How do 100 percent fruit juices differ from other fruit drinks and sodas? [*They have all of the vitamins and minerals from the fruit, have some fiber, but have no sugars added.*]
- Which products have the most sugar per serving? [*Compare packaged breakfast cereals, breakfast pastries, candies, and sodas.*]

Read Package Labels

Kids who are able to read can learn a great deal about sodas from food labels. Package labels give nutrition information in two parts: Nutrition Facts and ingredient lists, as shown in Figure 13.1. Find a 12-ounce can or bottle of Coca-Cola or Pepsi. Examine the Nutrition Facts panel:

- How many servings does this bottle contain? [*1*]
- How many grams of sugars? [*41*]
- How many grams of carbohydrates? [*41*]
- How come the sugars and carbohydrates are the same? [*Sugars are a type of carbohydrate. Starch is another. All the carbohydrates in sodas are sugars.*]
- What else does the drink contain? [*Nothing but 30 milligrams of sodium.*]
- What is sodium? [*Salt is 40 percent sodium; the rest is chloride.*]

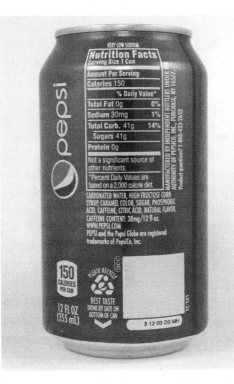

FIGURE 13.1 The Nutrition Facts panel from a 12-ounce can of Pepsi. Learning to interpret labels like this is a useful exercise for adults as well as children. Photo courtesy of Charles Nestle.

- Is that a lot or a little? [*It's only 1 percent of the amount recommended for a day.*]
- Do sodas provide any nutritional value? [*No, their calories are "empty," meaning that they do not contain any essential nutrients.*]

Next, observe the effect of portion size. Find a label for a 2-liter soda.

- How many servings in this bottle? [*8*]
- How many grams of sugars? [*27*]
- What does the 27 grams refer to? [*Only one 8-ounce serving.*]
- How many grams of sugars in the whole bottle? [*216 grams: 27 grams × 8 servings.*]
- How much soda will someone drink from this bottle at any one time? [*More than 8 ounces, most likely.*]
- Do bigger bottles have more sugar? [*Yes, they do.*]

Now ask kids to examine the list of ingredients on the label. For a Coca-Cola of any size, the ingredient list says: carbonated water, high fructose corn syrup, caramel color, phosphoric acid, natural flavors, and caffeine.

The FDA requires ingredients to be listed in order, beginning with the one present in the largest amount. Ask:

- Which ingredient makes up most of a soft drink? [*Carbonated water.*]
- Which ingredient is the second largest? [*HFCS.*]
- Where is sugar on this list? [*HFCS contains sugars made from cornstarch.*]
- If HFCS is really sugars, why don't the labels say so? [*Government labeling rules allow sugars to be called by many different names.*]
- Which ingredient is present in the smallest amount? [*Caffeine.*]
- How much caffeine does the soda contain? [*30 milligrams.*]
- Is that a lot or a little? [*A cup of coffee has about 150 milligrams, but sports and energy drinks can have more.*]
- Why do sodas contain caffeine? [*Caffeine is a stimulating drug that many people enjoy. It makes people want to drink sodas.*]

Count the Sugars

Sugars on food labels are measured in grams, but it is easier to think about them in teaspoons or packets. Ask kids to read the amount of sugars listed on soda cans or bottles per serving, convert grams to teaspoons, and consider what those amounts mean. One teaspoon contains about 4 grams of sugars.

- Read the number of grams of sugar on the package label.
- Divide by 4 to get teaspoons.
- For the 12-ounce soda (Figure 13.1): how many teaspoons of sugars? [*41 grams ÷ 4 = 10*]
- For the 2-liter soda, how many teaspoons of sugars per serving? [*27 grams ÷ 4 = 7*]
- For the 2-liter soda, how many teaspoons of sugars in the whole bottle? [*8 servings × 27 grams = 216 grams ÷ 4 = 54 teaspoons*]
- Is that a lot or a little? [*A lot!*]
- Do sodas taste that sweet? Think about how soda hides the taste of sugars, and why companies might want to make the sugars invisible.

Name the Sugars

While you are still in the supermarket, you can encourage kids to read the labels of other food products and see what else has sugars. Note the amounts of sugar listed in the Nutrition Facts label, and where sugars appear on the ingredient list. Sodas contain sugar, HFCS, or both. The official name of table sugar is sucrose. It is composed of two smaller sugars, glucose (the sugar in blood) and fructose (fruit sugar) in equal parts (50 percent, 50 percent). HFCS is also composed of glucose and fructose, but in somewhat different amounts, usually 45 percent glucose, 55 percent fructose.

But food companies are allowed to use many other names for sugar on ingredient lists, as shown in Table 13.2. All of these contain glucose, fructose, or both, except for lactose (which has glucose and yet another sugar, galactose).

Ask: Why do you think food companies use so many different names for sugars? [*Food companies might not want you to know how much sugar they add to food products, but you can usually figure that out by looking at total sugars on the Nutrition Facts panel and where sugars appear in the ingredient list.*]

Another activity: Go to the section of the store devoted to juice and other kinds of sugary drinks. Sodas are not the only drinks containing

TABLE 13.2 Some common names for sugars on food labels

Cane juice	Fruit juice concentrate	Molasses
Corn syrup	Glucose	Nectars
Dextrose	Honey	Pancake syrup
Evaporated cane juice	Lactose	Sucrose
Fructose	Maple syrup	Agave sugar

sugars. Other beverages can have just as much. Ask kids to look for sugars listed on the labels of energy drinks, sports drinks, bottled teas, lemonade, fruit drinks, flavored waters, and fruit juices.

- Which drinks have the most sugars?
- Do these drinks have any nutritional value? [*Some do, some don't. It depends on how much juice they contain.*]
- Why do food companies make so many sugary drinks? [*People like them and they make money for the companies.*]
- Why do fruit juices have so much sugar? [*Fruit is naturally sweet, but juices made from concentrate sometimes are diluted with less water to make them even sweeter.*]

HOME INVESTIGATIONS

Sodas consumed at home are the single largest source of sugars in kids' diets. The easiest way to discourage soda drinking at home is to declare the home a "soda-safe" environment. Make sure you have drinking water available, refrigerated if your kids like it cold. For treats, supply 100 percent fruit juices in small amounts. Because fruit juices have just as much sugar as sodas, the American Academy of Pediatrics recommends a limit of 6 ounces per day for children 1 to 6 years, and up to 12 ounces a day for children age 7 to 18.[5] A reasonable guideline for sweetened drinks other than 100 percent fruit juice is the USDA's standard for schools: no more than 60 calories per 12 ounces.

Do Some Experiments

While you are at home, you can have your kids do some experiments with sodas and their sugars.

1. The taste test. Add 10 teaspoons of sugar to a 12-ounce glass of water. Taste it. Does it taste as good as sodas?
2. What does ice do to the amount of sugar?
   - Measure the volume of an empty glass.
   - Put as much ice as you like in the glass.
   - Pour soda (or some other liquid) over the ice until the glass is full.
   - Take the ice out.
   - See how much soda is left.
   - How much sugar is that? You can assume that each ounce of soda contains one teaspoon of sugar even though this is a bit too much (soda companies say an ounce contains about 3.7 grams of sugar).
3. The tooth trick. Put a baby tooth in a glass of Coca-Cola and watch what happens after a week or so.
4. The sludge trick. Gently boil a Coke or Pepsi. Warning: be careful not to burn yourself or the pot.

Watch TV

Ask kids to count the number of times in a day or week that sodas are mentioned or shown on television, radio, Internet sites, Facebook or other social media sites, cell phones, or movies. Then ask:

- Why are soda ads so common? [*These are paid product placements.*]
- Why are sports, music, and TV celebrities shown with sodas? [*They are paid by soda companies to do this.*]
- How much do soda companies spend to try to get people to buy their products? [*The U.S. advertising budget for regular Coca-Cola alone was more than $250 million in 2013.*]
- How much does it cost to produce and place a thirty-second soda ad in prime time television? [*From a few thousand dollars for local stations to $4.5 million for the 2015 Super Bowl. The U.S. average was $112,100 in 2014.*][6]

Watch Ads Online and on Mobile Devices

Commercials for Coke and Pepsi are readily available on YouTube and company websites. Ask kids to watch them.

- How do the ads make kids want the products?
- How do sodas appear in the ads?
- What do the ads say about the sodas?
- What words and pictures do they use?
- How are the ads supposed to make kids feel about the products?

Watch for Marketing Aimed at African American and Hispanic Kids

As I discuss in Chapter 14, soda companies make special efforts to market to minority children, who are most at risk of health problems caused by obesity. Ask kids to look at advertisements and websites, and ask:

- How can you tell if a soda advertisement or website is aimed at African American or Hispanic kids?
- Why do soda companies use African American or Hispanic sports or music stars in advertisements?
- Why are some soda commercials available in Spanish?
- Is it fair for soda companies to aim commercials at minority children?
- What could minority children do to counter the effects of soda marketing?

RESTAURANT INVESTIGATIONS

Coke and Pepsi want kids to associate sodas with special occasions. If you take children to a fast-food outlet and order kids' meals, you can use the occasion to explain how soda companies partner with restaurants such as McDonald's. You can order kids' meals with milk, water, or a small portion of juice. You can ask kids to:

- Point to or count every soda advertisement in the restaurant.
- Look for soda advertisements on menu boards, walls, vending machines, napkins, and tray liners.
- Consider why these advertisements are there.
- Discuss why parents might want restaurants to stop including sodas in kids' menus.

If you would like kids to have a soda, you can ask for the smallest size, make sure it is filled to the brim with ice, and refuse refills. Explain why you are doing this by talking about or demonstrating the amount of sugars in sodas.

NEIGHBORHOOD INVESTIGATIONS

Take kids for a walk to your neighborhood stores. You can do this systematically by mapping out areas of a few square blocks. Go into every store, no matter what it sells. Observe whether sodas are available. Ask kids:

- How many places in this neighborhood sell sodas?
- Why do you think it is so easy to buy sodas in so many places?
- Can you buy fresh fruits and vegetables in as many places as you can buy sodas?
- Why is that?

This kind of activity can also teach kids about the effects of income inequality and targeted marketing. Take your kids to a high-income neighborhood, a low-income neighborhood, and a largely minority neighborhood and do some comparisons.

- Which neighborhood makes sodas more readily available?
- Which neighborhood makes fresh fruits and vegetables more readily available?
- Why do these differences exist?

INVESTIGATIONS WHILE TRAVELING

You can use the time while traveling in a car, bus, or train to ask kids to look at posters, billboards, and other signs where sodas are advertised.

- Count the number of soda advertisements. Analyze their content.
- How can you tell when advertising is aimed at kids?
- Why do so many soda advertisements feature famous people in sports or music?
- Do you think it is fair for soda companies to advertise to kids this way?

SCHOOL INVESTIGATIONS

A survey of soda drinking in Seattle, Washington, in 2012—before the new USDA nutrition standards went into effect—revealed that two-thirds of middle and high school students drank sodas, sports drinks, or flavored sweetened drinks while at school. Nearly a third of high school students drank soda in school every day, and about 10 percent drank two or more sodas.[7] Ask kids to:

- Count the number of vending machines in their schools.
- List all drinks sold. How much sugar do they contain?
- Determine if full-sugar sodas are available. [*If they are, the school is not following USDA standards.*]
- See if sodas are advertised in newspapers, on television, on posters, on vending machines, on drink cups, or anywhere else in the school.
- Compare soda ads to those for healthier items.
- Compare prices of sodas to those for healthier drinks.
- Think about why sodas are sold in schools. Why do schools allow this?
- Explore the difference between education (what schools are supposed to do) and advertising. How can you tell the difference?

Now take a look at the availability of full-sugar sodas within the area immediately surrounding the school. Map out a few blocks within easy walking distance. Note:

- The number of places that sell sodas
- The variety of sodas they sell
- The location and number of signs advertising sodas
- Whether healthier foods are equally available
- If healthier drinks are available, compare their prices relative to those of sodas

Ask: why are sodas so readily available near schools?

TAKE ACTION

If kids are interested in working to create a healthier food environment, you can suggest some actions they can take:

- Make your home a soda-free environment.
- Organize friends to petition your school to remove soda vending machines.
- Your school is supposed to supply clean drinking water at no cost. If it doesn't, petition to make sure it does. File a complaint with the school board or USDA.
- Petition your school to regularly maintain and clean all water fountains. You can take photographs of broken fountains and present them to the school board, for example.
- Demand healthy meals at school and at home.
- Organize your friends to ask the city council to ensure healthy food options in your neighborhood.
- Start a community garden.
- Boycott companies that market unhealthy foods to kids.
- Use social media to organize support for these actions.
- Write letters, op-eds, and position papers, and create videos and podcasts to promote your actions.
- Have fun working to make the world a healthier place for everyone.

USE THE RESOURCES

The American Heart Association has issued a toolkit for parents, the Rudd Center offers Advocacy 101 for parents, and the University of California. San Francisco, offers a toolkit through its Youth Speaks program. Kids have developed their own "Soda Sucks" campaign.[8] Other useful materials are produced by the organizations listed in Appendix 1.

Targeting Minorities
and the Poor

14

Marketing to African and Hispanic Americans

A Complicated Story

In 2013, the Hispanic Institute of Washington, D.C., issued a report about how sugary drinks affect the health of its community. The institute urged its Hispanic constituents to stop collaborating with soda companies. Its report, *Obesity: Hispanic America's Big Challenge*, called the community to action: "The negative effects of sugary drinks, other bad food choices and lack of regular exercise on the health of the fastest growing group in America will continue until Hispanics use their considerable political clout to influence public policymaking and their economic strength to influence purveyors of those products."[1]

In an interview, the institute's president, Gus West, said. "Of course, we're responsible for what we eat and drink . . . but we're also subject to the effects of massive advertising and misleading promotional campaigns—especially on our children and the poor." Community organizations, he said, need "to walk away from funding by the processed food and big sugary drink companies." Hispanic organizations "broke with tobacco companies" in the 1990s and now need to do the same with soda companies.[2]

Obesity, as the institute's report pointed out, changes the game. It forces Hispanic and African Americans to reexamine their relationships with soda companies. In the pre-obesity era, some members of these communities viewed targeted marketing as a testament to their rising economic and social status within American society. While these members of minority groups prized—and continue to prize—the efforts of soda companies to advertise in their publications and support their organizations, the rising prevalence of obesity in their communities led others to view such relationships as exploitative. To some community leaders, soda companies echo the actions of tobacco companies in the ways they market to groups most vulnerable to the harm caused by their products.

In this chapter, I examine the exceptionally complicated relationship of soda companies to racial and ethnic minorities in the United States. Soda company alliances are complicated not only historically but also because the African American and Hispanic communities are not monolithic; they are highly diverse in ancestry, appearance, culture, economic status, political views, and even what they expect to be called. In this book, I use the term *Hispanic* to describe the multiplicity of American groups who trace their ancestry to Spanish-speaking Latin America or Spain. I use it interchangeably with its synonym, *Latino*, the term preferred in Texas and other parts of the Southwest.[3] Similarly, I use the term *African American* (in preference to the more familiar but perhaps less respectful synonym, *black*) to refer to U.S. residents—also highly diverse—whose ancestry can be traced back to countries of sub-Saharan Africa.

Within minority communities, relationships with soda companies lead to diverse outcomes and produce winners and losers. The members of these communities most likely to benefit from soda industry marketing and philanthropy are usually those least likely to bear the burdens of soda-related health problems. This diversity—in income, social status, and outlook—complicates efforts to reduce soda intake in minority communities. The unequal distribution of costs and benefits within African American and Hispanic groups in part explains why some well-established and prominent minority organizations support the soda industry in its opposition to public health measures such as soda taxes or size caps. In this context, the Hispanic Institute's call to action broke new ground.

THE HEALTH ISSUES

African and Hispanic Americans drink more sodas and—no surprise—display a higher prevalence of obesity and type 2 diabetes than their white counterparts. As shown in Table 14.1, although 55 percent of whites say they routinely drink regular (sugar-sweetened) sodas, nearly 70 percent of African and Hispanic Americans report doing so, and these groups generally drink less diet soda. When asked, they say that their soda-drinking habits are strongly influenced by television advertising, especially when commercials feature celebrities of their own race or ethnicity.[4]

TABLE 14.1 Self-reports of soda drinking habits, adults, 2011

GROUP	DRINK DIET COLA, PERCENT	DRINK REGULAR (SUGAR-SWEETENED) COLA, PERCENT	NUMBER OF REGULAR COLAS CONSUMED PER WEEK
All	36	58	5
White	39	55	5
Hispanic	25	68	6
African American	22	69	7

SOURCE: Adapted from Mintel, "Carbonated Soft Drinks—US—February 2012."

TABLE 14.2 Prevalence of obesity and combined overweight and obesity in U.S. adults, 2009–2010*

GROUP	OBESE, PERCENT	OVERWEIGHT AND OBESE, PERCENT
All adults	36	69
White	34	68
African American	50	77
Hispanic American	39	77
Mexican American	40	80

* Percentages are rounded off. Overweight: BMI of 25–29.9. Obesity: BMI of 30 or more. BMI is weight in kilograms divided by the square of height in meters.

SOURCE: KM Flegal et al., "Prevalence of obesity and trends in the distribution of body mass index among US adults, 1999–2010," *JAMA* 2012;307(5):491–97.

Similar results might be expected for minority children, who consume more calories from sodas than white children and are often heavier, but few studies have examined soda consumption in children by race or ethnicity. One study found minority children to consume more sodas at home, but this pattern did not correlate with obesity. Among adults, links between sodas and obesity are easier to demonstrate. African and Hispanic Americans (particularly Mexican Americans) display a higher prevalence of overweight and obesity than their white counterparts. As shown in Table 14.2, the prevalence of obesity is highest in African American adults, but the combined prevalence of overweight and obesity is highest in Mexican Americans.[5]

Obesity is a principal risk factor for type 2 diabetes, and you might guess that its prevalence is higher among African Americans and Hispanics than in whites. You would be right. Its prevalence is nearly twice as high, as shown in Table 14.3. The table provides percentages for cases of diabetes that have been diagnosed by a doctor. Type 2 diabetes does not always come with symptoms that send people to doctors, and many people do not know they have the

TABLE 14.3 Diagnosed and undiagnosed diabetes among American adults, 2010

GROUP	DIAGNOSED, PERCENT	DIAGNOSED PLUS UNDIAGNOSED, PERCENT
All	8	11
White	7	11
African American	13	19
Hispanic American	12	Insufficient data to estimate

SOURCE: National Diabetes Clearinghouse, 2011.

condition. The figures in the second column represent an estimate of the percentage of the population with undiagnosed as well as diagnosed diabetes.[6]

TARGETED SODA MARKETING: THE PRE-OBESITY ERA

To discuss soda companies' relationships with minority communities, it is convenient to divide the history into two distinct eras: before and after the recognition of obesity as an especially acute problem for these groups. In the pre-obesity era, some members of minority groups considered access to soft drinks—and to soda companies' offers of employment, partnerships, endorsements, marketing, and philanthropic grants—to be prized symbols of acceptance by an otherwise discriminatory and exclusionist mainstream society. To the extent that members of minority groups perceive soda companies as supporters of their communities, such favorable views persist. Recent public health efforts to reduce soda consumption have forced a re-examination of these relationships, especially when prominent minority organizations strongly support soda companies' fights against public health measures (Chapters 25 to 27).

From the time sodas were invented in the late 1800s until the middle of the twentieth century, the American population was racially segregated in the North as well as the South. Soda fountains also were segregated. Once sodas were sold in bottles, however, anyone could buy them. During the Great Depression of the 1930s, Pepsi began selling its 12-ounce soda for the same nickel as a 6.5-ounce Coke, a strategy designed to appeal to the poor. When Walter Mack took over Pepsi in 1938, he deliberately set out to make Pepsi more widely available to the "Negro market." Pepsi recruited African American interns during World War II and, most remarkably, opened integrated canteens for those serving overseas, this at a time when U.S. military services were firmly segregated. After the war, Pepsi hired an Urban League staff member, allowed him to recruit a small staff of African American marketers to promote the drink at churches, schools, and sports events, and to place ads in African American publications featuring African American celebrities. In some circles, Pepsi became known as the drink for African Americans, whereas Coca-Cola remained the elite drink for whites.[7]

Although based in the South—and perhaps *because* it was based in the overtly segregated South—Coca-Cola did nothing special to appeal to African Americans until after World War II. Coke placed its first ad in African American newspapers in 1951 and soon began supporting community organizations such as the National Association for the Advancement of Colored People (NAACP). In Coca-Cola's version of this history, the company never discriminated against African Americans: "From the turn of the century to the mid-1950s the promise of a 'nickel Coke' made the product widely available to Americans of all means, with no barriers of race or class. . . . As early as 1914, there is documentation showing that Coca-Cola was being served in African American–owned soda fountains." Perhaps, but those fountains were segregated. Segregation, explains the company historian, "was not a policy of The Coca-Cola Company but of segregation laws in the U.S., which were generally enforced in the South."[8] Figure 14.1 provides a contemporary commentary on this history.

Looking back on this history, ironies abound. In 1949, despite threats from the Ku Klux Klan to disrupt the game, Brooklyn Dodgers team members Jackie Robinson and Roy Campanella broke Atlanta's baseball color bar in an exhibition game with the Atlanta Crackers—a team owned by the president of Coca-Cola.[9] During the late 1940s and early 1950s, members of the African American professional community began to advocate for more access to sodas, more advertising in African American publications, and more inclusion in the soda corporate world. They organized boycotts to induce Coca-Cola to begin hiring African American salesmen. When the Supreme Court desegregated schools in 1954, southern Coke bottlers who were serving on White Citizens Councils vowed to close the schools rather than integrate them. This created a dilemma: if Coca-Cola forged relationships with African Americans—who made up 30 percent of the southern market for its products—it might alienate its white customers.

Moss Kendrix, an African American public relations specialist, offered the company a way out of the dilemma: advertise directly to the African American community:

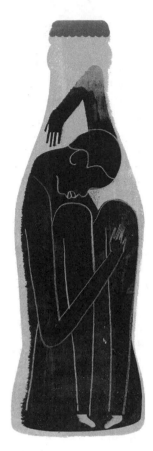

FIGURE 14.1 The artist Keith Negley takes a contemporary look at soda companies' relationships with minority communities. The drawing appeared as an illustration to a *New York Times* op-ed, "When Jim Crow Drank Coca-Cola," January 29, 2013. Used with permission of Keith Negley.

> Profits to the Coca-Cola Company and its bottlers would be immeasurable. . . . In addition to capitalizing on the current Negro market, the project would embrace a type of public relations involving youth which should tend to cultivate future markets. The Coca-Cola Company, in displaying interest in the children of the present Negro market, should note a type of appreciation on the part of Negro parents that would definitely pay dividends in increased sales of "Coke."[10]

Coca-Cola hired Kendrix as a roving ambassador. He induced the company to place separate-but-equal ads featuring prominent African American athletes. It did so, but only in African American publications.[11]

This project paved the way for soda companies' responses to the civil rights movement. With respect to sodas, this movement was about making the products accessible to African American customers, opening up jobs in the companies, and getting the companies to advertise and do business with firms owned by African Americans. It was not an accident that the civil rights movement began in earnest in 1960 when four African American college students sat down at a Woolworth soda fountain in Greensboro, North Carolina. The refusal to serve them Cokes was a powerful symbol of injustice— the denial of their ability to fully access the American way of life.[12] Atlanta, Coca-Cola's hometown, desegregated lunch counters the following year.

When Dr. Martin Luther King Jr. received the Nobel Peace Prize in 1964, Coca-Cola's president, Paul Austin, led the way in convincing other white businessmen to support a local celebration dinner in his honor. Reportedly, Austin said, "It is embarrassing for Coca-Cola to be located in a city that refuses to honor its Nobel Prize winner. We are an international business. The Coca-Cola Company does not need Atlanta. You all need to decide whether Atlanta needs the Coca-Cola Company."[13]

But when Coca-Cola did not respond to employment demands, King urged his followers to use their political power to boycott the company's products. In Memphis, Tennessee, the night before he was assassinated, King said:

> Now the other thing we'll have to do is this: Always anchor our external direct action with the power of economic withdrawal. . . . We just need to go around to these stores, and to these massive industries in our country, and say, "God sent us by here, to say to you that you're not treating his children right. And we've come by here to ask you to make the first item on your agenda fair treatment, where God's children are concerned. Now, if you are not prepared to do that, we do have an agenda that we must follow. And our agenda calls for withdrawing economic support from you." And so, as a result of this, we are asking you tonight, to go out and tell your neighbors not to buy Coca-Cola in Memphis . . . [N]ow we must kind of redistribute the pain. We are choosing these companies because they haven't been fair in their hiring policies.[14]

Coke's response was to increase philanthropic contributions to the African American community, a strategy designed to deflect criticism and elicit loyalty. The company made donations to historically black colleges, the

NAACP, and other civil rights groups. It began hiring African Americans into the lower ranks of its workers. By the early 1980s, African American employees constituted 24 percent of Coke's workforce—but included only one executive, Carl Ware, a vice president of "special markets." Coke's discriminatory hiring policies became the target of the Rev. Jesse Jackson's Operation PUSH (People United to Save Humanity) campaign. PUSH aimed to renegotiate the relationship of corporate America to the African American community. It called for a month-long "don't choke on Coke" boycott, politely framed as a "withdrawal of enthusiasm." The Coke CEO refused to meet with Jackson, instead sending Ware to do the negotiating. But the company eventually agreed to the PUSH campaign's terms. It appointed twenty African American wholesalers, made loans to African American entrepreneurs in the beverage industry, agreed to increase its advertising in African American publications, and committed to doing business with banks owned by African Americans.[15]

The company also began working on its relationship to the rapidly expanding Hispanic community. It hired Ogilvy and Mather, an advertising and public relations firm, to conduct a survey of Hispanic attitudes and concerns. In 1984, Coke used the survey results as a basis for creating a formal business agenda for the Hispanic community. Backed by a $10 million investment, the company hired Hispanic advertising firms, Hispanic executives, Hispanic sales and marketing representatives; established partnerships with Hispanic banks and vendors; and set up an education fund for Hispanic students in key cities.[16]

By the early 1990s, Pepsi and Coke were fighting for market share among minority groups. The head of Coca-Cola said "Our strategy is very simple, and it's to lead in the ethnic activities of America, to increase our coverage in ethnic stores—for example, in the inner city—and to leverage the brand strength that we already have with Hispanics and with African-Americans." Some minority groups welcomed the attention. An NAACP director said, "We favor companies diversifying their strategies and including a more balanced picture of [what] their consumer market is, rather than just picturing white families." The contradictions inherent in such marketing were already well understood by advertising executives: "If you don't market to minority groups, you can be accused of not caring about them. . . . If you do market to them, you can be accused of exploiting them."[17]

But well into the 1990s, Coca-Cola was still dealing with serious racial problems within the company. A report in 1995 observed that "Coke got whiter and chillier as one went up the ranks," and described the company as a "professional wasteland" for African American employees—institutionally racist from the top down. Stories of personal and financial discrimination—more than a 40 percent difference in salaries between white and black employees, for example—established the basis for a class-action lawsuit. The Labor Department investigated and found numerous violations of federal anti-discrimination laws; it asked the company to fix the problems. In 1999, current and former Coke employees organized the Committee for Corporate Justice, a group aimed at improving job inequities among minority employees. Its class-action suit against Coca-Cola involved twenty-two hundred current and former employees, who demanded compensation for systematic discrimination involving every aspect of their jobs: evaluations, promotions, terminations, and pay.[18] Figure 14.2 outlines the events related to this lawsuit.

Coca-Cola offered to increase its support for minority-owned suppliers, banks, and retailers, but employees continued the boycott. They stated,

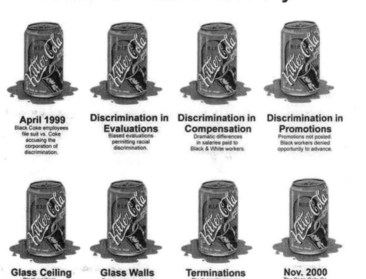

Coke's Black History

April 1999
Black Coke employees file suit vs. Coke accusing the corporation of discrimination.

Discrimination in Evaluations
Biased evaluations permitting racial discrimination.

Discrimination in Compensation
Dramatic differences in salaries paid to Black & White workers.

Discrimination in Promotions
Promotions not posted. Black workers denied opportunity to advance.

Glass Ceiling
Black workers blocked from equal opportunity to advance to top level positions.

Glass Walls
Company segregated into divisions where Black workers are leaders in less powerful areas.

Terminations
Black employees are terminated at higher rates than White employees.

Nov. 2000
The Coca-Cola Co. pays $192.5 million to settle a racial discrimination suit.

FIGURE 14.2 The reasons for African American employees' class-action discrimination lawsuit against Coca-Cola in 1999 and its resolution in 2000. From Stop Coke Discrimination, February 1, 2007. Courtesy of Ray Rogers.

with eloquence, that they were "disappointed, disturbed, and disgusted with a company that would disadvantage, disrespect, and disenfranchise some of its most loyal employees." They organized a "ride for corporate justice" from Atlanta to Washington, D.C., and camped out at a Coke shareholders meeting in Delaware.[19]

In 2000, mediation settled the class action suit for $192.5 million. The settlement required Coca-Cola to appoint a task force to oversee improvements in company policies toward minorities and women. Although employees continued to complain of discriminatory practices, the task force recognized "the significant progress The Coca-Cola Company has made in restructuring its personnel practices in the past five years." But the task force must have suspected that Coke's corporate culture had not really changed. In its final report, the group called on Coke's CEO, then Neville Isdell, to embed and sustain the fairness and diversity policies. Did the company succeed in doing so? In 2012, sixteen African American and Hispanic production workers in Coke bottling plants in New York City sued the company for forcing them to work in "a cesspool of racial discrimination." The workers complained of constant racial epithets, unfair assignments and disciplinary action, and retaliation when they objected.[20]

Pepsi, a company based in the North, has a somewhat better employment history, but not by much. In 2012, the Minneapolis office of the Equal Employment Opportunity Commission fined PepsiCo more than $3 million to resolve findings of nationwide hiring discrimination against black employees. In yet another irony, *Latino* magazine in 2013 named Coca-Cola and PepsiCo as among the top one hundred companies providing the most opportunities for this community.[21]

TARGETED SODA MARKETING: THE POST-OBESITY ERA

We have seen that marketing sodas to African and Hispanic Americans has long been a sales strategy, often demanded by members of the groups who stood to benefit from such relationships. But with the realization that levels of soda consumption, obesity, and diabetes are higher in minority groups than in the general population, targeted marketing practices have demanded reconsideration. Such practices and philanthropy can now appear manipulative rather than beneficial, especially when directed at children.

PepsiCo, for example, is one of the fifty leading advertisers in Hispanic media, spending $33.6 million on that market alone in 2013. Soda companies

TABLE 14.4 Soda company marketing initiatives aimed at minority groups, selected examples, 2013–2015

SODA COMPANY	MARKETING INITIATIVE
Coca-Cola	Sponsors Mexican soccer team at the Latino World Cup
	Sponsors Essence Festival
	Partners with the United Negro College Fund in Pay it Forward program, which offers apprenticeship experiences to youth
	Celebrates Hispanic Heritage Month through scholarships for Hispanic high school students
	Sponsors Ohio Hispanic Economic Development Summit
	Recruits artist to create portfolio of posters for black history month
	Issues special bottle commemorating the 50th anniversary of the civil rights movement.
PepsiCo	Sponsors Student Business Case Competition finale event for the National Society of Hispanic MBAs
	Sponsors 20th annual Black Enterprise/Pepsi Golf & Tennis Challenge
	Develops campaign, Familias de Campeones, to build relationships with Latino football fans
	Gives $1 million grant to Los Angeles Plaza de la Cultura y Artes to develop an edible teaching garden and culinary arts program
	Introduces "Pepsi Limon" in 2015

target Hispanic children through advertisements on Spanish-language television that feature soccer and Spanish-speaking celebrities. Hispanic children also see soda advertisements on English-language television, but more soda advertising is aimed at them than at non-Hispanic children. The same is true of advertising aimed at African American children. As a result, African American children visit soda websites more than do white children and see more soda commercials on television and elsewhere.[22] As for minority adults, soda companies reach them through advertisements and sponsored events featuring athletes and celebrities, and through music concerts, cultural festivals, dance competitions, and business and professional conferences. Table 14.4 gives a few examples of such marketing activities in 2013.

Soda companies also produce posters and publications aimed at promoting cultural values, as shown in Figure 14.3. Because these activities are typically sponsored by foundations established by Coca-Cola or PepsiCo, they appear as philanthropy, not marketing. But even these few examples reveal that the line between philanthropy and marketing is blurred. Both aim to promote brand loyalty and increase soda sales.[23] As discussed in Chapter 5, the connections between soda marketing, soda sales, soda consumption, increased calorie intake, and obesity are well established.

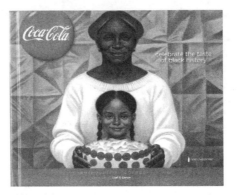

FIGURE 14.3 Coca-Cola's commemorative "black history" cookbook, 2011. The company produced the book to "celebrate the taste of black history…More than just a tribute to black history, this volume is a celebration of black present and our way of saying thank you for allowing Coca-Cola to be a part of your life."

Soda companies explicitly use philanthropy to forge relationships with African and Hispanic American community groups. As part of the settlement of the class-action lawsuit in 2000, Coca-Cola committed $50 million to support minority organizations and causes. Today it is difficult to imagine an African or Hispanic American organization or event that is *not* sponsored by Coke, Pepsi, or the American Beverage Association. In Table 14.5, I list a few selected examples of the great many such groups supported just by Coca-Cola.[24]

Let me give two examples of how such sponsorship works. In 2012, Pepsi gave $100,000 to the National Association of Hispanic Journalists, half for scholarships for journalism students. Pepsi announced the gift as part of La Promesa, a corporate social responsibility campaign focusing on "Latino empowerment and the issues that matter most to Hispanics." My second example: In 2013, the United Negro College Fund gave its president's award to Ingrid Saunders Jones, the African American Coca-Cola executive responsible for much corporate giving to minority groups. When she retired as chair of the National Council of Negro Women, the Coca-Cola Foundation surprised her with a $1 million gift to this group.[25] Under such circumstances, recipient journalists and community groups can hardly be expected to write stories or make statements criticizing soda companies for producing drinks that contribute to poor health in their communities.

Obesity, however, makes such sponsorship appear less favorable. In 2013, for example, Yale alumni protested PepsiCo's sponsorship of a speech

TABLE 14.5 Selected examples of minority community groups receiving philanthropic support from the Coca-Cola Foundation, 2011

100 Black Men of Atlanta
Abyssinian Development Corporation
Cesar Chavez Foundation
Chicago Urban League
Congressional Hispanic Caucus Institute
Hispanic Foundation of Silicon Valley
Hispanic Heritage Foundation
National Council of La Raza
National Alliance for Hispanic Health
National Association for the Advancement of Colored People (NAACP)
National Association of Hispanic Journalists
National Association of Hispanic Nurses
National Black Caucus of State Legislators
National Black Nurses Association
National Coalition of 100 Black Women
National Council of Negro Women
National Minority Supplier Development Council
National Puerto Rican Coalition

to be given by the first Supreme Court justice of Hispanic origin, Sonia Sotomayor. This protest prompted a reporter to comment that "a long-running dispute between Yale University and some of its alumni over the university's connections to PepsiCo...has—in a way—reached the Supreme Court."[26]

Another example involves the celebrated African American singer Beyoncé Knowles. As the most famous supporter of First Lady Michelle Obama's Let's Move! initiative, she has come under fire for her appearances in Pepsi commercials. In 2012, she accepted a $50 million, multiyear deal with Pepsi that put her face on soda cans (see Figure 14.4). Her explanation: "Pepsi embraces creativity and understands that artists evolve.... As a businesswoman, this allows me to work with a lifestyle brand with no compromise and without sacrificing my creativity." Although the Pepsi deal put her in conflict with the goals of Let's Move! and prompted calls for her to be "disinvited" from singing the national anthem at President Obama's inauguration, the White House continued to work with her.[27]

As soda companies compete more intensely for the minority market, they sometimes end up taking risks that get them in trouble. Pepsi, for example, recruited two rap musicians, Tyler the Creator and Lil Wayne, to make edgy Mountain Dew commercials that would "go viral." Objections that the commercials used vulgar, sexist, and racist language and images

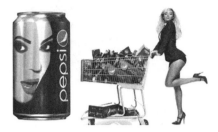

FIGURE 14.4 Pepsi ads featured Beyoncé in 2012. The singer had just accepted a $50 million deal to promote Pepsi, despite her role as a spokesperson for the White House Let's Move! campaign to reduce childhood obesity. This photograph appeared as an illustration in PepsiCo's Annual Report in 2012.

forced the company to withdraw them. Coca-Cola's 2013 Super Bowl ad, which depicted an Arab walking in the desert with a camel, provoked criticism that it perpetuated racist stereotypes.[28]

Despite these problems, the advertising industry rationalizes marketing aimed at African and Hispanic Americans as a sensible and meritorious business strategy. David Morse, the author of a book about how to market to race, ethnicity, and sexual orientation, argues that this kind of market segmentation builds brand loyalty:

> But let's face it. Hispanics and African Americans are much less interested in diet products. Sugary drinks—often the sweeter the better—do well with them.... And in my experience, the big soft-drink companies...have strong multicultural marketing efforts. And they are reaping the benefits...As a multicultural marketer, I applaud the leadership of the soft-drink industry in recognizing the changing face of America. Many of their African-American and Hispanic customers do too.[29]

Advertising Age seconds this view and urges marketers to sponsor emerging Hispanic musicians who can easily relate to speakers of both Spanish and English and connect with a broader range of Latino customers.[30]

The condescension and cynicism involved in targeting minority groups at high risk of obesity and its consequences does make some marketers uncomfortable. In his 2012 interview about the karmic debt owed for selling Coca-Cola, former marketing executive Todd Putman explained: "It was just a fact that Hispanics and African Americans have a higher per capita consumption of sugar-based soft drinks than white Americans. We knew that if we got more products into those environments those segments would drink more."[31]

A DILEMMA FOR ADVOCATES

Decades of soda company philanthropy have convinced many—but by no means all—African and Hispanic American groups that soda companies have their interests at heart, that philanthropic gifts are welcome contributions, and that efforts to tax sodas or cap soda sizes are modern-day manifestations of elitist white supremacy. These opinions leave advocates for minority health, who may view marketing targeted to minority groups as inherently racist and exploitative, with few options.[32] Their efforts to reduce soda intake and its health consequences in African and Hispanic American communities must begin by recognizing and building on the long history of minority-group efforts to desegregate and gain access to soda advertising, employment, and philanthropic partnerships.

If the disproportionate share of health burdens borne by minority groups is to be reduced, these groups must now fight equally hard—and more creatively—to help members of their communities recognize the connection between consumption of heavily marketed junk foods and sodas and the disproportionate health burdens they bear. Advocates must find ways to empower their communities to understand how soda company philanthropy and marketing are inextricably linked to business objectives. One way to reveal the primacy of business motives might be to suggest to soda companies that their grants to minority groups come with no strings attached: no press releases, no logos, and no in-kind contributions. Groups negotiating for soda industry funding might ask that all donations be anonymous, and take note of the response.

15

Selling to the Developing World

In 1975, shortly after President Richard Nixon's historic visit to China, a Pepsi vice president noted its significance for his company: "There are eight hundred million gullets in China and I want to see a Pepsi in every one of them." Sixteen years later, Roberto Goizueta, then chief executive of Coca-Cola, said much the same: "Willie Sutton used to say he robbed banks because that is where the money is. Well, we are increasingly global because 95 percent of the world's consumers are outside this country. It's that simple." By the early 1990s, Coke's international sales already accounted for 80 percent of its profits. Coke's president at the time, Donald Keough, told a reporter: "Our single and relentless focus has been internationalizing this business....To do so, we have become the most pragmatic company in the world....When I think of Indonesia—a country on the Equator with 180 million people, a median age of 18, and a Moslem ban on alcohol—I feel I know what heaven looks like."[1]

From the outset, Coke had its eye on foreign markets. The company made its first foreign sale in 1899 to a merchant in Cuba. Within the next decade, Coke sold syrup to countries such as Mexico, Puerto Rico, and the Philippines, and established its first international bottling plant, also in Cuba, in 1906. For the next twenty years it expanded its foreign franchises, and by 1930 it was supplying concentrate to bottlers in seventy-six countries. Even so, its foreign presence was quite limited by today's standards. World War II ended the limits. The company pledged to provide a Coke for 5 cents to every American in the armed forces anywhere in the world, a feat it accomplished with the full cooperation—and donated transportation—of the military. By the end of the war, it was supplying 155 international bottling plants, as compared to just one for Pepsi, and its global investments

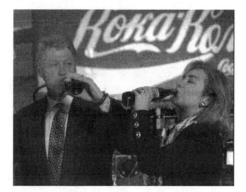

FIGURE 15.1 President Bill Clinton and his wife, Hillary, share a Coke in Moscow, 1995. On May 11, 1995, after a summit meeting with Russian president Boris Yeltsin, the President and First Lady took a break on the way to the airport to visit a new Coca-Cola bottling plant. Pepsi, which also had bottling plants in Russia, was not pleased. AP photo/Greg Gibson Photography. Used with permission.

continued to grow rapidly. The fall of the Iron Curtain in 1989 opened up further business opportunities. By 1995, Coca-Cola had invested $1.5 billion in Eastern Europe. Its $65 million bottling plant near Moscow achieved particular notoriety when President Bill Clinton and his wife, Hillary, stopped by for a visit and were photographed drinking Russian Cokes (Figure 15.1).[2]

Today, international sales continue to account for a large percentage of soda company profits and virtually all growth potential. As the president of Coca-Cola international stated in 2014, the half of the world's population who had not consumed a Coke in the last thirty days created a business opportunity worth $300 billion. Table 15.1 lists the leading worldwide markets for soft drink sales. The United States still generates the highest sales, although it and most of the other countries on this list are in mature stages of development where soda consumption is slow or stagnant. The figures in this table explain why the world's emerging economies of developing world are such attractive sales targets.[3]

Beyond the top ten, Coca-Cola sells products in what it claims is two hundred countries and continues to derive more than 80 percent of its sales from countries outside the United States, particularly China, Japan, and those in Latin America. In 2013, when the United States lifted decades-old trade sanctions against the military junta in Myanmar, only two countries remained under U.S. trade embargoes: North Korea since 1950, and Cuba, the site of Coke's first international sales since 1962. As one Coke executive put it, "The moment Coca-Cola starts shipping [to Cuba] is the moment you can say there might be real change going on.... Coca-Cola is the nearest thing to

TABLE 15.1 The leading world markets for soft drinks (all kinds), 2013

COUNTRY	SALES, $ BILLION
United States	176
Japan	86
China	67
Brazil	43
Germany	37
Mexico	37
United Kingdom	21
Italy	20
Spain	19
France	19

SOURCE: Adapted from Euromonitor International, 2013.

capitalism in a bottle."[4] President Obama's relaxation of Cuban trade restrictions in 2014 and terrorist nation status in 2015 seemed likely to leave North Korea as the last remaining country where Coca-Cola cannot be sold.

PepsiCo also says it sells products in more than two hundred countries, but its international sales account for only 35 percent of profits. It too invests in emerging and developing markets. It is the leading food and beverage business in Russia, India, and the Middle East, the second-leading business in Mexico, and among the top five in Brazil and Turkey.[5]

Investment analysts view the soda industry as straddling two worlds: the stagnating markets of North America and Europe and the rapidly emerging economies of Latin America and Asia. The biggest drivers of sales growth are countries with large populations in middle stages of development—Brazil, Russia, India, and China, four countries so critical that they are known collectively as BRIC or, with South Africa, BRICS. Soda companies view the Middle East and Africa, where per capita consumption is still very low, as the "new regional hot spots."[6]

Because of their enormous populations, China and India are obvious targets for soda marketing. In 2014, strong sales growth in China—especially from small, inexpensive bottles—helped Coca-Cola exceed its quarterly revenue estimates. The company announced plans to invest more than $4 billion in China from 2015 to 2017. In India, it had opened fifty-eight bottling plants by the end of 2013. It invested in research on how to reach consumers in Africa, and committed to spend $12 billion on marketing to that continent by 2020. PepsiCo also has promised to invest $5.5 billion in India and $5 billion in Mexico by 2020.[7]

TABLE 15.2 Top-ten emerging markets for foods and beverages, carbonated soda availability, and prevalence of obesity

RANK[a]	COUNTRY[a]	ESTIMATED SALES GROWTH, PERCENT, 2012–2017[a]	SODA PRODUCTION, 12-OUNCE SERVINGS, PER CAPITA, 2012[b]	OBESITY, PERCENT, 2008[c]
1	China	8	25	6
2	India	5	8	2
3	Russia	4	86	27
4	Brazil	2	240	19
5	Indonesia	4	10	5
6	South Korea	4	76	8
7	Malaysia	3	50	14
8	Mexico	2	413	32
9	South Africa	3	188	31
10	Turkey	2	133	28

SOURCES: [a] Food and Drink Europe, May 28, 2013.
[b] Euromonitor International, Total Volume Carbonates (includes diet and regular carbonated sodas).
[c] Central Intelligence Agency. The World Factbook, 2008: Obesity.

Concerns about obesity and its consequences do not enter into such investment decisions except to the extent that health campaigns might reduce growth in sales. The Indian public health community has already issued warnings about the potential effect of increased soda consumption on obesity. It and other Asian populations with low soda consumption still display relatively little obesity. But even small increases in body weight are associated with type 2 diabetes among Asians, and the prevalence of the disease is rising rapidly in those countries. Table 15.2 mixes data from different sources in different years to get an overview of how per capita soda production relates to the prevalence of obesity in the top-ten emerging international markets. The table shows that the more soda produced and available in a country, the higher its prevalence of obesity. Given its high soda consumption, Brazil would be expected to have a higher prevalence of obesity than it now displays. By all reports, it soon will.[8] At the very least, soda consumption reflects an overall dietary pattern that predisposes to weight gain.

International Marketing Methods

Although individuals in emerging and developing countries may have little money to spend, marketing to them makes good business sense. Small

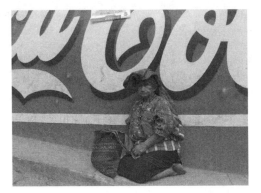

FIGURE 15.2 Street scene with Coca-Cola, Todos Santos, Guatemala, 2005. Courtesy of Emily Yates-Doerr.

increases in soda purchases among enormous numbers of people quickly add up. Soda advertising is so ubiquitous in developing countries that it has become a largely unremarkable part of the landscape, as shown in Figure 15.2.

But street signs are only the most visible indication of soda marketing to the developing world. Coke and Pepsi study how to reach people of different cultures and create effective business partnerships in each country. Coca-Cola, for example, was an early user of cell phone technology to advertise to young, tech-savvy customers in Japan.[9] It supports local concerts and sports teams, as well as international sporting events such as the Tour de France, World Cup soccer, and the Olympics. It also supports student scholarships, health programs, and women's empowerment initiatives, offers emergency relief in natural disasters, and encourages environmental causes. As I explain further in Chapter 17, such efforts encourage brand loyalty and promote sales.

Coca-Cola is particularly adept at using philanthropy to win friends and deflect critics. To cite just one example: in 2012, a Reuters investigative team looked into the partnership practices of Latin American health groups such as the Pan American Health Organization (PAHO), a subsidiary of the World Health Organization (WHO). PAHO had accepted a $50,000 gift from Coca-Cola. A Coke official sits on the steering committee of WHO's Pan American Forum for Action on Non-Communicable Diseases, a group that develops methods to counter obesity in Latin America ("non-communicable" is the international term for diseases that Americans call "chronic").[10] Given Coke's generosity, nobody should be surprised if these groups do not initiate or join campaigns to drink less soda.

PepsiCo employs a similar strategy. In 2013, it announced a partnership with the Asian Football Development Project (AFDP), a group with goals that extend beyond the game itself. The AFDP uses grassroots soccer teams to promote the health, social development, and empowerment of women and girls in forty countries, with a focus on the Middle East and India. As a PepsiCo representative explained, "We believe that the strength of the PepsiCo brand is in a community relations context...realizing dreams and giving opportunities to those who are less fortunate and PepsiCo is proud to be part of that." Pepsi runs similar projects in Egypt and Nigeria.[11] As with all such projects, the recipients benefit, but so does PepsiCo. The partnership exposes participants who might otherwise not be reached to Pepsi logos, builds brand loyalty, creates goodwill, and deflects concerns about the health consequences of its products.

The efforts of soda companies to reach international markets leave nothing to chance. If an opening exists, they move right in. Both companies use innovative and country-specific methods to sell sodas in the emerging economies of Asia, the Indian subcontinent, the Middle East, and Africa. In Dubai, for example, Coca-Cola placed Hello Happiness telephone booths in areas frequented by South Asian guest laborers, who often work under highly restrictive conditions. The booths accepted Coca-Cola bottle caps instead of coins for a free 3-minute international phone call, and the company videotaped a commercial featuring the workers' enthusiastic appreciation of this opportunity. The booths were dismantled a month later. A representative of Human Rights Watch termed the commercial "odious," on the grounds that Coca-Cola used the low-income workers to advertise its product while requiring them to buy Cokes to use the special booth.[12]

Table 15.3 gives additional examples of marketing innovations in developing countries from 2012 to 2014. Some are easily recognized as marketing. Others are more subtle and appear as philanthropy or social responsibility.

Undoubtedly as a result of such efforts, Coca-Cola scores high in international surveys of corporate public approval. Among sixty international companies, it received the second-highest favorable ranking in the Philippines. It was ranked fourth in India and South Korea, fifth in Thailand, seventh in Myanmar, and eighth in China.[13] But even within countries that welcome them enthusiastically, soda companies attract critics who, for reasons of politics or public health, view their marketing in a far less rosy light.

TABLE 15.3 Soda marketing initiatives in developing countries, selected examples, 2012–2014

COUNTRY	SODA MARKETING INITIATIVES
Brazil	Coca-Cola Brazil and the Coca-Cola Foundation invest $2.1 million in programs to expand opportunities for African-Brazilians. Coca-Cola sponsors the FIFA World Cup games, as it has since 1978.
China	Pepsi CEO opens new bottling plant in Zhengzhou; opens new food and beverage center in Shanghai; donates $1 million earthquake aid to Sichuan.
India	Pepsi spends $72 million to sponsor cricket tournament. Coca-Cola recruits Bollywood stars to promote "Share Happiness" campaign in films, digital media, merchandise, and on-ground initiatives in 1,000 communities; launches online store for product delivery.
Indonesia	Coca-Cola says it will spend $700 million on marketing among other big plans.
Kenya	Coca-Cola partnership sells solar power to rural kiosks.
Laos	Coca-Cola announces joint venture to open bottling operation by 2014.
Mexico	Coca-Cola partners with Nestlé to provide advice about nutrition as part of an anti-hunger campaign.
Myanmar	Coca-Cola develops marketing campaign based on consumer research; distributes free samples; donates $3 million to support women's economic empowerment. Pepsi signs with UNESCO to develop vocational training initiatives.
Nigeria	Coca-Cola partners with Lagos State Ministry of Women Affairs and Poverty Alleviation to establish Retail Kiosks Program as platform for women's economic empowerment. Coca-Cola Nigeria partners with International Finance Corporation to provide $100 million in financing to women microdistributors.
Pakistan	Coca-Cola creates "Happiness Without Borders" campaign to share drinks with customers in India.
Philippines	More than 6,000 women attend Coke-sponsored International Women's Day celebration.
Singapore	Coca-Cola pilots "phenomenally successful" cans that split in two for sharing.
Vietnam	Pepsi forms bottling and marketing partnership; considers Vietnam "linchpin" of campaign to expand in emerging markets.

The Marketing Challenges: Political

Soda companies engage in a broad range of marketing strategies not only to promote sales but also to reduce the considerable risks of selling products in cultures and political systems decidedly different from those of the United States. Any company that does business overseas has to cope with trade restrictions, political instability, and fluctuations in the value of the dollar, as well as profound cultural misunderstandings. In 2013, for example, Coca-Cola conducted a marketing campaign in Israel involving placement of 150 popular first names on its cans. Although about 1.5 million Arabs live in Israel, no Arab names appeared on the cans. The campaign did nothing to ease tensions in that country.[14]

Both Coke and Pepsi must confront views of their core products as emblems of American cultural, economic, and political domination if not imperialism. Although a great many people in developing countries view Coke and Pepsi as symbols of freedom and the most enviable aspects of American society, others view the companies as aggressive invaders intent on exploiting the local population—"Coca-Colonization," as the French called it in 1950.[15]

Historians record numerous instances of soda company interference in the politics of the countries in which they do business—in the name of protecting that business. In the early 1970s, the chairman of PepsiCo asked President Nixon to help protect the company's interests in Chile, which had just elected a government expected to be unsympathetic to U.S. corporations. Intervention by the United States led to the eventual overthrow and assassination of Chile's president, Salvador Allende. Pepsi did a similar intervention in Guatemala's internal affairs. In that country, Coca-Cola has long been accused of complicity in the murder in 1978 of a union leader who worked for the company. Coke's labor problems in Guatemala continued well into the 1990s and elicited boycotts protesting the company's alleged violence against union organizers.[16]

Similar events in Colombia led to creation of the Killer Coke campaign to stop Coca-Cola's ongoing and allegedly violent interference with union organizing—actions documented extensively in books and films but firmly denied by the company (see Chapter 28). Figure 15.3 illustrates an expression of that campaign. Killer Coke is active on college campuses, where it organizes student groups to try to end Coca-Cola's pouring rights contracts as a means to force the company to improve its international labor practices.[17]

Other examples abound. In 2003, demonstrators in Thailand poured Coca-Cola onto the streets in protest against the American invasion of Iraq. More recently, the president of Iran threatened to ban Coca-Cola in retaliation for economic sanctions imposed against his country, and the late president of Venezuela, Hugo Chávez, called on supporters to boycott foreign imports such as Coke or Pepsi. In India, more than a thousand Muslim-owned hotels and restaurants in Mumbai refused to serve Pepsi and Coca-Cola in protest over the United States' support of Israel in its conflict with Hamas in the Gaza strip. And in 2014, in retaliation against Western sanctions imposed when Russia took the Crimea from the Ukraine, the Russian Communist Party said that "similar measures should be extended

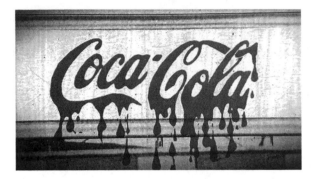

FIGURE 15.3 Graffito on a wall in Guatemala. This screenshot comes from a documentary film about Coca-Cola and labor rights in Latin America, *The Coca-Cola Case: The Truth That Refreshes*, by Carmen Garcia and Germán Gutiérrez, National Film Board of Canada, 2009.

to...the import, manufacture, and sale of carbonated beverages such as Coca-Cola, Fanta, Sprite, Pepsi-Cola, whose profits are sent to the corrupt West." In such situations, soda brands are perceived as symbols of U.S. aggression. Other international campaigns aim to change the practices of soda companies. A boycott campaign in Vietnam accused Coca-Cola of tax evasion and lack of social responsibility to its customers.[18] Coca-Cola's use of local water supplies has also evoked substantial international opposition, as I discuss in Chapter 22.

The Marketing Challenges: Obesity

Soda companies have every reason to be concerned about public health campaigns aimed at reducing consumption of their products. One U.S. campaign, conducted by a coalition of international nongovernmental organizations—the Sweet Enough Network—calls for bans on all sugary food products in schools, particularly soft drinks.[19] A broader effort comes from the Global Dump Soda campaign. This is a project of American and international consumer advocacy groups in countries such as India, Japan, Malaysia, and Mexico. The campaign's goals are to induce soda companies to:

- Stop marketing sodas to children under age 16
- Stop selling sodas in schools
- Only sponsor physical activity or health programs that do not feature corporate logos or brands
- Sell sodas in smaller portions[20]

The WHO supports such goals. In 2010, this agency called for reducing the marketing of high-sugar foods to children. Although its recommendations did not specify soft drinks, the report came with an accompanying resolution to reduce the marketing of nonalcoholic beverages (translation: sodas) to children. In 2012, the WHO identified key global strategies related to obesity prevention, among them community-based and policy actions to limit the marketing of unhealthy beverages to children. The most effective way to implement such recommendations, said the United Nations special rapporteur on the right to food, Olivier De Schutter, is to "impose taxes on soft drinks (sodas)."[21]

Perhaps in response to the WHO's leadership, more than thirty countries have instituted national or regional policies to restrict the availability of sodas in schools. In 2013, the WHO surveyed anti-obesity initiatives undertaken by its member nations. Most had instituted policies to reduce obesity and diet-related diseases, and about half reported restrictions on marketing sodas in schools. But only one-third regulated the marketing of sodas to children. Although American advocates might consider all of these policies to be major gains, the WHO report lamented that most countries considered obesity to be a problem demanding personal responsibility rather than government action. Thus, the most common policies were those aimed at

TABLE 15.4 Actions of developing countries to restrict soda marketing and reduce consumption, selected examples

COUNTRY	ACTION TO RESTRICT SODA SALES OR MARKETING
Brazil	Brazilian Front for the Regulation of Food Advertising supports resolution to eliminate promotional messages in any medium aimed at children and counter Coca-Cola's "Positive Energy" campaign. Dietary guidelines for the Brazilian population say to avoid "nutritionally unbalanced" soft drinks.
Chile	Policies recommend no more than 40 grams sugars per day. Companies cannot advertise junk foods or sodas to anyone under age 14. High-sugar products must be identified as such on food labels.
India	High Court rules that junk foods cannot be sold in schools; enacts 5 percent tax on sugary beverages.
Mexico	Researchers recommend against consuming sodas; 47 organizations demand taxes on soft drinks as part of a national "Crusade against Hunger;" taxes sodas and junk foods and does not permit them to be marketed to children (see Chapter 27).
Russia	Ministry of Health proposes restrictions on soda advertising, especially to children.

educating individuals through dietary guidelines, food labels, and media campaigns about healthy eating.[22]

Some countries, however, are taking more forceful steps to reduce soda marketing and consumption. Table 15.4 gives a few examples.

Such anti-soda policies are clearly having an effect. In India, for example, sales of Pepsi and Coke are not growing as fast as they used to, a situation attributed to increasing preferences for drinks that seem healthier—fruit drinks, nectars, juices, and energy drinks. This is one reason soda companies are committing billions to marketing in that country. In response to widespread condemnation of selling soft drinks in schools, soda companies have been forced to create "responsible marketing" campaigns. PepsiCo, for example, says it "commits not to engage in product advertising or marketing communications directed to students in primary schools," although with exceptions for fund-raisers and educational purposes, among others.[23]

It is difficult to know what such commitments mean in practice, especially in light of Pepsi's other marketing efforts. On this point, the Global Dump Soft Drinks campaign calls on soda companies to stop marketing to children in *any* form: print and broadcast advertising, product placement, Internet advertising, mobile phone messages, athletic event sponsorship, signage, packaging promotions, merchandising, and other means. Public health advocates have plenty of challenges to face in reducing soda intake in developing countries, but these precedents offer considerable cause for optimism.

16

Advocacy

Excluding Sodas from SNAP

The USDA's Supplemental Nutrition Assistance Program (SNAP, familiarly known by its former name, food stamps), might not seem an obvious target for health advocacy to reduce soda intake, but it has become one, and not for the first time.[1] Like any other welfare or food assistance program, food stamps elicit debate about a range of thorny issues: how to balance nutritional benefits against their costs, how to ensure against fraud, and—most important for our purposes—how to decide which foods and drinks are eligible for purchase by participants. Whether SNAP actually meets the food needs of recipients is a matter of much less urgency to Congress.

The origins of the current program date back to the Great Depression of the 1930s when masses of unemployed people, unable to afford the foods that farmers produced, formed "breadlines knee-deep in wheat." This is the phrase used to describe the ironic tragedy of that era: hungry people waited in long lines for food handouts while the crops and animals raised by farmers rotted or were destroyed for lack of money to buy them. To take care of both problems—protect the income of farmers and feed the poor—the government issued stamps that could be used like cash. Participants were permitted to use some of the stamps to buy any food *except* alcoholic beverages, drugs (and, therefore, dietary supplements), and items consumed on the premises. They could use others only for surplus commodities. This program lasted until the 1940s, when World War II greatly reduced both unemployment and farm surpluses.[2]

Following that war, changes in agriculture policy encouraged farmers to overproduce, and Congress began to consider how to use farm surpluses to address reemerging hunger in the United States. In part because the USDA viewed the hunger problem as exceptional and temporary, it opposed reinstitution of food stamps. But when John F. Kennedy became president in 1961, his administration initiated a pilot food stamp program. Although studies at the time showed the pilot to have little effect in reducing farm surpluses, it demonstrably improved the nutritional status of participants. It also increased retail food sales. On that basis, Congress considered instituting national food stamp legislation.

Congressional proponents of food stamps tended to come from northern states and urban regions, whereas those from farm states cared more about the effects of agricultural overproduction on prices paid to farmers.[3] The geographical differences suggested that coupling agricultural surpluses to food assistance might be politically expedient. By engaging in classic logrolling—you vote for my issue and I'll vote for yours—Congress passed the Food Stamp Act in 1964. In 1973, Congress permanently linked food stamps and agricultural supports when it transferred food stamp legislation to the farm bill, where it uncomfortably remains. In 2008, Congress changed the name of the program to SNAP on the grounds that the program's purpose was to improve nutrition and that the stamps had been replaced by Electronic Benefit Transfer (EBT) debit cards.

SNAP is an entitlement program: anyone who meets eligibility requirements can enroll. The level of participation closely tracks rates of poverty and unemployment. When the economy weakens, the number of eligible people increases, as happened rapidly following the recession in 2008. By the end of 2014, more than 46 million Americans were enrolled in SNAP for an average monthly benefit of $125. The program cost taxpayers nearly $74 billion in benefits and administration that year, a decrease from peak costs in 2012. Nevertheless, from its relatively modest beginnings, SNAP continues to overwhelmingly dominate the farm bill and to account for close to 80 percent of its total authorized expenditures.[4] Its enormous cost makes SNAP a sitting target for budget challenges. It also forces questions about how well the program promotes the nutritional status and health of its beneficiaries.

Unfortunately for getting answers to such questions, research examining the relationship of SNAP to obesity and its health consequences is extraordinarily difficult to do. Obesity-related health conditions are highest among low-income groups in general, and it is not easy to single out the particular influence of SNAP, let alone the specific contribution of sodas. Nevertheless, some studies demonstrate that SNAP participants consume more sodas, have lower scores on indices of healthy eating, and are more obese than low-income nonparticipants. Other studies find SNAP participants to have slightly higher levels of obesity and metabolic risk factors for chronic disease than their low-income non-SNAP counterparts. USDA researchers report that the overall diets of SNAP participants are less healthful than those of nonparticipants, in part because of higher sugar intake.[5]

The relationship of SNAP food purchases to obesity is a relatively new area of research, enormously impeded by lack of reliable information on how participants spend their SNAP dollars. Because all purchases are done electronically, such information ought to be easy to collect, but the USDA claims it is not authorized to collect data on SNAP purchases. Nevertheless, the evidence that is available suggests that the longer people are enrolled in SNAP, the more likely they are to be obese. This could happen because SNAP participants buy more food than they would if given cash, buy more of heavily advertised junk foods and sodas, or are affected by cycles of binge and deprivation brought on by inadequate benefits delivered only once a month. Among children, however, SNAP participation is associated with better nutrient intake with no effect on the prevalence of obesity.[6] The apparent shift in the overall condition of adult SNAP participants from nutritional inadequacy to overweight and obesity raises questions about whether SNAP dollars should continue to be permitted to pay for foods—particularly sodas—that contribute to poor health.

HOW SODAS GOT INTO SNAP

Why SNAP participants can buy sodas with SNAP benefits and why retailers can accept SNAP dollars for sodas requires explanation. In proposing the Food Stamp Act of 1964, Congress specified items that could not be purchased with public funds. At first, the House put soft drinks in the same ineligible category as alcohol, tobacco, and foreign agricultural products. The Senate, however, rescued sodas from the exclusion list because they were used in hospitals for medical purposes and "hungry persons will not spend much money for these items unless needed." Arguing against this rescue was Sen. Paul Douglas (D-Ill.):

MR. DOUGLAS.   I do not want to include Coca-Cola or Pepsi-Cola or any of that family. I like them myself, but I do not believe they should be permitted to be substitutes for milk. They are not valuable for the diet. They can be a waste of money especially for young people.... I [also] move to include carbonated soft drinks among the items for which food stamps may not be issued.

MR. ELLENDER.   [Allan Ellender, D-La.]. Mr. President, I hope the Senate will reject the amendment.... I believe it should be left to the people who have the stamps to decide what they wish to buy. We have excluded alcohol and tobacco; I think we have gone far enough.

MR. DOUGLAS.   Mr. President, I should like to speak concerning the proposal.... If we include them [carbonated soft drinks], this will be used as propaganda against an otherwise splendid and much needed measure. I want to help the poor and hungry and not sacrifice them for Coca-Cola. The Senator knows that these have no nutritional value—none at all.... I hesitate to use such language, but the only benefit I can see in the present language is that it will increase the sales of the Coca-Cola and other cola and soft drink companies.[7]

Douglas's objection failed. Today, SNAP participants may not use their EBT cards to buy beer, wine, liquor, tobacco products, pet foods, household supplies, dietary supplements, medicines, hot foods, or foods eaten in the store. They are free to buy these items anytime they like, but only with their own money. Soft drinks, along with candy, cookies, snack crackers, and ice cream, remain fully eligible. As discussed below, the soda industry continues to lobby against adding sodas to the SNAP-ineligible category, and every attempt to date has failed. Recipients are fully allowed to use their SNAP EBT cards for soda purchases.[8]

DO SNAP PARTICIPANTS BUY SODAS?

Indeed they do, although nobody really knows how much. Some stores keep track, but they are not obliged to reveal the data, and do not. Without data, we are forced to deal with estimates, and poor ones at that, not least because people who receive SNAP benefits can buy sodas either with the EBT cards or with their own money.

The most widely quoted estimate of the SNAP dollars spent on sodas is $4 billion, but other estimates range from $1.7 billion to more than $6 billion. Because such estimates are based on economic models, reports from single supermarket chains, conjecture, or hearsay, none can be considered reliable.[9] Nevertheless, it is a good guess that some SNAP participants use their benefits to buy sodas, and that the total amount they spend on sodas runs into the billions. In this sense, SNAP is a multibillion-dollar taxpayer subsidy of the soda industry.

Even more troubling, tax policies in many states give SNAP participants an *incentive* to buy sodas using their benefits. New York State, for example, imposes a sales tax on sodas. But SNAP rules do not allow states to collect taxes on purchases made with EBT cards. This makes sodas less expensive when bought with SNAP benefits than when purchased with the participants' own money.[10]

WHO BENEFITS FROM SNAP SODA PURCHASES?

Participants are not the only beneficiaries of SNAP benefits. The benefits also include a transfer of $70 billion (in 2014) from taxpayers to the particular retail establishments—more than 230,000 of them—authorized by the USDA to accept SNAP EBT purchases. Large supermarkets and chain stores collect more than 80 percent of SNAP dollars. The USDA actively recruits stores to participate in SNAP, and thousands of retailers apply to share in the benefits. If you were wondering why chain drugstores suddenly started to sell groceries, think SNAP. When Big Lots, the nation's largest closeout retailer, observed that more than six million potential customers had recently been added to SNAP rolls, it decided that "our business needs to provide customers multiple reasons to shop in our stores." The chain added coolers and converted registers to accept SNAP EBT cards.[11] Other stores have done the same.

The USDA uses two methods to authorize stores to accept SNAP EBT purchases. The stores either must prove that half their sales come from SNAP-eligible staple foods or must continuously offer for sale at least three varieties of each of four kinds of foods: meats, poultry, or fish; breads or cereals; fruits or vegetables; and dairy products. Of these categories, at least two must include perishable foods.[12] The bananas, apples, and oranges often sold in participating drugstores meet the perishable requirements, as do frozen chicken nuggets and ice cream.

Authorized stores advertise their acceptance of SNAP purchases and put "SNAP eligible" signs on coolers of such products and, of course, on those containing soft drinks (Figure 16.1). I asked the manager of a local Walgreens why his store put those signs on the cases for sodas, Red Bull, and ice cream. "SNAP recipients don't know they can use their cards to buy those foods," he told me. His explanation for the lack of such signs on fresh fruit: "They know they can buy fruit with EBT cards." He then added, "Profit margins are higher on the packaged items." Whether anyone actually buys the perishable fruit is irrelevant, which may explain why it is often displayed so unattractively.

Competition for SNAP dollars also explains the marketing practices of some of the smaller soft drink companies. Monster Energy drink used to be sold as a dietary supplement, which made it ineligible for SNAP purchases. In order to qualify, the company repositioned the product as a food with a Nutrition Facts label. Its chairman, Rodney C. Sacks, explained that he was doing this to "eliminate our competitive disadvantage in certain states, where energy drinks labeled as conventional food, like Red Bull, are exempt

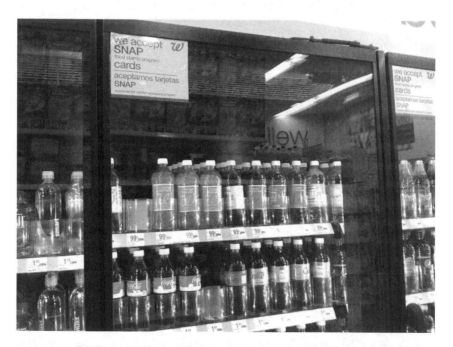

FIGURE 16.1 SNAP sign, Walgreens drugstore, Manhattan, 2013. The sign, still in use in 2015, advertises that SNAP benefits can be used to purchase sodas. Although similar signs are posted near ice cream and frozen meals, none appear near the fresh fruit. Courtesy of Daniel Bowman Simon.

from sales tax and are also eligible for redemption with food stamps, while energy drinks labeled as dietary supplements like Monster are not." This repositioning may be part of the reason Coca-Cola bought a 16.7 percent share of Monster Beverage in 2014.[13]

In many stores, SNAP purchases constitute a significant fraction of sales. The agricultural economist Parke Wilde estimates that SNAP dollars accounted for more than 17 percent of all food purchases for at-home use from food retailers, and 10 percent of such purchases from all stores. Food advocacy lawyer Michele Simon says food manufacturers and retailers profit so greatly from SNAP that the program really is more about what retailers sell than what participants receive. The dependence of retailers on SNAP dollars explains why soda and other food corporations insist on choice in use of benefits, and also why they generously support anti-hunger organizations, whose opposition to changes in SNAP eligibility requires discussion.[14]

THE STRANGE POLITICS OF SNAP SODA ELIGIBILITY

That businesses benefit from SNAP dollars also helps to explain why advocacy to remove sodas from SNAP so perfectly illustrates the adage "Politics makes strange bedfellows." Groups from widely disparate sectors of the political spectrum are allied on one side or the other for reasons of their own self-interest.[15]

Those in Favor of Making Sodas SNAP-Ineligible

Removing sodas from SNAP eligibility would not break precedent. In 1972, when Congress established WIC, the Special Supplemental Nutrition Program for Women, Infants, and Children, it specified that eligible foods must promote the health of pregnant women, breast-feeding mothers, and young children. WIC benefits cannot be used to buy sodas. But WIC is not an entitlement program, and its expenditures were less than one-tenth those for SNAP in 2012.[16]

How do SNAP participants feel about the idea of making SNAP choices more like those of WIC? In 2010, the Center for Science in the Public Interest (CSPI) asked SNAP participants and nonparticipants to say whether they agreed with the statement "Food stamps should *not* be allowed for buying sugary soft drinks." The unpublished survey found that nearly 60 percent of total respondents agreed, but only 30 percent of SNAP recipients. In 2011, New York City did its own survey: nearly two-thirds of SNAP respondents either supported the idea (49 percent) or did not care (16 percent). Among SNAP participants who said they typically consume sugary drinks, 59 percent either supported excluding sodas or said they did not care. Nearly half said they were likely to cut down on sodas if they could not use their SNAP benefits to buy them. Other surveys report similar percentages of participants favoring use of benefits for healthier foods.[17] One interpretation of these results is that a sizable proportion of SNAP recipients might appreciate some disincentive to unhealthful food choices.

In 2013, the mayors of eighteen cities wrote Congress, "It is time to test and evaluate approaches limiting SNAP's subsidization of products, such as sugar-sweetened beverages, that are contributing to obesity." The American Medical Association passed a resolution asking its members to work to "remove sugar-sweetened beverages from the SNAP program." Here's where the strange bedfellows appear: these groups were joined by the National Center for Public Health Policy, which, despite its name, is a highly conservative free-market think tank. The center owns stock in Coca-Cola and PepsiCo, and its staff members attend annual meetings where they raise questions about "why taxpayers are being forced by law to subsidize the sweet tooth of nearly 50 million [SNAP recipients]" and why soda companies are doing so much "lobbying against restricting food stamp use to items with at least some nutritional benefit."[18] The center interviewed PepsiCo's CEO, Indra Nooyi, and reported that she

> definitely understands our concerns about taxpayers subsidizing unhealthy lifestyles—she just prefers a different approach to curbing the problem...Ms. Nooyi thinks [the USDA]...should incentivize healthy purchases. While this is an interesting idea, it dodges Pepsi's role in food stamp lobbying, and there is no reason that the USDA and state governments can't incentivize healthy lifestyles and restrict soda purchases at the same time.[19]

In statements like this, Nooyi appears to admit that Pepsi products cause health problems, but wants the government to bear the burden of preventing them.

Those Opposed

As expected, the American Beverage Association (ABA) says:

> Education is at the core of changing behavior, not passing laws and regulations limiting choice. The bottom line is: it's not the government's job to grocery shop for our families; it's ours. Politicians should do what we elected them to do. We don't tell them how to build roads and bridges using our tax dollars, and they don't need to tell us what to put in our shopping carts.[20]

In making such arguments, soda companies are well aware that education and incentives, limited as they are, can do little to counter the impact of their massive marketing and philanthropy. Soda companies may insist that the government do nothing to interfere with food choice, but they expect taxpayers to pick up the costs of treating the health problems that result from poor food choices.

In 2011, the ABA hired a lobbying firm, Michael Torrey Associates, to deal with Congress about preserving choice in SNAP. The firm employs former officials of the USDA or staff of congressional committees dealing with SNAP legislation in the farm bill. During the 2012 election cycle, federal disclosure forms revealed substantial lobbying by soda companies on matters related to SNAP, especially because several states were considering bills aimed at removing sodas from program eligibility. The ABA reported that it lobbied federal officials on the need to "monitor efforts to restrict choice" and about "matters affecting preservation of choice" in SNAP. PepsiCo's lobbyists discussed "restrictions on use of SNAP for some foods," and Coca-Cola's worked to "promote choice and fairness in SNAP guidelines" and to "oppose programs that discriminate against specific foods and beverages in SNAP."[21]

Less expected, however, are the soda industry's allies on this issue—the USDA, for example. In 2007, the USDA released a position paper arguing against changing food eligibility requirements. Its reasons were the lack of unambiguous standards for defining a food as unhealthy, and program complexity and cost. It also cited the inadequacy of evidence that participation in SNAP contributes to poor diets or obesity, or that excluding certain foods would change purchase patterns. More recently, USDA researchers produced data demonstrating that if SNAP recipients could not use EBT cards to buy sodas, they would buy even more sugary drinks with their own money.[22] The USDA much prefers incentives for healthier options—carrots rather than sticks.

But the most unexpectedly vocal groups allied with the soda industry on this issue are advocates working to reduce hunger among Americans. Their objections rest on moral as well as practical grounds and are more difficult to dismiss out of hand. Such groups have a long and honorable history of advocating for the poor and defending federal food assistance programs against budget cuts. Yet they argue strongly against changes in SNAP requirements that might improve diets and prevent obesity. Such changes, they say, "would reintroduce the complexities, stigmas and confusion that we have all worked so hard to eliminate from SNAP (Food Stamps) in the last 30 years. It would be at cross-purposes with the basic intent...to reduce hunger, improve diets, and support families in difficult times."[23] The anti-hunger community prefers incentive programs to promote health through nutrition education and improved access to fruits and vegetables.

Perhaps, but it is difficult to disentangle the moral position of anti-hunger groups from their funding sources. When Ed Cooney, the executive director of the Congressional Hunger Center (CHC), told a reporter that changing SNAP eligibility requirements "will happen over my dead body," he insisted that "people have the smarts to purchase their own food, and we're opposed to all limitations on food choice." But the CHC lists PepsiCo among other food companies as a "major donor." When challenged to explain the potential conflict of interest raised by such donations, Cooney said: "At the Congressional Hunger Center, we do not accept funds that have any restrictions on them. Critics have indicated that this is an unholy alliance. I have no objection to that term. Those companies have access to members of congress that we don't have access to, people in the Republican leadership. We find this advantageous."[24]

The CHC is not the only anti-hunger group to actively oppose removing sodas from SNAP while accepting funds from soda companies. The largest of these groups, the Food Research and Action Center (FRAC), opposes even pilot projects to test the effects of excluding sodas from SNAP, and organized a coalition to lobby against such proposals. Coalition members include groups such as the CHC, but also Bread for the World, the Evangelical Lutheran Church, Feeding America—and the ABA. Coca-Cola contributed to the FRAC's annual fund-raising dinner in the early 1990s, and PepsiCo and the ABA do so today. Feeding America lists PepsiCo as a "leadership partner," and Coca Cola, PepsiCo, and the Dr Pepper Snapple Group are said to have contributed at least $100,000 each to that organization.[25]

With this kind of funding, it is understandable why anti-hunger groups appear unmoved by data demonstrating higher rates of soda consumption and obesity among SNAP participants. On the record, they argue that excluding sodas would stigmatize program participants. Off the record, they tell me—with considerable justification—that SNAP is highly vulnerable to congressional budget cuts and focusing attention on obesity makes the program even more vulnerable. To date, attempts to find common ground between anti-hunger and public health advocates on the issue of sodas in SNAP have been unsuccessful. I view this breach between two sets of passionate advocates for the poor as evidence for the soda industry's effective use of this particular divide-and-conquer strategy.

INCENTIVES: A POINT OF COMMON GROUND?

Other ways to improve the health of SNAP participants could be to "nudge" them toward healthier choices through education, and to reduce the cost of fruits and vegetables through federal or private farmers' market and other incentive programs. The largest of such programs is USDA's SNAP Nutrition Education (SNAP-Ed), funded at $401 million in 2014, but delegated to and split among the fifty states. The state programs aim to improve the likelihood that SNAP participants will choose foods consistent with the Dietary Guidelines and MyPlate. Although the guidelines say to "choose foods and drinks with little or no added sugars" and a MyPlate message is to "drink water instead of sugary drinks," SNAP-Ed messages do not mention sodas. Instead, they promote choosing more fruits and vegetables, whole grains, and low-fat dairy products; balancing calories; and being more active. Given the limited funding, I am not surprised that recent evaluations of SNAP-Ed show little or no association with improved food choices.[26]

Nevertheless, the USDA continues to push incentive programs rather than considering taking sodas off the SNAP-eligible list. As a result of apparently successful demonstration programs in New York and other states, the 2008 farm bill authorized the USDA to spend $20 million on Healthy Incentive Pilot (HIP) projects. The USDA chose Hampden County, Massachusetts, as the site for a year-long study. This involved 7,500 SNAP participants offered a bonus of 30 cents for every dollar they spent on targeted fruits and vegetables. They could use the bonus to purchase any eligible food. Preliminary results of the study showed a small but statistically significant increase in purchases of fresh fruits and vegetables among participants. How small? One-fifth of a cup.[27]

Farmers' markets have accepted food stamps for years. Although the value of redemptions increased from $4 million in 2009 to $21 million in 2013 and the increase helps local farmers, the amount spent at farmers' markets continues to be minuscule—less than 0.03 percent of the billions of SNAP dollars spent on other foods, mostly in supermarkets.[28]

Private groups also advocate for SNAP incentive programs. Wholesome Wave, a New England–based organization devoted to improving the ability of low-income communities to consume fresh, locally grown produce, does so through two programs. Its Double Value Coupon Program matches federal food assistance dollars, and its innovative Fruit and Vegetable Prescription Program underwrites the cost of directives from health care providers to buy more fruits and vegetables. Wholesome Wave reports that participants in these programs eat more fruits and vegetables. The programs reach thousands of SNAP participants a year, but at a cost of several million dollars. The Fair Food Network's similar Double Up Food Bucks program works in grocery stores as well as farmers' markets but is limited to Detroit and other Midwest cities. The double-value idea made it into the 2014 farm bill, which provided $100 million for this purpose. Getting this program into the farm bill was an impressive achievement and is wonderful for farmers' markets, but its ability to improve overall SNAP food purchases remains minimal.[29]

Another organization, SNAP Gardens, takes a different approach: educating SNAP participants to use their benefit cards to buy food-producing plants and seeds. Its founder, Daniel Bowman Simon, discovered a little-known provision in the 1973 food stamp legislation that permits this usage. Today, farmers' markets and community gardens throughout the country are partners in this effort (Figure 16.2).[30]

Taken together, these programs succeed in increasing fruit and vegetable purchases among a relatively few SNAP participants to a limited extent. They are expensive to run, reach thousands—not millions—of participants, and account for a tiny fraction of total purchases made with SNAP benefits. A study using mathematical models to compare bans on soda SNAP purchases with subsidies for fruits and vegetables concludes that subsidies are more likely to increase consumption of the subsidized foods, but that bans are far more likely to reduce obesity.[31]

FIGURE 16.2 Poster promoting use of SNAP benefits to buy seeds and food plants. The advocacy group SNAP Gardens encourages participants in the USDA's Supplemental Nutrition Assistance Program to grow their own food. Courtesy SNAPgardens.org.

ADVOCACY: NEW YORK CITY'S WAIVER ATTEMPT

In October 2010, New York State asked the USDA to waive its rules to allow a small pilot experiment in New York City: block the use of SNAP benefits to buy sodas. Specifically, city officials wanted to see what would happen if they excluded "sweetened beverages containing more than 10 calories per cup (exempting fruit juice without added sugar, milk products, and milk substitutes)." Based on Nielsen marketing data and other studies, the city estimated that its 1.8 million SNAP participants had used their EBT cards to buy $75 to $135 million worth of sugar-sweetened beverages in 2009.[32]

In an opinion piece in the *New York Times*, city health commissioner Dr. Tom Farley and state health commissioner Dr. Richard Daines pointed to the high prevalence of obesity and diabetes among New York City adults and children and their associated medical costs. They said:

> Every year, tens of millions of federal dollars are spent on sweetened beverages in New York City through the food stamp program—far more than is spent on obesity prevention. This amounts to an enormous subsidy to the sweetened beverage industry. . . . The city's proposed program would not reduce participants' food stamp benefits or their ability to feed their families a nutritionally adequate diet. They would still receive every penny of support they now get, meaning they would have as much, if not more, to spend

on nutritious food. And they could still purchase soda if they chose—just not with taxpayer dollars.[33]

The SNAP waiver request followed several other health proposals initiated by the city's health department with the backing of its mayor, Michael Bloomberg. During Bloomberg's first term in office, the city expanded its smoking ban to indoor public places, banned trans fats in restaurants, and established a national precedent in requiring chain restaurants to post calories on menu boards. The city imposed stricter rules on food sold in schools and supported the state's unsuccessful efforts to tax sodas (see Chapter 26). The health department created poster campaigns designed to reduce soda consumption, among them advertisements showing packets of sugar turning into fat in a soda cup, and others illustrating how much walking is necessary to work off soda calories and the health benefits of reducing portion sizes (see examples in Figures 17.1 and 25.1).

City officials believed their petition addressed issues that caused the USDA to reject a similar request from Minnesota in 2004. In denying the earlier attempt, the USDA stated that excluding junk foods from eligibility would stigmatize food stamp recipients, lead to confusion and embarrassment in the checkout aisle, and perpetuate the myth that participants do not make wise food purchasing decisions. New York health officials directly addressed concerns about stigma. They argued that numerous items are already excluded from purchase with SNAP benefits, and extending that list could hardly make a difference. They also intended to conduct a rigorous evaluation of the pilot project. Research, they said, is essential to resolve questions about stigmatization and whether excluding sodas could improve public perceptions of SNAP.[34]

The ABA objected: "This is just another attempt by government to tell New Yorkers what they should eat and drink." It encouraged trade associations for the snack food, candy, grocery retail industries—and anti-hunger groups—to lobby against the proposal. On the grounds that treating SNAP participants differently from other customers would be unfair, the ABA induced eighteen members of the Congressional Black Caucus to urge the USDA to reject the waiver. At this point, it will not surprise you to learn that Coca-Cola and PepsiCo contribute generously to the Congressional Black Caucus Foundation—Coke in the $250,000 to $500,000 range and Pepsi between $100,000 and $250,000. Caucus members, of course, deny that the contributions influence their opinions on such issues.[35]

In August 2011, the USDA denied the waiver request. It said the proposed pilot was too large and complex, did not resolve operational challenges, lacked a clear and practical means to determine product eligibility, and failed to include strong measures of soda purchases, consumption, and total caloric intake. Furthermore, because the USDA was already involved in the Massachusetts Healthy Incentives Pilot, it would be imprudent to reverse policy while the evaluation of that project was still ongoing.[36] Mayor Bloomberg's response was short but to the point:

> We think our innovative pilot would have done more to protect people from the crippling effects of preventable illnesses like diabetes and obesity than anything being proposed anywhere else in this country—and at little or no cost to taxpayers. We're disappointed that the Federal Government didn't agree and sorry that families and children may suffer from their unwillingness to explore our proposal. New York City will continue to pursue new and unconventional ways to combat the health problems that affect New Yorkers and all Americans.[37]

By the end of 2012, seven other states had made similar waiver requests. The USDA rejected all of them, arguing that only Congress has the authority to decide which foods are ineligible for SNAP purchases. By mid-2014, at least fifteen states had introduced bills to exclude sodas from SNAP purchases, but USDA secretary Tom Vilsack was not encouraging. In a speech in South Carolina he stated, "The alternative may not be to restrict, but to incent." He meant that his agency greatly preferred the far less controversial Healthy Incentives and double-value approaches, despite their minimal impact and high cost.[38] The goal of getting sodas out of SNAP remains wide open for advocacy.

ADVOCATE: REMOVE SODAS FROM SNAP ELIGIBILITY

Understand the Issue

- The contribution of sodas to poor health is well established.
- The WIC program sets a precedent in establishing foods eligible for purchase: it excludes sodas.
- Several foods and other items are already excluded from SNAP purchase.

- SNAP beneficiaries purchase more sodas than other low-income groups.
- SNAP participants are as overweight, perhaps more so, than other low-income groups.
- Soda companies and retailers specifically market sodas to SNAP participants.
- By permitting soda purchases, SNAP subsidizes disease-promoting behavior eventually paid for by taxpayers.
- Many SNAP participants favor creating a healthier environment for their food choices.
- Taxpayer-funded programs should promote health, not illness.

Engage in the Debate

Much of the debate about soda eligibility in SNAP is over the lack of data on purchases, the ethics of insisting that low-income recipients of taxpayer dollars eat more healthfully, and preferences for incentives rather than restrictions (Table 16.1).[39]

TABLE 16.1 Topic for debate: should sodas be excluded from SNAP eligibility?

OPPONENTS SAY	ADVOCATES SAY
We don't have enough data to support this policy.	We need data on SNAP purchases, but substantial research demonstrates that sodas are not good for health.
Poor people have a right to drink what everyone else drinks.	Yes, they do, and can buy sodas using their own—not taxpayers'—money.
SNAP participants will still buy sodas with their own money.	SNAP participants may think twice about whether they want to spend their own money on sodas.
A better policy would be to lower the cost of fruits and vegetables.	Both are good policies.
This policy would be complicated for stores to implement.	Retail technology helps stores manage such changes at low cost.
Restrictions on purchases are stigmatizing.	Obesity and poor health are stigmatizing. Existing SNAP restrictions do not stigmatize. WIC restrictions do not stigmatize and do not raise ethical concerns.
This is an example of the nanny state gone too far.	Regulations can help promote health and prevent diseases that are expensive for individuals and for society.
Anti-hunger advocates are against this proposal.	Anti-hunger groups are funded by soda and other food companies. Public health advocates support it. Soda company support for anti-hunger groups divides advocates for the poor who should be allies.

Take Action

SNAP is the most important food assistance program in the United States. No matter how advocates feel about soda eligibility, they want the program to be better funded and more effective. All advocates want to ensure an adequate safety net for those in need. While working to maintain adequate SNAP funding and to stave off congressional attempts to cut the program's budget, public health advocates can:

- Join and support organizations working on SNAP issues
- Require retailers to provide data on foods purchased with SNAP
- Promote city and state campaigns for SNAP waivers
- Encourage local farmers' markets to accept EBT payments
- Lobby Congress and the USDA to remove sodas from SNAP eligibility
- Build coalitions around this issue with health, medical, and anti-hunger advocacy groups
- Organize communities of SNAP participants to build support for soda exclusion
- Frame soda advocacy as part of a broader commitment to address the needs of the underserved

"Softball" Marketing Tactics: Recruiting Allies, Co-opting Critics

17

Marketing Corporate Social Responsibility

Companies such as Coca-Cola and PepsiCo must meet fiscal goals and answer to boards of directors and shareholders but also are expected to engage in corporate social responsibility (CSR), a term that I use here to refer to efforts to promote some social good—above and beyond legal requirements—aimed at benefiting employees, consumers, communities, or the environment. Soda companies publicize their CSR activities in annual sustainability reports. As Coca-Cola explains, the company's CSR initiatives "create value for shareowners while enhancing well-being for people and communities around the globe... [They grow] our business by making a difference wherever our business touches the world and the world touches our business."[1]

PepsiCo asserts that "what is good for society and what is good for business can and should be the same.... This is the cornerstone of our Performance with Purpose mission: that our long-term profitable growth (our Performance) is linked intrinsically to our ability to deliver on our social and environmental objectives (our Purpose)." As part of its philanthropic mission, Dr Pepper Snapple says it will "contribute a total of 100,000 volunteer hours and attain an annual giving level of $10 million in charitable cash donations, with the majority of support focused on fit and active lifestyles, environmental sustainability, emergency relief and hometown giving." The Coca-Cola and PepsiCo Foundations rank among the top fifty in the amounts given. In 2014, the Coca-Cola Foundation ranked number eleven (at nearly $70 million), and the PepsiCo Foundation ranked number thirty-one (more than $25 million).[2]

But, you may ask, aren't foundations different from and independent of the related corporations? At one time they may have been, but no longer. As some critics put it, "Corporate charity is no longer a garnish, an optional nicety, but instead sits at the center of the corporate plate, an integral element of a firm's core business strategy."[3]

As these chapters demonstrate, the corporation and its foundation operate as a single unit and their goals are indistinguishable. In any case, the amounts spent by soda foundations are dwarfed by the amounts spent on advertising. CSR disguises the primacy of corporate financial goals, allowing the American Beverage Association (ABA) to instead point to the soda industry's "longstanding commitment to its customers, consumers and communities."[4]

The return to soda companies from this generosity is considerable. CSR demonstrably creates a "health halo." Studies confirm that the public views food products marketed by firms with strong CSR reputations to be healthier. This halo effect is so strong that it induces people to underestimate the calorie content of products associated with CSR and to eat more of them—even when given objective nutrition information.[5]

This finding explains why CSR is such a critical component of the soda industry's business strategy, one driven by pressures to tax, restrict, or ban sodas as a means to reduce their impact on health and the environment. A basic commitment to CSR requires companies to monitor compliance with international ethical, legal, and economic standards of employment and operation, but soda companies do more. They engage in philanthropy and partnerships—"softball" tactics that link business objectives to social and environmental causes. Philanthropic partnerships are so important to industry growth that they have created a niche. There now exists a sponsorship industry made up of consultant groups whose entire purpose is to evolve "new and better ways for companies and brands to partner with organizations and events throughout sports, arts, entertainment, associations and causes—for mutual benefit."[6]

Although CSR philanthropy helps recipients engage in worthy causes, its underlying purpose is to create a favorable corporate image and promote sales. When considering the effects of soda company CSR, it helps to keep some caveats in mind:

- The business purpose of CSR is to win friends, promote brand loyalty, silence critics, head off regulation, and accumulate moral credit—and to create the illusion that the products are healthier.

- Soda companies may spend millions on CSR causes, but they spend *billions* to market their products and many more millions to protect business interests through lobbying and other "hardball" tactics, as explained in later chapters.
- If CSR programs do not lead to measurable sales increases, they are soon dropped.

Some years ago, Dr. David Ludwig, a pediatrician who specializes in working with obese children, and I had this to say about CSR:

> With respect to obesity, the food industry has acted at times constructively, at times outrageously. But inferences from any one action miss a fundamental point: in a market-driven economy, industry tends to act opportunistically in the interests of maximizing profit.... While visionary CEOs and enlightened food company cultures may exist, society cannot depend on them to address obesity voluntarily, any more than it can base national strategies to reduce highway fatalities and global warming solely on the goodwill of the automobile industry. Rather, appropriate checks and balances are needed to align the financial interests of the food industry with the goals of public health.[7]

I deal with the question of appropriate checks and balances in later chapters. For now, let's consider CSR as a marketing strategy, although one so complicated and extensive that it takes me six chapters to explain. Coca-Cola and PepsiCo discuss their CSR achievements in reports to investors and the public. These reports describe CSR activities so vast in number and scope that I must resort to a cliché: they leave no stone unturned. No possible recipient of soda industry philanthropy is too small or too local for soda companies to ignore as a potential ally.

For the purposes of this section of the book, I find it convenient to define soda CSR as indirect—"softball"—marketing linked to four socially responsible goals:

1. Promote health
2. Invest in communities
3. Support worthy causes
4. Protect the environment

TABLE 17.1 Big Soda CSR: strategic goals vs. marketing objectives

STRATEGIC GOAL	MARKETING OBJECTIVE
1. Promote health (this chapter) • Expand the portfolio of low- and no-calorie beverage options • Market smaller sizes • Educate the public about key concepts: energy balance, hydration, and physical activity	Deflect attention from the contribution of sodas to obesity and poor health. Shift responsibility for poor food choices and inactivity to consumers.
2. Invest in sponsorships and community partnerships (Chapter 18) • Promote sports and entertainment • Support local community initiatives • Provide community disaster relief	Gain brand loyalty. Win allies. Neutralize critics.
3. Support worthy causes (Chapters 19 and 20) • Partner with health professionals • Sponsor nutrition research • Recruit public health leaders	Enhance credibility. Neutralize critics. Influence policy.
4. Protect the environment (Chapters 21 and 22) • Reduce greenhouse gas emissions • Reduce package waste • Promote sustainable sugar production • Reduce water use	Deflect attention from the contribution of soda manufacture to exploitation of water resources, appropriation of land for sugar production, energy waste, and climate change, and from the linkage between soda consumption and package litter.

To me, this looks like "healthwashing" and "greenwashing"—cosmetic attempts to deflect attention from the harm to public health and the environment caused by soda production and consumption. In Table 17.1, I summarize and translate the four goals and subgoals of soda company CSR. In this chapter, I cover the first of these goals—promoting health. I deal with the others in subsequent chapters.

CSR STRATEGY #1: PROMOTE HEALTH

In 2010, executives of PepsiCo made a surprising announcement. The soda industry, they said, had a critical role to play in preventing chronic disease. Their company intended to expand its philanthropic and corporate initiatives to promote health through diet and physical activity programs that would encourage customers to make informed choices and live healthier lives. Among other commitments, PepsiCo promised to reduce the average amount of added sugar per serving in certain of its global beverage brands by 25 percent by 2020, and to "increase the range of foods and beverages that offer solutions for managing calories, such as reduced portion sizes." Today, through its Global Citizenship initiatives, the PepsiCo Foundation supports programs that "encourage healthy lifestyles and improve the availability of affordable nutrition." The foundation provided $1 million in grants for those purposes in 2012.[8]

In 2013, Coca-Cola similarly broke precedent and directly addressed linkages between its products and obesity. It produced advertisements stating the company's new position: "We'd like people to come together on something that concerns all of us, obesity. The long-term health of our families and our country is at stake, and...we can play an important role." To do so, Coke said it would:[9]

- Offer low- or no-calorie beverage options in every market
- Provide transparent nutrition information and list calories on the front of package labels
- Support physical activity programs in every country in which it does business
- Market responsibly, including no advertising to children under 12 anywhere in the world

As is evident from such promises, soda companies would like to be viewed as part of the solution to obesity rather than its cause. This takes some doing. They can and do produce artificially sweetened beverages and those with less sugar or packaged in smaller sizes, promote personal choice and physical activity, and emphasize the importance of hydration and calorie balance. What they do not do is commit to pulling back on the making and aggressive marketing of less healthful beverages or larger-size packages, or on their behind-the-scenes "hardball" activities to stave off regulation. Early in 2015, the ABA announced that in partnership with the U.S. Conference of Mayors it was awarding nearly half a million dollars to six cities—among them Lima, Ohio, and North Miami, Florida—for their "outstanding programs that encourage healthy weight through balanced diet choices and regular physical activity."[10]

For business reasons, soda companies must appear concerned about health, but investment analysts are dubious about the value of such initiatives. Calvert Investments, a fund management firm that uses "sustainability

as a platform to create value for investors," believes that Coca-Cola's commitments to combat obesity put its profits at risk. It says, "Stakeholders and investors will be monitoring the company closely to ensure that these pledges
are followed, and will pressure the company to make additional commitments. And while these commitments are robust, global sales of no- and
low-calorie sodas are also sharply down, calling into question the long-term
viability of this strategy."[11] With financial issues ever in mind, let's take a look
at some of the soda companies' health-promoting initiatives.

Expand the Portfolio of Low- and No-Calorie Beverage Options

Coca-Cola says that "for consumers who want low- or no-calorie options,
we offer more than 800 options—nearly 25 percent of our global portfolio.... Since 2000, our average calories per serving have decreased by 9
percent globally." Dr Pepper Snapple states that "in 2012 we exceeded our
goal to have 50 percent of our innovation pipeline dedicated to health and
wellness, with a full 55 percent of the pipeline focused on reducing calories,
offering smaller sizes and improving nutrition. At DPS, we firmly believe
consumers have the right to make beverage choices that fit their lifestyles."[12]

Pepsi, as I noted earlier, promises a 25 percent reduction in sugars in its
drinks, but only in certain brands in certain countries, and not until 2020.
Nevertheless, Pepsi works hard to position itself as a wellness company. It
publishes a guide to weight management through energy balance focused
on a "small changes" approach to weight loss: "Since drinking a diet beverage can save about 100 calories per 8 oz serving...diet beverages are a
useful way to reduce calorie intake." By Pepsi's interpretation of the science,
diet drinks help you lose weight, and any suggestions to the contrary are
mistaken, although its guide does admit that "more research is needed to
examine the role of low calorie sweeteners in preventing weight gain in
normal weight subjects." Fortunately for Pepsi, Coca-Cola comes to the
rescue. The company sponsors research studies designed to prove how well
low-calorie sweeteners help prevent and manage obesity-related diabetes
(Chapter 19 has more to say about soda-sponsored research).[13]

Diet drinks can be a hard sell. Artificial sweeteners are not natural
components of foods and convey bitter aftertastes; none of them tastes as
good as sugar. Although most studies confirm that artificial sweeteners are
safe in amounts commonly consumed, the chemicals continue to raise endless suspicions about their potential harm to health. In 2013, in an effort to

counteract declining sales, Coca-Cola embarked on a campaign to defend the safety of its sweeteners: "Time and again, these low- and no-calorie sweeteners have been shown to be safe, high-quality alternatives to sugar. In fact, the safety of aspartame is supported by more than 200 studies over the last 40 years." Lest scientists question the safety of these chemicals, the ABA sponsors breakfast sessions at meetings of the American Society of Nutrition to set "the record straight on low- and no-calorie sweeteners."[14]

The soda industry has reason to be concerned about negative perceptions of diet drinks. Sales of artificially sweetened sodas in the United States have been falling even faster than those of sugar-sweetened drinks, leading companies to scramble to find sweeteners perceived to be healthier. One such sweetener is stevia, a chemical extracted from the leaves of *Stevia rebaudiana*. In 2013, Coca-Cola introduced Coca-Cola Life to Chile and Argentina. This drink, sweetened with stevia, has "only" two-thirds the calories in regular Coke, is marketed as natural, and is sold with green labels and green cans. A year later, the company launched the product in Britain and the United States. PepsiCo introduced its own stevia-sweetened version, Pepsi NEXT, in Europe, but it is sweetened with sucralose (Splenda) in the United States. Skeptics suggested that Coca-Cola and PepsiCo had ulterior motives in marketing these products, at least in the United Kingdom. Nobody expected them to sell well. Their purpose was to make the companies appear to be responding to promises to reduce the calories in soda.[15]

Market Smaller Sizes

Every chance I get, I point out that smaller portions have fewer calories—something not intuitively obvious, as I discussed earlier. Smaller portions fit with "eat less" weight-loss strategies, and most people do not consume multiples of small containers at the same occasion. So I was happy when both Coke and Pepsi introduced 7.5-ounce minicans with fewer than 100 calories in 2009. Both companies set the selling price higher than the cost per volume of larger cans, but low enough to encourage sales—about 50 cents each, although always in multipacks. The minicans sold well, and by 2014, this strategy was contributing nicely to corporate profits. Business analysts, however, fretted that repositioning sodas as occasional treats to be consumed in small amounts would not do much for long-term corporate growth: "For all their adorableness, the petite containers are never going to replace the jumbo sizes in the grocery aisle, or the 50-ounce Double-Gulps at 7-Eleven. Regular cans and 2-liter bottles still account for 75 percent of Coca-Cola's soda sales in the U.S."[16] This last point explains why soda companies so fiercely opposed New York City's attempt to set a cap on soda sizes (Chapter 25).

Educate the Public About Key Concepts

In Chapter 8, I talked about how soda companies responded to the threat of obesity by reframing the issues to deflect attention from the harm caused by their products. Here are some ways they promote those frames.

Energy balance. In 2012, Coca-Cola gave the city of Chicago a $3 million grant for a wellness initiative offering nutrition education and exercise classes to help fight obesity. The company sponsors more than 280 such programs in more than 115 countries, and plans to provide similar programs in every country in which it does business by 2015. What do these programs teach? "Balance, variety and moderation are the fundamentals of good nutrition. All calories count."[17] As Coca-Cola explains:

> We agree with the widespread consensus that weight gain is primarily the result of energy imbalance—too many calories consumed and too few expended. No single food or beverage alone is responsible for people being overweight or obese. But all calories count, regardless of the source—including those in our beverages. All of our products can be part of an active, healthy lifestyle that includes a sensible, balanced diet and regular physical activity.[18]

In 2014, a Coca-Cola advertisement emphasized that it only takes 23 minutes of riding a bicycle to work off the 140 calories in a 12-ounce Coke (if you weigh 140 pounds).[19] Pepsi's weight management guide also emphasizes that "energy balance is the critical factor regardless of the food or beverage sources."

Strictly speaking, these assertions are correct. As a nutritionist and co-author of a book called *Why Calories Count*, I thoroughly agree that balance, variety, and moderation are fundamental principles of healthful diets, and that weight gain results from caloric imbalance. But soda companies are using these principles to make you forget about their marketing of sugary drinks and the overconsumption that results, actions that override normal physiological controls of hunger and satiety.[20]

Coca-Cola websites and advertisements say things like "We promote active, healthy living. We are committed to bringing real choice to consumers

TABLE 17.2 Coca Cola's international nutrition education programs, selected examples, 2012

COUNTRY	EDUCATION PROGRAM
Canada	$100,000 foundation grant to Boys and Girls Club of London, Ontario, for Youth ABCs (Ability to Bring Change!) to educate about the benefits of activity and healthy eating
China	Balanced Diet—Active Living: delivers science-based health information to the public in cooperation with China's Ministry of Health
France and 14 other countries	EPODE: a public-private partnership committed to promoting active, healthy lifestyles through community-based programs and family education
Italy	The Modavi Project: A Scuola inForma program to educate high school students about the importance of balanced nutrition and exercise
South Korea	Coca-Cola Health Camp: teaches healthy behaviors to students at risk for obesity

everywhere and to educating them on the role our variety of beverages can play in sensible, balanced diets as well as active, healthy lifestyles." Through its philanthropic foundations, Coke sponsors nutrition programs to educate consumers about "real choice" in balanced diets.[21] The company does this internationally as well as in the United States, as the examples in Table 17.2 indicate.

Hydration. People need fluids to maintain health. Why not Coke or Pepsi? As early as 1922, Coca-Cola told its stockholders that "a business as Coca-Cola must rest on some fundamental human desire. Coca-Cola was conceived to scientifically satisfy thirst, without the need of a glass of water afterwards." A pamphlet produced in the 1960s by the American Bottlers of Carbonated Beverages, the forerunner of the ABA, describes the critical role of water in the body—digestion, excretion, circulation, temperature regulation, lubrication—and the urgent need to maintain adequate fluid intake. Guess what: sugar-sweetened carbonated beverages are at least 86 percent water (see Figure 1.2).[22]

The soda industry still talks about hydration this way. In 2014, the ABA's statement on hydration science pointed out that "water is the predominant ingredient in carbonated soft drinks. Regular soft drinks are made up of 90 percent water and diet soft drinks with zero calories are 99 percent water.... Adults and children can consume a wide variety of fluids each day, including water, milk, juice, tea, sports drinks and soft drinks to meet their hydration needs. For all the appeal beverages generate from a taste standpoint, it's easy to forget they exist for an essential reason." Soft drinks, by this argument, are *essential*.

A pamphlet using the same arguments, written by Spanish physicians and "published with the collaboration of Coca-Cola," was distributed at the annual meeting of the Academy of Nutrition and Dietetics in 2013. Aimed at health and nutrition professionals, the pamphlet, *Hydration in the Workplace*, advises people doing heavy work in hot weather to replace fluids with cold water and soft drinks every twenty minutes.[23] In its annual sustainability report, Coke says, "We provide hydration choices and educate consumers about them." By this, Coke means that when you are thirsty, you can drink any of its beverage products—from bottled water to full-sugar Coke—and any one of them will be more fun to drink than tap water. PepsiCo distributed a similar pamphlet at the academy's annual meeting in 2014.

Education about calorie balance and hydration focuses squarely on personal choice. The companies provide beverage options; the choice is yours. To help you choose, both Coke and Pepsi list calorie information on the front of cans and nonreturnable bottles. Sizes up to 20 ounces list total calories. Above 20 ounces, the packages display the much less helpful calories per serving. In 2012, the ABA launched its Calories Count Vending Program. This puts a reminder that "calories count" on vending machines, and adds calorie labels to selection buttons. Dr Pepper Snapple also promotes nutrition education and choice: "DPS has a responsibility to our consumers to be transparent about our product ingredients and provide nutritional facts at their fingertips. It's one of our top priorities to help consumers, especially parents, make informed decisions while they shop."[24]

Physical activity. Coca-Cola says: "We are committed to being part of workable solutions to the problems facing society related to obesity. We seek to do this by assisting our associates and their families, as well as the communities that we serve, in promoting active, healthy living." Coca-Cola's television commercials use the slogan "Happiness is movement," and the company also sponsors a great many activity programs in countries throughout the world. It targets such sponsorship to health professionals, not only in the United States (Chapter 19) but also globally. In 2014, for example, it sponsored the fifth International Congress on Physical Activity and Public Health in Rio de Janeiro. Its thirty-four-country Exercise Is Medicine program encourages doctors and other health care providers to include exercise when designing treatment plans for patients. You can guess that these programs do not raise the possibility that drinking less soda might be a useful weight-loss strategy. The Coca-Cola Foundation says that about one-third of its philanthropic contributions go to organizations working to counter obesity, especially through promotion of physical activity. Table 17.3 gives some examples from the last half of 2013. About these programs, an editorial in the *Lancet* says: "This partnering is disgraceful. Health and medical conferences must raise their ethical standards and avoid such financial links."[25]

Dr Pepper Snapple also promotes the "calories out" part of energy balance. It sponsors a $15 million initiative to build or improve two thousand playgrounds in the United States, Canada, and Mexico. It partners with Good Sports to provide sports equipment, and with Canada Dry Mott's to produce the wonderfully named Random Acts of Play program that sponsors sports teams and activities throughout eastern Canada. And through its Let's Play community partnership with the nonprofit KaBOOM!, it builds playgrounds to help meet America's "play deficit."[26]

Body weight is about calorie balance, and physical activity is a major contributor to optimal health. But upping the level of physical activity without also reducing calorie intake is rarely enough to compensate for calorie overload

TABLE 17.3 Activity programs sponsored by Coca-Cola, selected international examples, 2013

COUNTRY	DONATION	ORGANIZATION, PHYSICAL ACTIVITY PROGRAM
Bolivia	$45,000	Fundacion Emprender, Let's Play
Denmark	$950,000	International Sport and Culture Association, MOVE Activation
Hungary	$250,000	Energy Balance Study and Active Living Communications Campaign
Indonesia	$307,000	Exercise Is Medicine program
Israel	$80,000	Special Olympics: Organizing Sport Competition for Individuals with Intellectual Disabilities
Japan	$190,000	Japan Running Promotion Organization, Improving Running Ability for Healthy Active Lifestyles
Taiwan	$120,000	John Tung Foundation, 2013 Rope Skipping for Healthy Lifestyles
Ukraine	$50,000	National Olympic Committee of Ukraine, Do Like Olympians
Uruguay	$15,000	Let's Play

SOURCE: Coca-Cola Foundation, 2nd and 3rd quarter reports, 2013.

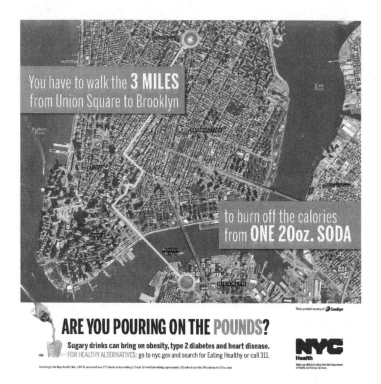

FIGURE 17.1 Poster from the New York City Department of Health and Mental Hygiene's 2011 subway campaign to encourage New Yorkers to drink less soda. The poster makes the point that it takes a hike of three long miles to compensate for the calories in just one 20-ounce soda.

when trying to lose weight. The need to reduce calories—eat less—to take off pounds is obvious from the math. On average, it takes about a mile of walking to expend 100 calories (more for people who are heavier and move more quickly, fewer for those who are smaller, lighter, and slower). This means that a 275-calorie, 20-ounce soda requires nearly three miles of walking to compensate. This was the point of a New York City health department campaign in 2011 (see Figure 17.1).[27] The difficulty of compensating for large numbers of soda calories induced Australian health advocates to protest Coca-Cola's advertisements as a "smokescreen." The ads promoted smaller portion sizes, low-calorie products, and physical activity but said nothing about the weight-promoting effects of soft drinks or their marketing. Soda company sponsorship of physical activity programs, conclude health advocates, is public relations in disguise.

QUESTIONING CSR

I am not alone in raising skeptical questions about CSR. In 2013, a study of Fortune 500 companies found that firms engaging in CSR are more likely to also engage in illegal and unethical behavior—what the authors call "corporate social irresponsibility"—toward recipients at some later point. Engaging in CSR activities apparently makes corporate leaders believe they have accumulated enough moral credit to justify less ethical behavior later on. The authors view the consequences of CSR-induced feelings of moral superiority to be so potentially risky that it advises corporations to institute special governance structures to counter them. Corporations, they say, should take firm steps to prevent executives from becoming morally complacent and should hold them accountable for unethical or illegal behavior that might occur as a result.[28]

In light of that research, the contradictions of CSR are more understandable. In 2011, public health researchers noted that soda company sponsorship of physical activity programs in Latin America may appear altruistic, but their true purpose is "to improve the industry's public image and increase political influence in order to block regulations counter to their interests. If this industry wants to contribute to human wellbeing, as it has publicly stated, it should avoid blocking legislative actions intended to regulate the marketing, advertising and sale of their products."[29]

I once made a similar point quoted by a reporter in an otherwise laudatory *New Yorker* article about PepsiCo's claims to have a leading role in public health issues: "The best thing Pepsi could do for worldwide obesity would be to go out of business."[30] This is a harsh statement, offered somewhat facetiously; long-standing soda companies are unlikely to stop making products that so many people like. But surely soda companies would enhance their credibility if they stopped marketing their products as essential for hydration, stopped marketing to children, and stopped actively opposing and undermining public health efforts to address obesity (Chapters 25–27).

I think it is fair to question whether soda company CSR should include health messages at all. Soda company "healthwashing" is invariably designed to promote goodwill, legitimacy, and health halos, and to mask the underlying profit motive. But even from a strictly business standpoint, the value of CSR is controversial. Although some business analysts believe CSR to be essential for long-term corporate development and growth, others are deeply skeptical. Corporations must produce returns for investors. If promoting social causes raises profits at all, it does so indirectly. I have discussed how Coke and Pepsi dropped their school rewards programs when sales failed to increase and how business analysts severely criticized PepsiCo for allowing Pepsi's rank to fall to number three, with shareholders forcing the company to put more resources into marketing its core, sugar-sweetened products.[31] A skeptical business professor, Aneel Karnani, wrote in the *Wall Street Journal*:

> Where private profits and public interests are aligned, the idea of corporate social responsibility is irrelevant: Companies that simply do everything they can to boost profits will end up increasing social welfare. In circumstances in which profits and social welfare are in direct opposition, an appeal to corporate social responsibility will almost always be ineffective, because executives are unlikely to act voluntarily in the public interest and against shareholder interests.... The danger is that a focus on social responsibility will delay or discourage more-effective measures to enhance social welfare in those cases where profits and the public good are at odds. As society looks to companies to address these problems, the real solutions may be ignored.[32]

In the final analysis, Karnani adds, "social responsibility is a financial calculation for executives, just like any other aspect of their business. The only sure way to influence corporate decision making is to impose an unacceptable cost—regulatory mandates, taxes, punitive fines, public embarrassment—on socially unacceptable behavior." Sodas, of course, are classic examples of Karnani's "profits and the public good at odds." They have no nutritional value, and excessive consumption is harmful. Soda companies use CSR to gloss over the conflict in these goals.

To health advocates, soda company CSR seems no different from the "socially responsible" actions of tobacco companies. Like tobacco companies, soda companies use CSR to head off regulation and refocus attention on personal choice. They use "moral credits" as a cover for the lobbying and other "hardball" strategies I cover in later chapters. The parallels suggest that advocacy might focus on "denormalizing" soda consumption—making it socially unacceptable to consume sugary drinks in anything other than minicans.[33]

18

Investing in Sponsorships and Community Partnerships

Big Soda spends fortunes on sports, entertainment, and community initiatives to, as one consulting firm states, "establish an emotional connection with consumers and drive sales volume." The companies do this through sponsorships and partnerships that appear to be (and sometimes genuinely are) philanthropic, although their underlying purpose is always to promote the brand.

SPONSORING SPORTS

Coca-Cola spent more than $290 million on sponsorships in the United States alone in 2013, PepsiCo spent more than $350 million, and Dr Pepper Snapple spent more than $40 million. Although some of the money is spent on entertainment, such as PepsiCo's $50 million deal with Beyoncé, discussed in Chapter 14, most sponsorship expenditures—64 percent—go for sports. Outside the United States, of Coca-Cola's global $300 million sponsorship spending and PepsiCo's $390 million, 84 percent goes for sports events. Coca-Cola, for example, has sponsored the Olympic Games since 1928 (including those in Nazi Germany in 1936) and has been an official sponsor of the World Cup since 1978. Table 18.1 gives some examples from 2013.[1]

These kinds of sponsorships demonstrably increase sales. They also earn business awards for the companies.[2] In response to criticism of its use

TABLE 18.1 Coca-Cola and PepsiCo top sports sponsorship deals, 2013

COCA-COLA	PEPSICO
International Olympic Committee	International Cricket Council
FC Barcelona	Manchester United Football Club
Real Madrid Club de Fútbol	Indian Premier League
Fédération Internationale de Football Association	Asian Football Confederation
Paris Saint-Germain Football Club	Confederation of African Football
Union of European Football Associations	National Football League
International Ice Hockey Federation	Major League Baseball
National Basketball Association*	National Hockey League

* In 2015, PepsiCo replaced Coca-Cola in this partnership.

of sports figures and sponsorship of premier sporting events, Coca-Cola invokes physical activity:

> The Coca-Cola Company promotes exercise as vital to everyone's health and well-being. By supporting physical activity and nutrition education programs in the communities it serves, Coca-Cola is working to help provide workable solutions to the problem of obesity and support efforts to increase physical activity worldwide. Coca-Cola sponsors more than 280 physical activity and nutrition education programs in more than 115 countries.[3]

Sponsorship of sports heroes and sports events advertises the brand, gives sodas a health aura, and makes them seem as cool as can be. Athletes too would be healthier drinking less soda.

PARTNERING WITH COMMUNITIES

As part of their commitments to corporate social responsibility (CSR), soda companies spend money in communities, although much less than on sports. PepsiCo explains: "PepsiCo is building brighter futures in the communities where we operate, through strategic grants provided by the PepsiCo Foundation and through employee volunteering and community service. We are making a difference every day by investing in our communities." Through its Global Citizenship initiatives, PepsiCo targets philanthropy to improving health, the environment, and communities. It specifically funds international community programs aimed at enabling job readiness and empowering women and girls. The PepsiCo Foundation spent $3 million on such programs in 2012.[4]

Coca-Cola says that since 1984 it has donated $650 million to support community initiatives worldwide, with a goal of giving back "1 percent of its prior year's operating income annually." The company's "enduring commitment to building sustainable communities…is focused on initiatives that reduce our environmental footprint, support active, healthy living, create a safe, inclusive work environment for our associates, and enhance the economic development of the communities where we operate."[5] In 2013, Coke invested $143 million in philanthropic contributions aimed at three priority areas: the economic empowerment of women, access to clean water, and active healthy living. Its foundation also supports arts and culture and economic development in the United States and HIV/AIDS prevention and awareness programs in Africa and Latin America.

PepsiCo funds community programs as well, but Coke provides more detailed listings in its various reports. Table 18.2 provides a few examples.

TABLE 18.2 Community initiatives funded by Coca-Cola, selected examples, 2013

COUNTRY	AMOUNT DONATED	COMMUNITY INITIATIVE
Australia	$77,000	Australian Indigenous Mentoring Experience
Azerbaijan	$100,000	Debate in Civil Society Public Union, Youth Inc. Program
France	$260,000	UNIS CITE, Booster Dropout Prevention Program
Indonesia	$104,000	The Ancora Foundation, Vocational Studies Scholarship
Israel	$40,000	Young Business Leadership, Young Business Leadership Program
Pakistan	$75,000	Kashf Foundation, Mainstreaming Female Entrepreneurs Through Microfinance and Capacity Building
Palestine	$50,000	INJAZ Palestine, NBC/INJAZ Palestine—Leadership
Spain	$187,440	Cruz Roja Espanola, Building Bridges Between the Job Market and Unemployed Young People
United States	$10,000	Portland, Oregon, park improvements
	$25,000	New Jersey Performing Arts Center, arts education
	$50,000	Georgia Charter Schools Association, Georgia Charter School of the Year Award
	$3 million	Garfield Park Conservatory Alliance, Park Families Wellness Initiative to create jobs for veterans, Chicago

SOURCE: Coca-Cola Foundation reports, 2nd and 3rd quarters, 2013.

The programs listed in Table 18.2 are just a small sample of those funded by soda companies over the past few years. But these examples indicate the breadth of funding and the inherent worthiness of the funded causes. For many of these groups, the money from soda companies surely makes a critical difference in what they are able to accomplish. Coke, as we see, is an equal opportunity funder. It funds programs in Palestine as well as in Israel. People in both places drink Coca-Cola.

The company calls its flagship community program "5 by 20." The numbers refer to the program's stated aim—to promote the economic empowerment of 5 million women entrepreneurs by 2020. The company aims to accomplish this goal by training women in business skills and providing access to financial services and networks of mentors and peers. Coke reports that the program reached 550,000 women in forty-four countries by the end of 2013. For women enrolled in 5 by 20, Coke funding provides an entry point into the entrepreneurial world. The company enables women who may have no other options to start small businesses throughout the Coca-Cola value chain—from fruit farmers to small retailers selling Coke and Coke products to artisans creating items from Coke packaging materials.[6]

Coke is not the only soda company to use community philanthropy as part of its CSR initiatives. PepsiCo reports $99 million in citizenship contributions in 2012. Dr Pepper Snapple's ACTION Nation program promotes "physically active, engaged and sustainable communities through volunteering and local sponsorships." DPS expects its employees to donate time to nonprofit organizations, and says that by 2015 they will have performed a total of 100,000 volunteer hours and provided $10 million annually in charitable cash donations. This company wants community efforts focused on four areas: fit and active lifestyles, environmental initiatives, celebrations, and emergency relief.[7]

These exemplary-sounding efforts mask their underlying business purposes. Grants to groups engaged in worthy causes facilitate the work of recipients but also encourage them to be grateful—and eager to do anything necessary to keep the funding coming, even to the extent of supporting the soda industry when it opposes public health measures. If nothing else, community grants buy silence about the health consequences of excessive soda consumption.

Sometimes, if philanthropy does not bring immediate returns on investment, the effort gets dropped. The most poignant example of this reality is the Pepsi Refresh Project, initiated in 2010. Pepsi offered millions of dollars in grants for community projects nominated and voted on by the public through a dedicated website. Many millions of people voted, and the winning projects received from $5,000 to $250,000. *GOOD Magazine*, whose mission is to "support and celebrate creative solutions to critical issues," partnered with Pepsi Refresh and worked closely with funding recipients.[8]

But the program soon ran into trouble on two counts. Because PepsiCo was unable to monitor the integrity of submitted programs in advance, it had to deal with questions of fraud. It also had to deal with questions about core values. A Harvard Business School case study on the project quoted a critic: "What do Pepsi and Coke actually sell? Soft drinks; liquid with a lot of sugar and no vitamins. And now they want to get associated with health, planet, art and culture, food and shelter, neighborhoods, and education? Using social media? I am very sorry, but I think there is a value clash somewhere."[9]

More telling, the Pepsi Refresh program had no discernible effect on Pepsi sales. When the sales gap became evident, the company introduced bonus voting points for people who showed proof of Pepsi purchases. When that action also failed to increase sales, the company ended the program and refocused its strategies on celebrity endorsements. One business analyst asked, "What *are* we to think about a brand that promises to make the world better and then drops everything when the going gets tough?... [I]t's hard to see the Pepsi Refresh Project as anything but a well-intentioned, innovative experiment that nonetheless siphoned a lot of money and focus from building the brand's core equity."[10]

In its 2013 analysis of food company philanthropy, the Center for Science in the Public Interest (CSPI) noted how closely philanthropy is linked to marketing, so much so that CSPI has a name for this strategy: "philanthro-marketing." The report produced this telling statistic: for every $1 that Coca-Cola donated to community causes in 2010, it spent $170 marketing its sugar-laden beverages. And PepsiCo's $2.3 million contribution to sustainability programs in 2011 was "dwarfed by the company's $60 million sponsorship of just one television show—*The X Factor*."[11]

PROVIDING COMMUNITY DISASTER RELIEF

But surely disaster relief is free of anything but altruistic motives? Soda companies are indeed quick to join relief efforts, usually in partnership with relief organizations. They often, if not always, provide in-kind contributions of sodas or branded bottled waters. In the company's 2011/2012 Performance with a Purpose report, PepsiCo noted that it contributed millions of dollars in disaster relief through organizations such as the Red Cross, Feeding America, and the World Food Program. As examples, PepsiCo cited $1 million in relief to victims of an earthquake in China's Sichuan province, $1.4 million—and thirty truckloads of foods and beverages—to victims of Hurricane Sandy, and $950,000 to the World Food Program for disaster relief in Pakistan.

Coke listed recipients of its disaster relief dollars and in-kind beverage contributions in its 2013/2014 Sustainability Report. Some of the donations were gifts to local Red Cross chapters. Table 18.3 gives a few examples.

I have no doubt that the victims of such disasters are grateful for whatever help they can get. They need and can use the bottled water. Whether they need sodas in these situations is another matter, but international victims of disasters are likely to enjoy donations of Coke or Pepsi products with which they were previously unfamiliar or had been unable to buy because of the cost. The in-kind contributions create substantial goodwill and can fill a genuine need. But they invariably come with strings. For soda companies, disaster relief has an additional purpose: it presents opportunities for introducing branded products into markets that might otherwise be difficult to penetrate. As the Pepsi Refresh example suggests, the marketing objectives remain paramount, and do so even in desperate situations.

TABLE 18.3 Coca-Cola's contributions to disaster relief, selected examples, 2013

COUNTRY	DONATION, CASH	DONATION, BEVERAGES	DISASTER RELIEF
Argentina	$100,000	120,000 liters	Flooding in Buenos Aires province
Central Europe	Unspecified	Unspecified	Heavy rain, flooding, landslides
China	$1.3 million	2.4 million bottles	Earthquake in Sichuan province
Mexico	$700,000	Unspecified	Hurricanes
Philippines	$2 million	$500,000 worth	Typhoon
United States	$100,000	Unspecified	Flash floods in Colorado
	$100,000	10,000 cases	Tornado in Oklahoma

SODA COMPANY PHILANTHROPY: A DILEMMA FOR ADVOCATES

In talking to people who work for international development or health agencies, I can see how conflicted they feel about soda company sponsorship of their projects. They tell me that small businesses and kiosks funded by soda companies enable poor people, particularly women with limited options, to earn a living by selling Coke and Pepsi products or otherwise working in the soda production chain. They are well aware that the kiosks sell high-fat and high-sugar packaged snack foods along with the sodas. But what other options are available to these women? Hence the dilemma.

The programs do bring some women out of poverty, but at a cost. They force the women to depend on soda companies and to push products that customers do not need and often can hardly afford. The benefits to participating women rarely extend beyond immediate sales and are not necessarily sustainable if the women want to advance. The benefits to the companies are much better defined. The programs expand soda sales to hard-to-reach populations. They induce brand loyalty. And they protect soda companies against criticism that their products promote obesity and type 2 diabetes among populations especially vulnerable to these conditions.

19

Supporting Worthy Causes

Health Professionals and Research

In this chapter, I focus on one particular expression of the "support worthy causes" strategy of corporate social responsibility—the soda industry's partnerships with health professionals and their associations, and its sponsorship of research studies in support of soda company objectives.

PARTNERING WITH NUTRITION AND HEALTH PROFESSIONALS

Soda companies expend considerable effort and expense to convince health professionals that sodas are merely beverages to enjoy and can be ignored as contributing in any special way to obesity or other health conditions. This strategy goes way back. In 1950, Cornell professor Clive McCay—famous for, among other things, dropping teeth into glasses of Coca-Cola and watching them dissolve—testified to Congress that the combination of sugar and acids in soft drinks caused tooth decay. The Coca-Cola company appointed a committee to respond to McCay and his fellow "food faddists, communists, crackpots, and the like." It gave a $5,000 grant and, later, other grants to Dr. Fred Stare (1910–2002), then chair of nutrition at Harvard Medical School. Stare wrote letters stating that Coke did not cause cavities. In 1954, he wrote an article on teenage diets for *McCall's* magazine recommending "soda, ice cream, or a Coke" as appropriate midafternoon snacks (thereby distinguishing Cokes from other sodas). Coke also funded the research of a prominent clinician at Emory University who demonstrated that sodas had no effect on teeth, and gave him a $12,000 annual stipend when he retired.[1]

Today, you might expect researchers, physicians, and nutritionists who work with overweight patients to be among the most vociferous critics of soda companies, and many are. But others, alas, are not. The soda deniers may view sugary drinks as only a trivial part of much greater diet-and-exercise or social problems. Some even extol the virtues of sodas as potential vehicles for improving the nutritional status of desperately poor populations.[2] Others may consider soda companies to be good corporate citizens whose iconic brands merit no special concern. Soda companies work hard—and spend generously—to institutionalize the view that partnerships, alliances, and personal friendships between health professionals and soda companies and their executives should raise no concerns about conflicts of interest.

But my interpretation is that these relationships are conflicted, and deeply so. To explain why, let me give four examples from 2014 and 2015. The first is the appointment of cardiologist Victor Dzau, former chancellor for health affairs at Duke University, to the presidency of the Institute of Medicine (IOM). During his time at Duke, Dzau came under scrutiny for his membership on the boards of directors of several corporations, PepsiCo among them, and the failure of the university to fully disclose these memberships. Dzau joined the PepsiCo board in 2005. In 2009, his compensation as director amounted to $260,000. By the time he accepted the IOM position in 2013, he owned 32,592 shares of PepsiCo stock, valued at about $2.5 million. Despite IOM committees having produced reports recommending reduced soda consumption, the IOM search committee evidently did not view financial connections with a soda company as a deal breaker. The IOM simply announced that "Dr. Dzau had already decided to step down from corporate boards before he accepted the position."[3] Whether the IOM under his leadership will continue to examine how sodas affect health remains to be seen, but Dzau's long and lucrative relationship with PepsiCo appears to be a potential conflict, at least until proven otherwise.

My second example comes from Great Britain, where a professor from Nottingham University, Ian Macdonald, was appointed to head a committee to propose a new dietary guideline for the nation's sugar consumption despite having disclosed that he received an annual consulting fee of £6,100 from Coca-Cola for advice about diet, obesity, and exercise. Five out of the seven members of his committee also received funds from Coca-Cola, other food companies, or a lobbying group, Sugar Nutrition. The British Department of Health issued a statement: "Professor Ian Macdonald has fully declared his conflicts of interest in accordance with the Code of Practice. He is a highly respected figure within the public health community and has made a valuable contribution to research into obesity and nutrition."[4] This agency also stated its disbelief that financial relationships with Coca-Cola might influence opinions about sugar intake. But as with Dzau, Macdonald arrived at his new and sensitive position with at least the appearance of a potential conflict.

The third example has to do with the Robert Wood Johnson Foundation (RWJF), the leading U.S. funder of anti-obesity initiatives—including those aimed at reducing soda consumption. Nevertheless, the head of the foundation, Dr. Risa Lavizzo-Mourey, seems to have close ties to PepsiCo's CEO, Indra Nooyi. In 2010, the RWJF-funded Trust for America produced an annual report on obesity that included a two-page statement from Nooyi on PepsiCo's role in fighting obesity; she was one of several "policy-makers and experts in the field of obesity" invited to offer perspectives on the topic. This was an opportunity for Nooyi to quote the playbook: "We firmly believe companies have a responsibility to provide consumers with more information and more choices so they can make better decisions."[5]

In 2014, Lavizzo-Mourey and Nooyi were interviewed together at a press event to celebrate the fulfilling of a pledge made by food and beverage companies to cut 1.5 trillion calories from their products. RWJF funded the study that validated the reduction. Although critics termed the pledge a "marketing ploy" and a "sham," not least because the reduction amounted to just a few calories a day per person, Nooyi used the occasion to demand applause for industry progress, to express frustration with the "endless criticism from activists who blame obesity on the food industry," and to invoke the blessing of the RWJF: "If we can pass the RWJF screens, I think we've done pretty good." On the matter of taxes and other regulatory efforts, Nooyi quoted the playbook: "I don't think we want to become a nanny state.... Freedom of choice is very important." When asked whether the RWJF supported such views, Lavizzo-Mourey said that the foundation had published reports unfavorable to industry, but when the industry did something right, it was important to "pause and say, 'We met that goal.'"[6] In that instance at least, having a connection to the head of a health foundation was good for PepsiCo's reputation and business interests.

My final example: In February 2015, Candice Choi, a reporter for the Minneapolis *Star Tribune*, revealed that Coca-Cola had recruited dietitians to write articles and blog posts on the theme "Heart Health and Black History

Month." Each of the posts described or illustrated a minican of Coke as an appropriate snack. Most—but not all—of the articles disclosed that the author "consulted" for Coca-Cola, but only one said the article was "sponsored." A spokesman for Coca-Cola explained that the company has "a network of dietitians we work with... Every big brand works with bloggers or has paid talent."[7]

At this point, I must confess to my own experience with soda company generosity. I have attended sessions at annual meetings of the American Society for Nutrition (ASN) sponsored by PepsiCo, subscribed to and read professional journals supported in part by grants from Coca-Cola, given lectures in the PepsiCo auditorium in Cornell University's food science department, visited soda company exhibits at annual meetings of the Academy for Nutrition and Dietetics, and once attended Coca-Cola's glamorous, supermodel runway presentation of red dresses, held during New York City's Fashion Week. This last event is part of Diet Coke's ongoing partnership with the National Heart, Lung, and Blood Institute, from which I have acquired a small collection of souvenir red dress pins. Unless I never leave my office, cancel my subscriptions to professional journals, and resign memberships in professional organizations, it is impossible for me to avoid benefiting from soda company largesse, given the ubiquity of its presence.

From these examples and the others I discuss in this chapter, I conclude that the reach of soda companies—personally and financially—goes deep into the health professional community, but these connections are hardly ever noticed, let alone elicit the level of critical scrutiny and ethical analysis that I believe they acutely deserve.

PARTNERING WITH NUTRITION AND HEALTH ASSOCIATIONS

The ASN is the premier professional association for nutrition researchers in the United States. It is supported by Coca-Cola and PepsiCo, among many other food companies, as sustaining partners. A session at its annual meeting in 2013 suggests why such partnerships merit critical attention. The Corn Refiners Association (CRA), which represents producers of high-fructose corn syrup, sponsored a session entitled "Sweetened Beverages and Health: Current State of Scientific Understanding." Speakers who reported consulting for Coca-Cola and PepsiCo gave talks on soda facts, solid vs. liquid calories, sugar addiction, and the metabolic consequences of sugar and soda consumption. Their statements were so utterly dismissive of health concerns about caloric sweeteners that I was not surprised when the CRA posted videos of the talks on its sweetener research website. You can watch the presentations and judge for yourself whether they reflect unbiased accounts of the research.[8]

Food and beverage company sponsorship is deeply embedded in the activities of the Academy of Nutrition and Dietetics (AND), the organization of professional dietitians formerly known as the American Dietetic Association—so much so that it became the subject of an investigative report by Michele Simon in 2013. Her report described soda companies' exhibits at AND's annual meeting, as well as their sponsorship of continuing education activities. The organization provides continuing education credits to members who attend lectures by sponsored speakers who explain why sugar is not harmful to children and why school nutrition standards that exclude sodas are unnecessarily restrictive. AND gives its corporate partners "the right to co-create, co-brand an Academy-themed informational consumer campaign." Through this mechanism, AND endorses Diet Coke's Heart Truth Campaign, featuring the red dresses and souvenir pins. A reporter who interviewed dietitians attending an AND convention in California found hardly any who realized that scientific sessions were sponsored by food companies.[9]

Both Coca-Cola and PepsiCo are "premier" sponsors of AND. Coca-Cola engages with AND through the company's Beverage Institute for Health and Wellness (BIHW), which AND authorizes to provide continuing education credits for dietitians and nurses. As Coke explains, the Beverage Institute

> is part of The Coca-Cola Company's ongoing commitment to use evidence-based science to advance knowledge and understanding of beverages, beverage ingredients, and the important role that active healthy lifestyles play in supporting health and wellbeing... [It] supports the educational needs of health professionals by sponsoring free continuing professional education (CE/CPE) programs led by recognized experts in fields such as nutrition, medicine, nursing, physical activity, behavior change, toxicology and various food science disciplines. All BIHW-sponsored CE/CPE programs meet the professional education standards of the Commission on Dietetic Registration (CDR).[10]

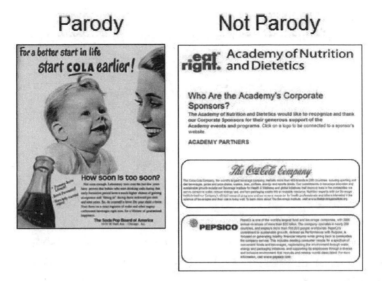

FIGURE 19.1 That soda companies sponsor the Academy of Nutrition and Dietetics is fodder for satire. The Soda Pop Board of America is entirely fictitious, but Coke and Pepsi's "wellness" partnerships with the academy are not. Courtesy of Robert Hutkins, University of Nebraska. The parody advertisement is from marketing executive R. J. White, used with permission.

The cozy relationships between Coke, Pepsi, and the academy are so blatant that they inspire satire. An example is shown in Figure 19.1.[11]

In 2013, PepsiCo's exhibit at the AND conference promoted a "mobile-based, interactive game that will challenge your wits and give you the chance to win fantastic rewards. All you have to do is visit the Check-In kiosk...and immediately start earning points to win amazing prizes." Coca-Cola's BIHW offers a long list of programs available for continuing professional education credits. Among them are sessions on topics such as these (with my translations of the take-home messages):[12]

- Energy balance [*soda calories don't count*]
- Mindful eating [*soda companies are not responsible for what you eat; you are*]
- Physical activity [*you can ignore soda calories*]
- Hydration [*sodas are an excellent substitute for water*]
- Myths about children's dietary recommendations [*sodas are fine for kids*]

- Translating scientific information into public health advice [*the evidence linking sodas to health problems is so flawed that you can ignore it*]

ASN and AND, of course, are not the only health professions organizations to accept soda company sponsorship. Table 19.1 provides some additional examples.

How do AND members view such involvement? In 2011, researchers at Simmons College surveyed nearly three thousand of the academy's members. In response to the question "Some professional associations accept funding from corporate sponsors. Do you believe the [academy] should also accept funding from corporate sponsors?" only 10 percent answered yes. The vast majority, 68 percent, said that the answer depended on the sponsor, and almost as many (66 percent) said that neither Coca-Cola nor PepsiCo was an acceptable sponsor. Some AND members, concerned that sponsorship affects their credibility, created their own advocacy group, Dietitians for Professional Integrity, aimed at ending financial ties with food and beverage

TABLE 19.1 Soda company sponsorship of other health and nutrition professional organizations, selected examples, 2012–2013

COMPANY	SPONSORED ORGANIZATION, PROGRAM
Coca-Cola	Juvenile Diabetes Research Foundation, Spring for a Cure campaign
	International Union of Nutritional Sciences, quadrennial International Conference on Nutrition
	Institute of Food Technologists, annual meeting career fair
	American Academy of Pediatrics, HealthyChildren.org website
	American College of Cardiology, CardioSmart program
	American Diabetes Association programs for education and outreach to the Latino community
	Ensemble Prévenons l'Obésité Des Enfants (EPODE, Together Let's Prevent Childhood Obesity) international network
	Flemish Professional Association of Food Experts and Dietitians advertising campaign, "Sugar Can Be Part of a Healthy Diet."
	Obesity Network Summit, Canada
	Monell Center, fellowship in taste biology
	Boston Medical Center, Drucker Award for nonprofit innovation
	Obesity Society, early career investigator travel grants
	International Hydration Conference, Spain
PepsiCo and Coca-Cola	The Sackler Institute for Nutrition Science, New York
	Institute of Food Technologists Student Association, Fun Run & Walk
PepsiCo	Yale alumni conference on women's leadership

companies: "We are a group of concerned dietetics professionals advocating for greater financial transparency, as well as ethical, socially responsible, and relevant corporate sponsorships within the Academy of Nutrition and Dietetics.... We do not think Coca-Cola, PepsiCo, Kellogg's, and other Big Food giants should sponsor the country's largest nutrition organization."[13]

Other sponsorships also have incited organized protest. When Coca-Cola gave a grant to the American Academy of Family Physicians (AAFP) to pay for its educational website (FamilyDoctor.org), family practice doctors in Contra Costa County, California, publicly tore up their membership cards (Figure 19.2). In his statement of resignation, the director of the Contra Costa County Health Department, Dr. William Walker, asked, "How can any organization that claims to promote public health join forces with a company that promotes products that put our children at risk for obesity, heart disease and early death?" Other physicians also view such alliances as counter to the ethical standards of family practice.[14]

You don't have to think hard to understand why soda companies might be eager to sponsor health professionals and their associations. They want to head off advice to consume less soda and to encourage neutral positions

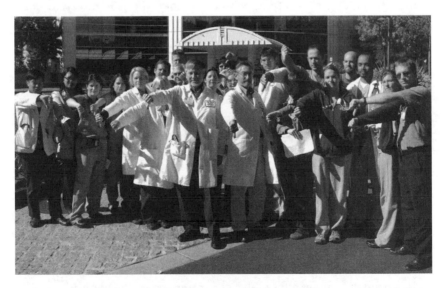

FIGURE 19.2 Family physicians demonstrate against Coca-Cola's partnership with their professional society. Twenty doctors in Contra Costa County, California, resigned their memberships in the American Academy of Family Physicians to protest its acceptance of an educational grant from Coca-Cola, 2009. Courtesy of Dr. William Walker, director, Contra Costa County Department of Health Services.

on soda consumption—to buy silence, if nothing else. Sponsorship leads to "corporate capture," the term used to explain the undue influence of corporations on public institutions or, in this case, on health professionals whose major concern ought to be public health.[15]

It is difficult to document silencing, but examples occasionally surface. A report on soda industry sponsorship by the Center for Science in the Public Interest cites several instances of how "reputable health organizations with financial ties to the beverage industry have echoed industry talking points, remained silent on soda issues, or actually opposed policies that the industry opposes." More recently, the president of the sixteenth World Congress of Food Science and Technology in Brazil cancelled a debate on the causes of childhood obesity explicitly because it might drive away food company sponsors.[16]

SPONSORING NUTRITION AND HEALTH RESEARCH

You can most easily observe corporate capture by food and beverage companies by looking at what happens when they sponsor research. Soda companies actively encourage scientists to apply for grants to conduct research studies, and some scientists are willing, perhaps eager, to take advantage of such opportunities. It is no coincidence that the conclusions of sponsored studies almost invariably favor the sponsor's interest. An examination of this non-coincidence in 2007 found industry-funded studies, many of them dealing with sodas, to be nearly eight times more likely to produce results favorable to the sponsor than studies with no industry funding. More recently, a review of reviews of the effects of sodas on weight gain found soda-sponsored studies to be five times more likely to find no effect. The investigators said 83 percent of soda-funded reviews showed little or no evidence for a link between sodas and weight gain, whereas the same percentage of independently funded studies observed strong associations. In general, reviews funded by soda companies rarely find evidence for negative health effects of soda consumption. In contrast, reviews funded by independent sources almost always demonstrate such connections.[17]

The discrepancy between the results of soda-funded and independently funded studies is so strikingly consistent that anytime I see a report of a study exonerating sodas from harmful effects, my first impulse is to look to see who paid for it. It isn't that I view industry-funded science as "bought."

This situation requires a more nuanced explanation. Industry-funded scientists tend to believe that such funding is appropriate and has no influence on how they design or interpret their research. The evidence, however, strongly suggests otherwise.

Research design involves choices of questions, assumptions, methods, and controls. It is not difficult to conduct a study that appears to meet high scientific standards, yet fails to include necessary controls that might lead to more critical conclusions or interpretations. Well-trained scientists know that for every study they do, they must take special care to control and compensate for unconscious bias. Industry-funded researchers need to do this even more. But controlling for unconscious bias is possible only when researchers recognize unconscious bias as a possibility, which many do not. By now, most scientific journals are so acutely aware of the biases introduced by industry sponsorship that they require authors to disclose funding sources and other potential conflicts of interest. Disclosure makes it easier to check for sponsorship, but it is not sufficient to dismiss concerns about such conflicts.

To illustrate this point, I provide in Table 19.2 some examples of sponsored studies on sodas and health published in medical or health journals, most of them peer-reviewed. Most journals demand that authors disclose such information, and they do. But in my reading of editors' summaries of peer review comments, the reviewers, who are nearly always anonymous, rarely pay attention to sponsorship, let alone consider soda company sponsorship to be a sufficient cause for rejecting a paper. On the basis of the examples in the table, I think they should. The studies listed here were either paid for by soda companies or the American Beverage Association, or conducted by investigators who reported financial ties of one kind or another with soda companies. Their results firmly support industry values and business interests.

Some of these researchers consult for and have close ties to soda companies. But even more distant connections—doing research at a university that accepts soda industry grants, for example—seem to produce results consistently favorable to industry. At the very least, the connections give the appearance of conflict of interest and call for some skepticism.

Researchers who accept food and beverage industry sponsorship defend the practice with little discomfort, in part because they do not view it as influential or conflicting. This issue was discussed at the 2013 annual meeting of the ASN at a session devoted to industry funding of nutrition research. The session, however, was sponsored in part by the International

TABLE 19.2 Selected examples of studies funded directly by Coca-Cola or the American Beverage Association, or conducted by investigators with financial ties to these groups, 2012–2014

TOPIC OF STUDY	CONCLUSION (MY TRANSLATION)	SPONSORSHIP*
The cause of the worldwide increase in body weight	"Declining trends in energy expenditure explain the obesity pandemic"[a] (*What you eat doesn't matter*).	Coca-Cola supported publication and gave unrestricted research grants to three of the six authors.
Methods for measuring effects of sodas on health	"We found considerable variability... which renders these studies difficult to interpret collectively"[b] (*You don't need to believe meta-analyses suggesting that sodas cause health problems*).	The study was funded by Coca-Cola.
Validity of the National Health and Nutrition Examination Survey (NHANES)	"Methodological limitations compromise the validity... and the empirical foundation for formulating dietary guidelines and public health policies"[c] (*Dietary advice to drink less soda has no scientific basis*).	Coca-Cola funded the study and provided grants or fees to two of the three authors.
Interpretation of findings linking sodas to health problems	"Overreaching in presenting results in studies focused on nutrition and obesity topics is common in articles published in leading journals"[d] (*The link between sodas and health is exaggerated; you can ignore it*).	Coca-Cola originally funded the project.
Will reducing soda intake reduce obesity?	"Evidence to date is equivocal"[e] (*Pay no attention to it*).	The senior author's university receives grants from Coca-Cola and PepsiCo.
Metabolic implications of consuming sodas	"Great caution must be used when suggesting adverse health effects of consuming these sugars"[f] (*Sugars in soft drinks are harmless*).	Author consults for Coca-Cola and PepsiCo
The role of sugars in diabetes	"No unequivocal evidence that fructose intake at moderate doses is directly related with adverse metabolic effects or contributes excess energy to diets"[g] (*The sugars in sodas are not harmful to health*).	Coca-Cola supported the study's publication and provided grants to the senior author, who also consults with the company.
Sodas and cancer risk	"Overall, the findings are reassuring in terms of the association between soft drinks, including colas, and cancer risk"[h] (*You don't need to worry about the effects of sodas on health*).	Although Coca-Cola paid for the study, the authors reported, "There are no conflicts of interest."

TABLE 19.2 Continued

Ethical implications of obesity interventions	"Do not assume that achieving a health benefit overrides respect for other values and ethical principles"[i] (*Public health measures to prevent obesity raise serious ethical issues*).	Coca-Cola provided grants to both authors.
Health benefits of diet sodas	"Water is not superior to NNS [non-nutritive sweetened] beverages for weight loss."[j] (*Diet sodas are good for health*).	Study fully funded by the American Beverage Association; two of the investigators received consulting fees from Coca-Cola.
Is soda industry self-regulation effective?	"Self-regulation can be a powerful tool in the fight against obesity"[k] (*Public health measures to regulate soda consumption are unnecessary*).	The American Beverage Association financed the data collection.

* Journals require authors to disclose this information; it usually appears on the first page or just preceding the reference list. [a] Shook RP, et al. US Endocrinology, *2014;10(1)*:44–52. [b] Althuis MD, Weed DL. AJCN, *2013;98*:755–68. [c] Archer E, et al. PLoS ONE, *2013;8(10)*:e76632. [d] Menachemi N, et al. Am J Prev Med, *2013;45(5)*:615–621. [e] Kaiser KA, et al. Obesity Rev, *2013;14,620–633.* [f] Rippe JM. Advances in Nutr, *2013;4*:677–686. [g] Cozma AI, Sievenpiper JL. US Endocrinology, *2013;9(2)*:128–138. [h] Boyle P, et al. European J Cancer Pre, *2014*; doi: 10.1097/CEJ.0000000000000015. [i] Brown AW, Allison DB. Virtual Mentor, *2013;15*:339–346. [j] Peters JC, et al. Obesity, *2014;22*:1415–1421. [k] Wescott RF, et al. AJPH, *2012;102(10)*:1928–35.

Life Sciences Institute, which is funded largely by food manufacturers, among them Coca-Cola and PepsiCo. It was hardly a debate. The speakers, one of them employed by PepsiCo, emphasized the benefits of sponsored research and ignored or dismissed concerns about conflicts of interest. Public-private research partnerships (PPPs), they said, "are necessary for the progress of science. Industry can and should contribute extensive expertise, data sets, biological samples, funding, and a sound business perspective to partnerships. PPPs can help generate a common language and high-quality consensus science while addressing important unmet public health needs."[18] Objections to the biased nature of industry-sponsored "debates" are routinely ignored by ASN staff, for whom fund-raising is a high priority.

Industry-sponsored investigators explain the practice as essential at a time of scarce government research funding. They view it as harmless. At least some respond to suggestions that industry funding might influence their research as highly offensive personal attacks on their scientific integrity. The lead author of the sponsored NHANES study listed in Table 19.2, for example, explained to a reporter who had interviewed me about conflicts in nutrition science, "I'm criticizing the federal government, and it's not going to give us money for research, so I have to go outside....Coke doesn't know what we're doing. I guess when you can't attack the science, attack the scientist."[19]

Beyond such defenses, sponsored scientists criticize the motives and ethics of independently funded investigators whose research concludes that sodas do affect health. Such investigators, they charge, are victims of "white-hat bias," abbreviated WHB. This syndrome, they say, leads public health researchers to ignore studies with negative findings. Researchers affected by WHB, they assert, are "fueled by feelings of righteous zeal, indignation toward certain aspects of industry, or other factors. Readers should beware of WHB, and our field should seek methods to minimize it."[20]

The authors who made this charge admit that they consult for Coca-Cola and PepsiCo and are paid to advise the companies. They also disclose receiving "grants, honoraria, donations, and consulting fees from numerous food, beverage, dietary supplement, pharmaceutical companies, litigators and other commercial, government, and nonprofit entities with interests in obesity and nutrition." One of them was the subject of an ABC television report probing the effects of food industry sponsorship on nutrition science. The ABC investigators emphasized the parallels between the attack-the-science tactics of Big Soda and those that had been used for years to great effect by Big Tobacco.[21]

In a review of studies that link funding source to the outcome of research on the effects of pharmaceutical drugs, tobacco, and bisphenol-A (BPA, the endocrine-disrupting plasticizer), the bioethicist Sheldon Krimsky concluded that the correlation between research outcome and funding source may not be "definitive evidence of bias, but is prima facie evidence that bias may exist."[22] When you read studies funded by industry, he suggests, the default hypothesis always needs to be that the results are due to bias. The ethicist Jonathan Marks notes that private-public partnerships with food companies are especially perilous because when they frame obesity concerns solely as matters of personal responsibility, they inevitably undermine the mission, integrity, and credibility of the public or health professional partner. The consistently favorable-to-industry results of soda-sponsored research provides ample evidence for such concerns.

Independently funded scientists may have biases of their own, but their overarching research goal is to produce high-quality, reproducible results that will lead to improved public health. In contrast, the goal of soda companies is to use research as a marketing tool or to cast doubt on the science that links sugary drinks to obesity and chronic diseases. That is why soda company sponsorship of research at universities should concern everyone who cares about scientific integrity and credibility. PepsiCo, for example, funds a public-private partnership with universities in the Netherlands to conduct research on nutrition and muscle function in athletes and the elderly. Surely the purpose of this sponsorship is to focus attention on the output side of calorie balance. PepsiCo also funds a project at the Yale University Bioethics Center to establish guidelines for nutrition research using human subjects and to train PepsiCo research staff in research ethics. Is this center likely to host a debate on the ethics of marketing sugary soft drinks to children? I doubt it. PepsiCo funds a nutrition fellowship in Yale's Medical Scientist Training Program (MD/PhD) for a trainee whose work focuses on diabetes, obesity, and metabolic syndrome. It seems unlikely that any Pepsi-sponsored fellow will be engaged in research adding to the existing body of evidence that soda consumption raises risks for these conditions.[23] As Michele Simon explains:

> When food companies such as PepsiCo (even when speaking through their own scientific experts) opine on a major public health problem, we are not about to hear the entire story, but rather one filtered through the corporate agenda, which by definition must promote its bottom line, and thus omit the less flattering aspects. That's why no matter how many MDs or PhDs the company hires, or how many public health reports it infiltrates, PepsiCo should never be looked to as an expert on anything other than what it does best: marketing and selling highly processed food and beverage products to the world.[24]

SHOULD NUTRITION AND HEALTH PROFESSIONALS ACCEPT FUNDING FROM SODA COMPANIES?

Although in theory food company financial support should not necessarily bias results, opinions, or actions, in practice it appears to or does. The biasing comes as a result of corporate imperatives to increase shareholder value. For the soda industry, partnerships with health organizations provide substantial benefits: they give credibility, increase consumer loyalty, engage researchers' cooperation, and silence criticism that the products cause harm.

The soda industry's "healthwashing" strategies should remind you of those used by the tobacco industry. That industry was well aware that sponsored researchers do not—and, perhaps, cannot—recognize their loss of objectivity. This failure of recognition is best observed in the reactions of sponsored researchers to the slightest suggestion that the funding source might influence how they design, conduct, or interpret research. Because the goals of health and nutrition professionals and researchers are not the same as those of food and beverage companies, conflicts of interest must always be considered a strong possibility in industry-funded research.[25]

At the twentieth International Congress of Nutrition (ICN), held in Granada in 2013, industry sponsors played prominent roles. Investigators from the World Public Health Nutrition Association (which refuses all industry funding) used this situation as an opportunity to probe attitudes about corporate funding. They compared the responses of speakers at an ICN scientific session funded and organized by Coca-Cola to those of speakers in unsponsored scientific sessions. As expected, the sponsored speakers generally favored food industry sponsorship and judged the benefits to be greater than the risks. In contrast, independently funded speakers were more skeptical and generally agreed on several points:

- Big Food uses its links with scientists and officials to distort science, confuse professionals and the public, provoke false debates, and distort reputations.
- The public, the media, and policy makers are unlikely to respect information or advice that comes from researchers sponsored by Big Food.
- The need for science to be funded independently is compromised when industry is encouraged to support scientists.
- Overt and covert links with Big Food are against the interests of public health and nutrition professionals.[26]

In an ideal world, such issues would never arise. But given the limited funding available from independent sources, researchers concerned about the role of industry sponsorship sometimes feel that the best they can do is to recognize the potential for conflicts of interest, take steps to minimize such conflicts, and keep public health at the forefront of their professional actions and opinions. They know they must take special precautions to ensure that the purpose of their sponsored research is more to advance knowledge in the public interest than to help sell sodas.[27]

The United Nations Standing Committee on Nutrition (SCN) has established its own "principles of engagement" with food company donors. Before accepting funding, it assesses, among other items:

- Relevance of the partnership to SCN's vision and mandate
- Effectiveness of the partnership in meeting SCN's goals
- Management of conflicts of interest
- Transparency of the arrangements
- Safeguards to protect public policy making from corporate influence
- Respect for principles of human rights[28]

Are "the best they can do" and engagement principles like these sufficient? I don't think so. I agree with the Canadian physicians who maintain that "health organizations, even when desperate for money or resources, should avoid co-branding with the food industry.... When they partner, health organizations become inadvertent pitchmen for the food industry. They would do well to remember that corporate dollars always introduce perceived or real biases that may taint or distort evidence-based lifestyle recommendations and health messages."[29]

When young investigators ask me whether they should accept research funding from Big Food, I am forced by experience to advise them that doing so will put their academic credibility at risk. If they publish research favorable to the interest of the sponsoring company, they run the risk that colleagues will not believe their results or respect their scientific integrity.

20

Recruiting Public Health Leaders

Working from Within

In its recruitment materials, Coca-Cola says, "When pride, passion and drive come together, you get the people of The Coca-Cola Company. We're looking for experienced professionals who want to make a difference, develop and inspire others, drive innovative ideas and deliver results, and who live our values." Nutrition and health professionals take jobs with soda companies, and not only because such jobs pay well. Some—perhaps many—also take such jobs because they care deeply about improving health and nutrition and believe they can have a greater impact working from the inside corporations to influence policies and practices. Given the demands of corporate investors, I and others have doubts about the value of trying to make meaningful changes from within.[1] To be meaningful, some of us think, changes must go deeper than just promoting reduced-sugar drinks and lower-salt snacks. Truly meaningful changes such as those in marketing practices, for example, are likely to reduce profits, elicit complaints from investors, and, therefore, be unsustainable.

To illustrate the complexities and contradictions of working from within a soda company, this chapter draws on a single example, that of Dr. Derek Yach, a South African national trained in medicine and public health. I think it fair to do this not only because of Dr. Yach's prominence in the public health community but also because he continues to speak for the value of working from within food companies to address diet-related health problems. I am basing this chapter on Dr. Yach's published writings and on my personal experience with some of the events described here. I also gave him an earlier draft of this chapter to review as well as a final draft. He returned both with exceptionally gracious comments, from which I quote. It is worth hearing what he has to say.

Let's begin this account in February 2007, when Dr. Yach shocked the international public health community by taking a job with PepsiCo as director and later vice president of global health policy. Why shock? Just a few years earlier, he had left his position as director of non-communicable (chronic) disease at the World Health Organization (WHO) in Geneva after a change in administration left him with minimal staff and authority—a situation widely understood as a consequence of his vigorous opposition to sugar industry marketing and lobbying.[2]

Public health advocates considered Derek Yach to be nothing less than heroic for his attempts to counter the marketing strategies of tobacco and food companies. I certainly do. He was the guiding force behind the WHO's Framework Convention on Tobacco Control, an international treaty to curb cigarette marketing, and he continues to call for stronger controls on tobacco. In his writings about tobacco industry practices, he has been especially critical of the companies' funding of scientists and research projects and of the industry's deliberate attempts to create scientific doubt and controversy. "The goal of the tobacco industry's 'scientific strategy,'" he once wrote, "was not to reveal the truth but to protect the industry from loss of revenue and to prevent governments from establishing effective tobacco control measures."[3]

To reduce the worldwide prevalence of chronic disease, he would also have to take on the food industry. In leading WHO's efforts to develop a global strategy for prevention of chronic diseases, Dr. Yach had to deal with food company executives concerned that an international public health agency would suggest eating less of their products. He assured them that they would be included in discussions: "We want to tap their expertise and reach and send a dual message that physical activity and optimal diet are very important." While keeping those lines of communication open, he organized international meetings and commissioned reports aimed at setting limits on the marketing of junk foods and sodas to children. I attended such meetings at WHO headquarters in Geneva and in Treviso, Italy, at which participants explored ways to counter the marketing of soda and junk foods to children.[4]

At the time, Dr. Yach was also supervising the production of a consultation report aimed at establishing a research basis for a global strategy to reduce obesity and other chronic disease risk factors. The report, published in 2003, advised restricting intake of "free" (added) sugars to 10 percent or less of daily calories. Although this percentage had been recommended for decades by U.S. and other national agencies (see Chapter 4), it had never been proposed by so prominent an international agency. Sugar industry groups immediately went into action. They enlisted senators from sugar-growing states to induce the Department of Health and Human Services (HHS) to threaten to withdraw U.S. funding from WHO. They convinced the HHS chief counsel, appointed by President George W. Bush's industry-friendly administration, to send WHO a detailed critique of the report, conveniently drafted by sugar industry lobbyists. When released in 2004, WHO's Global Strategy on Diet, Physical Activity, and Health said to "limit the intake of free sugars" but omitted any mention of "to 10 percent of calories" or even of the research report behind the recommendation.[5]

Nevertheless, WHO relieved Dr. Yach of his non-communicable disease directorship. He gave his version of what happened in an interview with the BBC's Betsan Powys:

POWYS: The man behind the *Strategy* is Derek Yach. It should be a big week for him. Instead, even before the *Strategy* is discussed, he's packing his bags and moving on. Removed from his job leading the assault on obesity and sidelined, he has few doubts that taking on the food and sugar lobbies marked him out.

YACH: I was physically shifted out of an office with strong secretarial and administrative support, and management of about 250 staff, and the next day moved into an office which was very obscurely placed, difficult to find, no secretarial support, impossible [to] find my mail. Colleagues, friends, people in government [said] that there were pressures, particularly from some of the US interests which preferred to have me no longer as close to the food-related issues as I had been.

POWYS: Just this week came evidence he was right. A leaked email revealed how the World Sugar Research Organisation planned to make the most of Derek Yach's departure. With the man they described as "hostile" gone, they now hoped sponsorship would buy them influence in Geneva. But whether Derek Yach was in or out, the fight over the *Strategy* report was still on.

YACH: They must have paid millions to lobbyists to try and stop the report [from] ever coming out. They went to the director generals

both of WHO and FAO [Food and Agriculture Organization] almost
on the eve of its release and threaten[ed] that WHO would lose some
of their funds—large amounts of their funds—and got US senators to
sign their names onto the letters where those threats were made.[6]

Yach took a position at Yale and, later, at the Rockefeller Foundation. In his
comments on the earlier draft of this chapter, he explained that while still at
WHO he knew he had to "talk to the food industry in a sustained dialogue
aimed at seeing where we might find common cause...I knew we had to
work differently with food companies versus tobacco companies and did
so."[7] In 2005, I attended a meeting he organized in Johannesburg, South
Africa, aimed at achieving "truth and reconciliation" between food industry
executives and food advocates.

PepsiCo announced Dr. Yach's appointment in 2007 with this statement: "With health and wellness as our primary growth opportunity, we are
investing in senior talent who will actively engage external partnerships
and government and non-government organizations to arrive at policies
that positively impact our strategy."[8] PepsiCo, in Yach's view, had been committed to wellness since the late 1990s, when it sold off its interests in Taco
Bell, KFC, and Pizza Hut and acquired two companies making healthier
products, Quaker Oats and Tropicana.

In 2008, the British professional journal *Public Health Nutrition* published an editorial by Dr. Yach discussing his move to PepsiCo. In an invited
commentary on that piece, Dr. Ricardo Uauy, head of the International
Union of Nutritional Science, said he believed "Derek is genuine in his motives and he has chosen this job as a new challenge and opportunity to influence the private sector from within." Uauy said he had asked PepsiCo's
CEO, Indra Nooyi: "'Why have you taken our standard bearer in the fight
against chronic diseases? Some say he has now joined the enemy.' Her reply
was instant and to the point: 'We have asked Derek to change this company;
in five years we want to have most of our product line meet the international standards supporting life-long health...if he fails we fail.'"[9]

It is easy to understand why PepsiCo would want to recruit a distinguished public health scientist of Derek Yach's experience and credibility,
but I can only speculate about why he accepted the job. The pay was undoubtedly generous, but, as he told a reporter, "his mother worried that he'd
lost his mind. Didn't he realize, she asked, that they sell soda and chips, and
these things cause you to get unhealthy and fat?' Yes, he said, he knew what

Pepsi made. But he wanted to help guide the $43 billion snack food multinational toward a more balanced product menu.'"[10] In his emails to me, Yach also cited "the inspiring vision of a new CEO with a proven track record...[an] agreement to pursue external relationships with leaders who sought change...the potential to reach almost 2 billion consumers touched by PepsiCo products...and yes a reasonable salary."

In his *Public Health Nutrition* editorial, Yach explained: "I have been privileged to work with the most committed colleagues in the public sector. Now I am finding equally committed colleagues in the corporate sector who share the public health community's desire to make a difference in the lives of consumers. Let us work together to make that difference."[11]

But what difference could he make in a company whose first priority necessarily must be selling and profiting from salty snacks and sugary drinks? Within a month of Yach's appointment, the *New York Times* was writing about the soda industry's new focus on healthier options. It noted that because of concerns about obesity, sales of traditional sodas were falling in the United States, and healthier drinks were now seen as the industry's growth opportunity. A few months later, PepsiCo announced that it, along with ten other companies, would stop marketing non-nutritious products on television to children under the age of 12. Its rival, Coca-Cola, had already withdrawn such commercials. PepsiCo stated its philosophy of health and wellness in a brochure in 2007: "We recognize our responsibility to encourage people to adopt healthier lifestyles—beginning with the products that we offer." The brochure promoted physical activity, restated the company's promise not to advertise to children under age 12, reiterated its commitment to voluntary self-regulation, and emphasized the growth opportunities in health and wellness.[12]

These actions might have been in place before Dr. Yach began working for Pepsi, but he surely must have had a hand in the 2008 letter signed by the CEOs of Pepsi, Coke, and six other food companies in response to the WHO's Global Strategy. The companies restated their commitments to marketing healthier products and to continuing "our efforts with respect to portion control." They promised to provide nutrition information on package labels even when not required, and to continue their self-regulation of marketing to children: "We recognize...we should apply our individual marketing and advertising commitments on a global basis. This year, we therefore intend to finalize and announce plans and timetables to achieve this, together with appropriate independent mechanisms to monitor their delivery." The companies also said they would continue to promote physical activity and healthy lifestyles and "support public-private partnerships to accomplish the objectives of the WHO in this area."[13]

Because none of these pledges broke new ground, it is difficult to assess what Dr. Yach was able to achieve in his role at PepsiCo. By 2011, the *Wall Street Journal* was quoting Pepsi's CEO, Indra Nooyi, as "trying to reassure Wall Street that soda and potato chips aren't taking a backseat to nutrition" and promising that she was only putting $50 million in direct corporate funding into Pepsi's nutrition business that year. A few months later, when sales of Pepsi fell to third below Coke and Diet Coke, investment analysts became "impatient over PepsiCo's anemic stock price" and complained that Nooyi's vision to sell nutritional products—water, diet sodas, and lower-calorie drinks—was more about public relations than reality. The company, investors insisted, had to refocus its attention on selling the core products, Frito-Lay and Pepsi. Nooyi soon made management changes and announced that PepsiCo would devote $500 million to $600 million in new marketing for its core brands.[14]

Although Dr. Yach's name was not mentioned in the management changes, he left PepsiCo in October 2012 to take a position with the South Africa–based Vitality Group, which designs, promotes, and implements comprehensive worksite wellness programs. From that base, he continues to work closely with PepsiCo as an advisor on its ongoing health and agriculture initiatives. When asked, Yach rated his success at PepsiCo at 65 percent. PepsiCo was not the problem, he said. The *public* was the problem. "What I never knew was the power of consumer demand. They just want this unhealthy stuff."[15] In his comments to me, he pointed out "two reasons for slow progress. Consumer demand was one—the other was/is the high price of commodities (like fruits, vegetables) required to build a healthier portfolio relative to heavily subsidized corn and soy." He also noted that "the timing of the changes introduced at PepsiCo coincided with the start of what would become the worst global recession in living memory."

In his speeches and published articles, Dr. Yach stressed and continues to stress the importance of food industry efforts to promote global health, sustainable development, and sufficient nutrient intake. The industry, he says, deserves credit for providing nutritious, safe, and affordable foods that support health and promote improvements in economic development. In combatting nutritional problems, he points out, "voluntary action in the private sector, specifically by the food and drinks industry, can complement public policies and is, in some cases, more effective than government restrictions."[16] With respect to obesity in particular,

> PepsiCo's pledge to remove and eliminate the direct sale of full-calorie sodas from all schools worldwide has made progress and is in effect in 100 countries around the world. In the U.S., the total volume of PepsiCo beverages sold that are in the mid- and low-calorie range has sharply increased from 25 percent five years ago to 50 percent today and is likely to reach 75 percent within the next five to eight years.... [This is] happening even in a recession, and it's happening even where the pressures are high for short-term gains.[17]

I do not know whether PepsiCo is making such changes because it must in order to compete in today's global marketplace or because of Dr. Yach's intervention. But by recruiting him, PepsiCo gained a distinguished, eloquent, and highly credible champion of the company's business interests in the United States and internationally.

In the 2008 exchange in *Public Health Nutrition*, Dr. Kaare Norum, a Norwegian nutrition professor who was a key participant in the team that developed WHO's Global Strategy, expressed skepticism about PepsiCo's motives for recruiting Dr. Yach and suggested that his taking the job might have done more harm than good:

> The acquisition of notable health experts and political advisors provides a 'halo effect'—or perhaps less charitably a smokescreen—behind which to hide. This strategy has been adopted not only by PepsiCo, but by many Big Food companies which seem to think that engaging a few advisers to give their blessing to some modified products offers a solution in responding to the challenge of improving diet and tackling obesity. In fact, it may undermine greater efforts to bring about real change.[18]

Real change, Norum argued, would mean a commitment from PepsiCo to adhere to an international code—mandatory, not voluntary—to stop marketing to children under age 18. Given how far the company's actions fall short of this objective, I score Derek Yach's five-year stint as a clear win for PepsiCo.

DEREK YACH'S RESPONSE

As mentioned earlier, I invited Dr. Yach to comment on drafts of this chapter. He wrote that he "would really hope you change this ending to take a broader view and ask what really could be learnt not just re sodas but about overall change in a massive food company—and what would have happened if the external world had been more supportive of internal efforts! In reality I suffered an academic boycott by many leading journals who refused to even send out papers for peer review on the ground they were too pro industry."

Although he manages to find prestigious outlets for publication of many articles, I can confirm at least one instance in which his participation was rejected on the grounds of pro-industry bias. In 2008, Dr. David Ludwig and I invited Dr. Yach to collaborate on a commentary for *JAMA* (the Journal of the American Medical Association) on the food industry's role in obesity. The journal's editors said no, and we wrote the piece without him. We titled it "Can the Food Industry Play a Constructive Role in the Obesity Epidemic?"[19] Our conclusion: not likely, in view of the discrepancy between the goals of industry and public health. In retrospect, I doubt we could have come to this conclusion had he been a co-author.

Nevertheless, in assessing his accomplishments at PepsiCo, Dr. Yach says he was able to:

- Play a leading role with others at PepsiCo to build a global research and development program "that placed salt, sugar and saturated fat reduction at its core"
- Establish internal nutrition guidelines for long-term development and reformulation of foods and beverages, and metrics to monitor progress
- Build PepsiCo's internal capability to bring nutrition and agriculture together and provide greater support for sustainable agriculture
- Initiate a range of partnerships to advance business and health goals
- "Cajole and negotiate within industry for major efforts aimed at addressing obesity in the USA"
- Engage in academic discussions about constraints on industry progress and about the value of well-designed partnerships, and "do so through participation in often hostile conferences and through efforts to publish in peer review publications"

With regard to this last point, Yach said he was able to highlight "several realities that NGOs [nongovernmental organizations], WHO and academics rarely consider when calling for change: the relatively small contribution of multinationals to the total intake of foods and beverages in developing countries; the weakness of regulatory enforcement in most developing countries; the importance of addressing total dietary change and not just specific nutrients and products; and more." His publications, Yach wrote, "provided insider perspectives to the academic world rarely seen or documented."

I appreciate and respect Dr. Yach's viewpoint, but I continue to believe that working from within industry ends up doing more for industry and its marketing than it does for public health.

More "Softball" Tactics: Mitigating Environmental Damage

21

Advocacy

Defending the Environment

In 2012, Coca-Cola sold about twelve *billion* bottles and cans of sodas, waters, and other products.[1] These containers—and their contents—have to be constructed from raw materials, cleaned, transported, refrigerated, and, eventually, consumed or discarded. All of this requires vast amounts of energy and water, and releases vast quantities of greenhouse gases, pollutants, and trash into the environment. Soda company officials are well aware that their products deplete and contaminate water supplies, contribute to climate change, and generate garbage. Cleaning up the mess they create is a major focus of soda company corporate social responsibility (CSR). Both Coke and Pepsi routinely win congratulations and national and international prizes for such efforts.

All three Big Soda companies have established impressive goals for environmental protection. Dr Pepper Snapple's are the most specific and immediate. By 2015, DPS says it will:

- Improve energy efficiency and reduce carbon dioxide emissions by 10 percent per gallon of product.
- Increase the quantity of products shipped per gallon of fuel by 20 percent.
- Replace 60,000 vending machines and coolers with equipment that is 30 percent more energy-efficient.
- Reduce water use and wastewater discharge by 10 percent per gallon of finished product.

- Recycle 90 percent of the solid waste caused by manufacturing processes.
- Conserve more than 60 million pounds of plastic through weight trimming and recycling.[2]

Pepsi's environmental goals also address conservation of water and energy and reduction of greenhouse gas emissions and package waste, but add promotion of sustainable agriculture. Coca-Cola's goals do all this and even more. The company pledges to help protect fragile environments such as that of the Arctic.[3] Notably absent from these pledges, however, is even a hint of a commitment to bottle deposit laws—incentive regulations that add a price penalty to the retail cost of a drink, refundable when customers return containers to a collection center. Such laws demonstrably improve recycling rates. But recycling, according to Big Soda, is not its or government's responsibility; it is the *consumer's* responsibility.

In this chapter, I examine soda company efforts to reduce greenhouse gas emissions, reduce package waste, and promote sustainable agriculture and environmental initiatives—and the efforts of advocates to hold companies accountable for doing so. Because efforts to conserve water supplies and protect water quality are essential for soda production and raise their own issues, I deal with water separately in Chapter 22.

Soda companies spend hundreds of millions of dollars annually to fix the environmental problems they created in the first place. Environmental CSR earns them praise, moral credits, and public applause. But behind the scenes, soda companies lobby relentlessly to shift environmental burdens to users and taxpayers, and they oppose all attempts to require bottle deposits or to ban soda bottles and cans from protected areas. I begin this discussion by addressing issues related to soda companies' environmental promises.

UNDERSTAND THE ISSUES: SODA COMPANIES' ENVIRONMENTAL PLEDGES

Reduce Greenhouse Gas Emissions

Greenhouse gases—mainly carbon dioxide but also fluorocarbons used in refrigeration—contribute to climate change. The production of sodas generates greenhouse gases through combustion of fossil fuels to run manufacturing plants, trucks, and cold-drink equipment. Out of concern about this problem, the industry commissioned a study to examine the production of carbon dioxide in soda supply chains. Published in 2012, the study estimated the total carbon emissions, or "carbon footprint," created by producing two sugar-sweetened soda products: a shrink-wrapped six-pack of 1.5-liter PET (polyethylene terephthalate plastic—"polyester") bottles produced in Europe, and a cardboard twelve-pack of 12-ounce aluminum cans from the United States.[4] The results:

- Each 1.5-liter PET-bottled drink in a six-pack creates a carbon footprint of 251 grams (1.5 kilograms for the pack).
- Each 12-ounce canned drink in a twelve-pack creates a carbon footprint of 195 grams (2.3 kilograms for the pack).

Translated into pounds, these drinks generate a carbon emission of about half a pound each (3 to 6 pounds for the packs). This may seem like a lot but is much less than the 8,900 grams (8.9 kilograms or about 20 pounds) of carbon dioxide produced by one gallon of gasoline. Even so, the Sierra Club estimated that Coca-Cola alone generated 5.32 million metric tons of carbon dioxide in 2011, and that the combined emissions of Coke, Pepsi, and Dr Pepper Snapple amounted to more than 11.7 million metric tons that year.[5] That's 2.6 *billion* pounds, with Coca-Cola alone accounting for close to half.

The soda industry study also examined how each component of the supply chain contributed to the carbon footprint. Table 21.1 shows the results. Producing the container generates the greatest percentage, followed by production of the sweetener, either sugar or high-fructose corn syrup (HFCS).

TABLE 21.1 Sources of carbon dioxide emissions in the soda supply chain, percent of total

SUPPLY CHAIN COMPONENT	SODA IN 1.5 LITER PET BOTTLE, PERCENT	SODA IN 12-OUNCE ALUMINUM CAN, PERCENT
Container	35	71
Sweetener	33	10
Distribution transportation	17	9
Gas and electricity, retail	7	6
Other	8	4

SOURCE: Beverage Industry Environmental Roundtable, 2012.

Such percentages must be considered estimates, as they are based on unverifiable assumptions and models. Nevertheless, they pose a challenge to soda companies. The companies can try to reduce the carbon emissions caused by their use of gas and electricity, transportation, and production of containers, but they have virtually no control over the energy cost of sugar or HFCS production. The sweetener problem explains Coca-Cola's modest goal: a 5 percent reduction of carbon emissions from the 2004 baseline by 2015. Nevertheless, its efforts to reach this goal were enough for the U.S. Environmental Protection Agency (EPA) to rank the company as one of its top Green Power Partners in 2013. Coca-Cola's rapidly expanding sales in developing countries, however, create high demands for electricity and gasoline, and its carbon footprint in those countries was 11 percent *higher* in 2011 than in 2004. In some countries, South Africa, for example, it did better. There, Coca-Cola improved its energy efficiency by 33 percent, an accomplishment that earned it a Climate Change Hero Leadership Award.[6]

To reduce the footprint, Coca-Cola can and does attempt to control emissions from delivery trucks and refrigeration. The company is switching to more energy-efficient fuels such as electricity, natural gas, and biodiesel, incorporating diesel-electric hybrid vehicles into its fleet, and retrofitting trucks to switch off automatically rather than idling. In developing countries, it encourages use of alternative fuels. In rural Africa, for example, it funds projects to bring solar power to Coke kiosk owners. Such projects help the company by encouraging brand loyalty. Coke also promises to have all of its new cold-drink equipment free of fluorocarbons by 2015. For such efforts, the company ranked twenty-sixth on Corporate Knights' Global 100 Sustainability Index in 2015.[7] Similarly, PepsiCo pledges to reduce greenhouse gas emissions from its manufacturing plants and transport fleet by 20 percent by 2015. The EPA gave PepsiCo its Energy Star Partner of the Year Award for Sustained Excellence in 2012.

Reduce Package Waste

Generating billions of bottles and cans every year creates a monumental disposal problem that leaves soda companies with limited choices for remediation. Short of selling fewer sodas, all they can do is to reduce the size and weight of the packaging, or recycle and reuse the plastic and metals. A better option might be biodegradable packaging, but that technology is not yet available. In the meantime, soda companies do what they can to reduce package weight and to recycle materials used in production (although not consumption). Pepsi reports that it reduced the weight of its packages by more than 350 million pounds in a recent five-year period, mainly by thinning its PET bottles. The company says it recycles or reuses more than 90 percent of its solid waste, and many—although by no means all—of its plants send less than 1 percent of their waste to landfills.

Coca-Cola increasingly uses a PET "PlantBottle" with 30 percent plant-based materials such as sugarcane and molasses, and is working with biotechnology companies to develop bottles that are fully plant-based. It promised to source 25 percent of its PET plastic from recycled or renewable material by 2015. Irony alert: it is nowhere near meeting that target. Why? Because the supply of recyclable PET bottles is too low. Although the shortfall is due in part to China's demand for PET bottles to recycle into clothing and furniture, the most important reason is the low level of PET bottle recycling. As a British report found, five *billion* PET bottles went to landfills in 2013.[8]

Why don't citizens recycle soda bottles? Because soda companies and their trade associations have lobbied for decades against bottle deposit laws that might provide incentives for recycling. Here's another irony: Coca-Cola invented bottle deposit laws. Way back in the early 1900s, the company's glass bottles were too expensive to be thrown away. The company required a small deposit on the bottles, redeemable upon return. By the late 1920s, about 80 percent of Coke bottlers used a deposit system. As late as 1948, the return rate was an astonishing (in retrospect) 96 percent. But soon after, the companies realized that one-way cans and, later, plastic bottles would be more profitable. They would no longer have to collect, transport, and clean the returned containers. Instead, these jobs could be outsourced to local municipal garbage collection agencies—and paid for by taxpayers. Today, Coca-Cola reports lobbying to "highlight company innovations in recyclable packaging and work to grow packaging recovery" (translation: get consumers to recycle the bottles and cans they use).[9] The dismal result of soda company opposition to deposit laws is that the average content of recycled plastic in Coke's PET bottles was only 6 percent in 2014, according to Coca-Cola's annual Sustainability Report.[10]

Get Consumers to Recycle

Coke's alternative strategy has been to encourage users of its products to recycle. Indeed, the company and its foundation invest in community cleanup and recycling initiatives throughout the world, as shown in Table 21.2.[11]

TABLE 21.2 Coca-Cola funding of community recycling initiatives, selected examples, 2011–2013

COUNTRY	DONATION	RECYCLING PROGRAM
Brazil	$950,000	Instituto Coca-Cola Brasil: Recycling Cooperative Management Capability
Canada	$50,000	The Great Canadian Shoreline Cleanup
Colombia	$72,965	Strengthening Recyclers Production Units
Ecuador	$20,000	Fundacion Galapagos Ecuador, Coastal Clean Up program, Galapagos Islands
Mexico	$100,000	Junior League of Mexico City, Recycle for Nature, schools
New Zealand	$170,000	Keep New Zealand Beautiful
United States	$350,000	Keep America Beautiful, recycling bins to community groups and college campuses
	$50,000	Save the Harbor/Save the Bay, Youth Environmental Education Programs
	$2,590,000	Earth Day grant to Chicago to install 50,000 recycling carts (with photos of Coke logos) in Chicago

SOURCES: Coca-Cola Foundation's 2nd and 3rd quarter reports, 2013, and contemporary news accounts.

To encourage consumer recycling, Coke funds education programs. In 2011, for example, its bottler in Israel used online advertising, radio, Facebook, and even "pop-up stores" to promote sales of handbags, T-shirts, hats, and other items made from discarded bottles. This campaign also introduced ten thousand recycling receptacles for the bottles. In North America, Coke worked with NASCAR at racetracks to divert more than 11.5 million beverage containers into recycling streams. Coke's consumer recycling initiatives are especially noticeable in Great Britain. The company said, "We will encourage visitors to London 2012 to recycle their empty packaging. Recycling bins will be provided around the park and we will use fun ways to prompt people to recycle." For this recycling campaign during the London Olympics, Coca-Cola won an Environmental Initiative of the Year award. In 2013, the company ran a "Don't Waste; Create" campaign offering discounts to people who recycle or find clever ways to reuse plastic bottles; it also placed a label on Coke bottles saying "Plastic, Widely Recycled." In Vietnam, Thailand, and Indonesia, Coca-Cola distributes special bottle caps that "upcycle" plastic bottles as water squirters, lamps, pencil sharpeners, and baby feeding bottles.[12]

Not to be outdone, PepsiCo has entered into a five-year partnership with the Nature Conservancy. Their Recycle for Nature program expands the availability of recycling bins in the United States at places such as gas stations and convenience stores. For every percent increase in recycling per year, PepsiCo has committed to increasing the size of its contribution to the Nature Conservancy for water conservation projects. The ABA celebrates the soda industry's efforts to promote recycling: "The beverage industry's bottles and cans are among the most recycled consumer packaging in the U.S. We work hard to package our products with materials that are widely accepted in recycling programs and are designed to be recycled with other, similar materials. . . . And we are always looking for ways to do more."[13]

I would find it easier to believe the companies' altruistic motives for recycling if they did not persist in opposing environmental protection measures involving discarded cans and bottles. The ABA states its position unambiguously: "What is the most important factor in recycling? It's not the bottles and cans—it's you! Nothing happens unless you take the first step and get those recyclables to the bin."[14] The association's position on container deposit laws is equally clear:

> Do deposit systems work?
>
> No. The biggest problem is that deposits focus on such a small part of the solid waste or litter problems. Relying on deposits to solve these broad and complex problems is overly simplistic and just won't work. Furthermore, deposit laws effectively require that a whole new system be established to collect and manage beverage container materials—something that existing recycling infrastructure has already in place. Requiring the establishment of duplicative, new systems is bad public policy.[15]

As summarized by one Coca-Cola regional manager, "We are not in the recycling business, we are in the beverage business."[16]

An example of how this opposition plays out in practice involves Coca-Cola and the Grand Canyon. During the past forty years, Coca-Cola has donated at least $13 million to the national park system, whose concessions sell sodas and bottled water. In 2011, Grand Canyon park officials discovered that discarded water bottles accounted for 30 percent of recyclable waste in the park. They announced that they were banning sales of bottled water and would instead provide water filling stations. The ban affected Coke's Dasani water but not sodas. Even so, the company was widely reported to have exerted intense pressure on park officials to withdraw the ban. By one report, a spokeswoman for Coca-Cola, Susan Stribling, said, "Banning anything is never the right answer. . . . If you do that, you don't necessarily address the problem." Bottle bans, she said, limit personal choice. "You're not allowing people to decide what they want to eat and drink and consume."[17]

Nevertheless, park officials enacted the ban a year later. In response, Ms. Stribling said that although her company did not condone such bans, it would "continue to work to 'find a solution that is in the best interest of the parks and the public.'" Coca-Cola, she said, "favors 'constructive solutions' such as creating more recycling programs."[18]

Produce Sugar Sustainably

PepsiCo publishes a brochure devoted to its efforts to promote agricultural sustainability. Its pledge: "We are committed to minimizing the impact that our business has on the environment with practices that are socially responsible, scientifically based and economically sound."[19] Its guiding principles are to preserve and conserve soil and to sustainably manage water, energy, land, and agrochemicals. PepsiCo, of course, makes snack foods as well as sodas. Although the brochure has plenty to say about efforts to lessen the environmental impact of producing corn, wheat, potatoes, and sorghum, it says nothing about sugar, an omission that I find rather conspicuous.

Sugar poses acute environmental problems for soda companies. The companies do not produce it themselves. Instead, they obtain it from worldwide suppliers, in effect outsourcing the environmental hazards of sugar production. Sugar, as the World Wildlife Fund (WWF) once put it, "has arguably had as great an impact on the environment as any other agricultural commodity." Growing sugarcane and sugar beets involves many highly polluting practices. Producers of sugarcane burn fields before harvest, clear wildlife habitats, use and waste huge amounts of water, apply agrichemicals intensively, and discharge mill effluents. Indeed, the environmental impact of sugar production is so overwhelming that entire books are devoted to describing the full extent of the damage it causes.[20]

From an environmental perspective, the most important contribution soda companies could make to agricultural sustainability would be to use less sugar. Without that as a viable option, the companies do what they can to reduce the environmental consequences of soda production. Coca-Cola covers its vulnerability in this area by partnering with WWF and other international organizations to attempt to sustainably source cane sugar, beet sugar, and HFCS. Its principles for sustainable agriculture deal with management of water, energy, soil, and climate protection, and with conservation

of habitats and ecosystems. Its commitment to achieve international Bonsucro production standards for its sugar supply by 2020. Bonsucro standards
require companies to measurably reduce the undesirable environmental and
social effects of sugarcane production and processing. But progress toward
achieving such standards is slow. In 2015, both Coca-Cola and PepsiCo
achieved higher scores than they had in earlier years on a Sustainability
Scorecard produced by Oxfam as part of the Behind the Brands campaign
described later in this chapter. Nevertheless, Coca-Cola's score was still only
54 out of 100 and PepsiCo's only 43.[21]

Coca-Cola funds many projects to mitigate the environmental damage
from sugar production. In Australia, for example, it engages in a Project
Catalyst partnership with WWF, the government, and sugar farmers to
reduce fertilizer and pesticide effluents from sugarcane farms in the north.
These effluents flow into local waterways and, eventually, into waters surrounding the Great Barrier Reef, where they destroy coral. Such projects,
useful as they are, barely address the extent of environmental harm caused
by sugar production.[22] But they help Coca-Cola to position itself as an environmental protector. In July 2014, the company's two-page advertisement in
National Geographic depicted a rugged, third-generation sugarcane farmer:
"Since 2007, The Coca-Cola Company has helped protect natural ecosystems like the Great Barrier Reef in Australia by supporting farmers like
Gerard, who test, validate, and embrace innovative practices that help reduce
the environmental footprint of sugarcane production."

Promote Environmental Causes

The ABA advertises that "our industry is leading the way and doing our part
to reduce our environmental impact.... Ours is an industry standing together in pursuit of solutions to environmental challenges in communities
throughout America."[23] To that end, Coca-Cola funds solar energy, ecology,
and "green" projects throughout the world. By far the largest of such projects is Arctic Home, a cause-marketing campaign aimed at protecting the
polar bear—the company's advertising icon—and its Arctic habitat. As the
company explained in its 2011/2012 Sustainability Report, "We packaged
Coca-Cola in white cans...for an urgent cause: the plight of polar bears,
whose habitat is seriously threatened by climate change. The white Coke
cans were just part of our five-year 'Arctic Home' program and a five-year
commitment initiated with our longtime conservation partners at WWF."

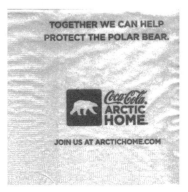

FIGURE 21.1 Napkin distributed with airline refreshment service. Coca-Cola's Arctic Home program involves a $2 million donation over five years and the solicitation of public donations to a campaign by the World Wildlife Fund to protect the habitat of polar bears.

In 2011, Coca-Cola committed $2 million to WWF's polar bear conservation program. WWF's Arctic Home website and advertisements solicited donations online or by text message; the campaign collected another $3 million in public contributions by the end of 2013. An Arctic Home video promotes Coca-Cola's support of WWF scientists and advertises the company's environmental philanthropy. In 2014, I picked up an element of that campaign on an airplane (Figure 21.1).

As can be seen from these examples, beverage companies are most likely to promote environmental initiatives when they promote business objectives. If the initiatives do not help increase profits, the companies cannot do much to achieve environmental goals. Corporate environmental philanthropy shifts attention away from the problems created by soda production and consumption and as much as possible transfers the burden of cleaning up environmental damage to the public.[24] In the absence of government regulation to prevent such damage, advocates have created campaigns to hold soda companies accountable for their pledges and to induce them to initiate and adhere to environmental protection measures.

ADVOCATE: PROTECT THE ENVIRONMENT FROM SODA-INDUCED DAMAGE

In this section, I introduce advocacy campaigns for bottle bans and container deposit laws, but also for two other environmental causes related to soda production: the damage caused by extracting oil from tar sands and the consequences of land acquisition for sugar production— "land grabs."

Promote Bottle Bans and Deposit Laws

Engage in the Debate

In Table 21.3, I summarize the Container Recycling Institute's suggestions for how to respond to soda industry arguments against bottle-deposit laws.[25]

Join the Campaigns

Advocates in many countries have created organizations working to reduce the impact of soda consumption on the environment and to hold soda companies accountable for the pollution they cause.

Container Recycling Institute: bottle deposits. Studies unambiguously demonstrate that container deposit laws improve recycling rates. In the United States, these laws typically call for adding 5 or 10 cents to the cost of a drink, refundable when the container is returned to a collection center. The Container Recycling Institute publishes data indicating that among the eleven states with container deposit laws in 2010, overall recycling rates

TABLE 21.3 Topic for debate: should governments pass laws requiring recycling of soda bottles and cans?*

THE SODA INDUSTRY SAYS	ADVOCATES SAY
Container deposit laws address only a small proportion (7–25 percent) of total litter.	Beverage containers account for 40–60 percent of litter; deposit laws significantly reduce container litter as well as other types of litter by large percentages.
Deposit laws are not needed. Curbside recycling takes care of the problem.	Both systems are needed, but materials collected through deposit programs are of better quality than those collected at curbside.
Deposit return is inconvenient; consumers prefer curbside recycling.	Curbside recycling is only available to half the U.S. population; people return to stores to shop anyway.
Deposit programs are expensive to run.	Deposits are more effective than other recycling and waste reduction programs; recovery rates in deposit states are more than 2.5 times higher than in states without bottle bills.
Deposits are a tax and increase the price of beverages.	Deposits are a refundable tax. No-deposit containers are a corporate subsidy and, therefore, a hidden tax; they shift to taxpayers the cost of disposal and of curbside recycling programs.

* Adapted from Container Recycling Institute, Bottle Bill Myths and Facts.

ranged from 66 percent to 96 percent. In sharp contrast, recycling rates in states without deposit laws averaged about 30 percent. For PET bottles, the rates were lower but the difference was still striking: 48 percent in deposit states as compared to 20 percent in non-deposit states.[26]

As noted earlier, the ABA disagrees. It views recycling laws as "a misguided policy choice" because they increase costs, are inconvenient, and require transport to recycling centers. Targeting such a small part of the waste stream, it says, is hardly worth the trouble.[27] The ABA's public relations materials do not mention that deposit laws increase the retail price of sodas and might reduce sales.

Greenpeace: Cash for Containers. The leading ABA member, Coca-Cola, actively opposes bottle deposit laws to the point of filing lawsuits. In 2013, it took the lead in opposing such bills in Vermont and Australia. In Australia, it sued to prevent a Cash for Containers initiative developed by the environmental group Greenpeace—and won.[28] Of Coca-Cola's actions Greenpeace said:

> Coke's so-called "alternative" to a Cash for Containers scheme is to install more bins (LOTS of bins) with the aim of making it easier for people to recycle their rubbish. The trouble is, this National Bin Network would only be installed in places like shopping centres and main streets, but not on beaches, parks and other places where plastic pollution is having deadly effects on marine life.... If Coke wants to pay for more bins, that's great. They should also offer to pay for the emptying of these bins which is actually much more costly and is paid for by us, the taxpayers, through local councils. And they should drop their opposition to Cash for Containers.[29]

Greenpeace was so incensed by Coke's stance that it created a satirical "Coke Refunds" website to publicize the company's opposition to recycling incentives. It also linked discarded Coke bottles to the death of seabirds.[30]

As You Sow: corporate accountability. In 2011, As You Sow, a group advocating for holding corporations accountable for the damage they cause, issued a scorecard on recycling efforts by major companies. It gave both Coke and Pepsi grades of B-minus. Even so, its expectations must be low. As You Sow said the most important development since its last survey was that soda companies had agreed to take responsibility for collection and recycling of used bottles and cans—if the United States passes new laws requiring them to do so. Apparently, soda company willingness to comply with legal requirements is considered a major step forward.[31] The companies' actions make it clear that they will not support bottle deposit or recycling bills unless they have to.

Take Action
The Container Recycling Institute publishes a toolkit for advocacy for container deposit laws.[32] This provides information, strategies, materials, and guidelines to support advocates who want to get the facts, build support, recognize and counter opposition arguments, and use available resources.

Stop Oil Extraction from Tar Sands. In 2013, the environmental advocacy groups Sierra Club, ForestEthics, and many others sent an open letter to ten leading corporations, among them Coca-Cola and PepsiCo, warning that fuels derived from Canadian tar sands produce three times the carbon emissions of cleaner fuels. Extracting oil from tar sands is especially hard on the environment because it involves open-pit mining, large water withdrawals, and discharge of highly contaminated water. The climate movement, the groups said, "has largely given big corporate oil consumers a free pass. Those days are over.... [T]he Sierra Club and ForestEthics will shine a bright spotlight on the need for corporate leadership to head off a climate crisis, starting with oil consumption."[33]

Although recognizing the efforts made by soda companies to reduce carbon footprints, the groups singled out Coke and Pepsi for their own special campaign—Tastes Like Tar Sands (see Figure 21.2). Why soda companies? The Sierra Club and ForestEthics say the soda industry is one of the biggest oil users in the United States and its trucks run on "one of the dirtiest oils on Earth, [from] carbon-intensive Canadian tar sands." Coke and Pepsi, they say, use so much oil that they could—and should—require transportation providers to use fuel from refineries that do not process tar sands. The campaign involved newspaper ads and online calls for signatures on petitions demanding that Coke and Pepsi raise the fuel efficiency of their trucking fleets.

Stop Sugar "Land Grabs". Oxfam, an international anti-poverty and human rights organization, created the Behind the Brands campaign mentioned earlier to improve the agricultural sourcing and sustainability policies of the world's ten largest food and beverage companies, including

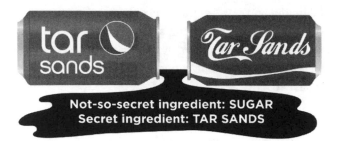

FIGURE 21.2 Illustration from an advocacy campaign against soda companies' use of oil extracted from tar sands. The Sierra Club, ForestEthics, and other environmental groups campaigned to get Coca-Cola and PepsiCo to stop allowing their trucking fleets to use crude oil from Canadian tar sands. Their "Tastes Like Tar Sands" campaign ran in 2013. Image courtesy of the Sierra Club.

Coca-Cola and PepsiCo. Oxfam wants these large food producers to improve the impact of their production methods on women, farmers, workers, climate, and water, and to be openly transparent about doing so. In assigning sustainability scores, Oxfam considers the companies' awareness, knowledge, commitments, and supply chain management.[34]

Because demands for sugar production in developing countries often lead to violations of land rights and takeovers of land that occur without the free consent of farmers and rural communities, Oxfam wants companies to create and adhere to policies that protect farmers from such "land grabs." In 2013, Oxfam published a policy brief explaining how sugar production drives land acquisitions that hurt small farmers, violate human rights, and contribute to hunger, especially among women. The report gave many examples, some of them involving production facilities that supply sugar to Coke and Pepsi. Oxfam recognizes that soda companies do not necessarily have legal responsibility or control over land grabs, but it argues that they ought to take responsibility for protecting land rights in their supply chains:

> Land grabs happen when local communities that rely on land to feed their families and earn a living are evicted without consent or compensation. Oxfam's "Behind the Brands" campaign has warned that the world's ten biggest food and drink companies, including Coca-Cola and PepsiCo, lack strong enough policies to prevent land grabs and land disputes in their supply chains. Oxfam is calling on Coca-Cola and PepsiCo... to become leaders in their industry

by making a commitment to zero tolerance of land grabs in their supply chains, to publicly disclose from whom and where they source their commodities, and take other measures to prevent land rights violations.[35]

Soon after this report appeared, Coca-Cola pledged to engage with its sugar suppliers to adhere to principles of informed consent when acquiring land across its operations, disclose its suppliers, publish human rights assessments, and work with international governments to support responsible land rights practices. In 2013, Oxfam gave Coca-Cola a score of 6 out of 10 ("fair") on land rights issues, compared to only 2 ("poor") for Pepsi. Unable to get Pepsi to budge on this issue, Oxfam increased the pressure. It created a "Take Action" website: "Tell Pepsi to make sure their sugar doesn't lead to land grabs."[36] To drive the point home, Oxfam organized a demonstration at PepsiCo's headquarters in Purchase, New York, in November 2013 (see Figure 21.3).

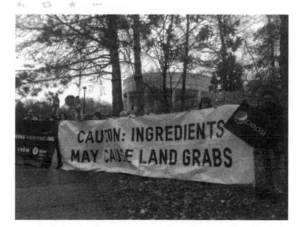

FIGURE 21.3 Tweet from Oxfam America members demonstrating at PepsiCo's headquarters in Purchase, New York. They were urging Twitter followers to tell the company to stop taking over the land of indigenous communities for sugar production, November 22, 2013. This action was part of Oxfam's Behind the Brand and Stop Land Grabs campaigns. Courtesy of Will Fenton/Oxfam America.

This tactic worked. Early in 2014, Oxfam announced that PepsiCo had committed to examining the social and environmental impact of its supply chains, beginning with its most important sugar-sourcing country, Brazil. Pepsi also established policies of zero tolerance for land displacements, fair and legal negotiations for land acquisitions, and use of appropriate grievance mechanisms for resolving future disputes. In 2014, Oxfam gave Pepsi a score of 7 ("added plenty of fizz on land issues") and an 8 to Coca-Cola ("leads the way"). Oxfam will, no doubt, continue to hold the companies accountable for these promises and for supporting United Nations guidelines on responsible governance of land tenure.[37] Other groups will too.

Overall, soda companies are making some progress in some environmental areas over which they have control. Whether these limited environmental efforts deserve the prizes they are awarded is debatable, especially in light of the industry's unyielding opposition to recycling and deposit laws. The efforts of the industry to externalize as much as they can of the environmental costs of soda production and consumption are also apparent in their dealings with water resources, as discussed in Chapter 22.

22

Advocacy

Protecting Public Water Resources

The planet's fresh water supplies are limited, but sodas are mostly water and require fresh water to produce. It is deeply ironic—again—that Cola-Cola and PepsiCo, both producers of bottled waters as well as sodas, win prizes for water conservation. In 2012, the Stockholm International Water Institute honored PepsiCo for having reduced its water usage by 16 billion liters since 2006. This industry jury praised PepsiCo for its watershed management systems, and for its programs to help farmers use water more efficiently. The jury noted that PepsiCo was one of the first companies to recognize the human right to water and to establish public-private partnerships to increase access to safe water in developing countries.[1]

Coca-Cola wins similar awards. In 2013, the Carbon Trust honored the company with its annual Water Standard award. This recognized Coke's leadership in measuring, managing, and reducing water use in Western Europe. In that uniquely water-efficient region, Coca-Cola used only 1.4 liters of water to produce one liter of soda—a water-use ratio or footprint of 1.4.[2] As this chapter explains, soda production in other regions results in higher water footprints, and the 1.4 ratio greatly understates the full water cost of producing sugary drinks.

Soda companies make award-winning efforts to reduce water use for one basic reason: they have to. How they use water affects their business and their reputations. Coca-Cola ranks water as the second-most-prominent risk to its potential profitability, just after obesity. "Water," Coca-Cola states in its disclosure to the U.S. Securities and Exchange Commission, "is the main ingredient in substantially all of our products and is needed to produce the agricultural ingredients on which our business relies. It is also a limited resource in many parts of the world, facing unprecedented challenges from overexploitation, increasing pollution, poor management and climate change."[3]

Coca-Cola notes that in many of the locations in which it does business, the demand for water already exceeds its supply. Population growth, urbanization, and climate change place further demands on water use, most acutely in regions of the developing world most actively targeted for sales expansion. In 2008, investment analysts at JP Morgan warned that water scarcity was more than just a supply-and-demand problem. It could ruin a company's reputation: "As water becomes more precious, companies' real and perceived behavior with respect to water consumption and discharge is also likely to have greater consequences in the marketplace, with an increased risk of consumer backlash against companies judged to be profligate or irresponsible."[4]

Here, I deal with the problems water poses for soda companies and describe how Coke and Pepsi—for the most part successfully—deflect criticism of their extensive water use not only through laudable conservation efforts but also through strategically placed philanthropic partnerships. Advocates want to hold soda companies accountable for such efforts but also to counter the troubling matter of soda companies' acquisition of international water rights.

HOW MUCH WATER DOES SODA REQUIRE?

The JP Morgan research analysts applauded food and beverage companies for recognizing water scarcity as a genuine operational risk and openly communicating that risk. But, they warned, companies need to do a better job of disclosing the true extent of the risk. Water use for sodas can be categorized as direct or indirect. Usually, the companies report only direct water use—the amount that goes into the final soda product. They tend to ignore or understate the amounts needed to produce the sugar, other raw materials, and the bottles—the indirect use. They also understate the risks involved in locating production facilities in water-stressed areas.

The JP Morgan analysts observed that the combined direct water use of just five food companies—Nestlé, Unilever, Kraft, Danone, and Coca-Cola—came to nearly 600 billion liters per year, an average of about 95 liters for every single person on the planet. Coca-Cola alone used 288 billion liters of water in 2006, nearly half the total for the five companies (it used more than 305 billion liters in 2013). The researchers estimated that

Coca-Cola's global water footprint was 2.4 liters of water per liter of product. Coca-Cola reported reducing its direct footprint to 2.16 liters by 2011, and to 2.08 by 2014.[5]

Water use varies by region, as shown in Figure 22.1. In 2011, Coca-Cola's water footprint was 1.74 for North America but 2.76 in the Pacific. Its footprint in Western Europe, as noted earlier, had fallen to the exemplary 1.4 by 2013.[6] Soda companies continue to do whatever they can to reduce direct water-use ratios everywhere they operate.

The International Bottled Water Association (IBWA) also is concerned about water-use ratios. It did its own study based on data from nine companies representing 40 percent of bottled water consumption in the United States. For flat water, the IBWA estimated that it takes 1 liter of water to produce each liter of product, and another 0.4 liter for processing (ratio: 1.4). Carbonated water requires 1.02 liters for processing, for a direct ratio of 2.02.[7] But advocates—and soda companies concerned about their reputations—want to know how much water is needed to produce the bottles and packaging, clean the production plants, and produce the sugars and other ingredients—in addition to the amount used in the drink itself. In 2011, investigators from the University of Twente Water Centre in the Netherlands conducted a careful assessment of the total direct and indirect water footprint of a specific soda: a half-liter bottle of a hypothetical carbonated beverage sweetened with beet sugar. They based their assessment on a systematic method developed specifically for this purpose.[8]

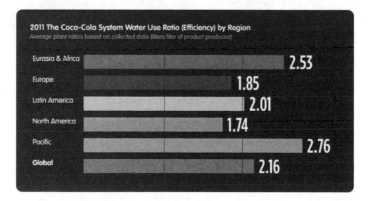

FIGURE 22.1 Coca-Cola's direct water-use ratios in 2011, by region. The ratios express the volume of water required to produce one liter of soda. These ratios underestimate water use, as they do not account for the indirect amounts needed to produce the bottles, packaging, sweeteners, and other ingredients.

The result: 170 to 310 liters per half-liter soft drink. But we don't care about half liters. We care about full liters. For that, we need to double these figures, giving us astonishing water-use ratios of 340 to 620 liters per liter of soda. The range varied with the type of sweetener and the country growing the sugar. The 620 water-use ratio applied to a soda made with cane sugar grown in Cuba, whereas the 340 ratio applied to a soda sweetened with beet sugar produced in the water-efficient Netherlands. Sodas sweetened with high-fructose corn syrup grown in the United States required 360 liters per liter. These amounts, enormous as they seem in comparison to the prize-winning 1.4, are on the low side of water use for food production; figures for meat and dairy production, for example, are higher.

Water scientists obtain the ratios by adding up separate estimates for the amounts of what they call green, blue, and gray water sources:

- Green: soil water from rain or seepage, some of which is used by plants and some lost by evaporation
- Blue: water in freshwater lakes, rivers, and groundwater aquifers, some of which gets taken up and used by plant crops or for irrigation
- Gray: water used to dilute pollutants to meet water quality standards[9]

That the *lowest* water-use ratio for a soda might be as high as 340 liters per liter alarms soda companies, as well it should. In 2007, Coca-Cola recruited the Nature Conservancy to help it see what could be done to fix the water-footprint problem. In a pilot investigation, the Nature Conservancy and its consultants chose to estimate the green, blue, and gray water footprints of another specific example, this time a half-liter plastic (polyethylene terephthalate or PET) bottle of Coca-Cola, sweetened with beet sugar, and produced in the Netherlands—the sweetener and the country already known to have the lowest water footprints.

The Nature Conservancy's study estimated the amount of water needed to produce the ingredients, make the packaging, and clean the bottles and plants. Its results: growing the beets and extracting the sugar accounted for fully two-thirds of the total water footprint. Sugar is highly water intensive. It takes 429 liters of water—375 green and 54 blue—to produce one kilogram (2.2 pounds) of beet sugar. Overall, 80 percent of the water use came from producing the soda ingredients, and packaging accounted for another 19

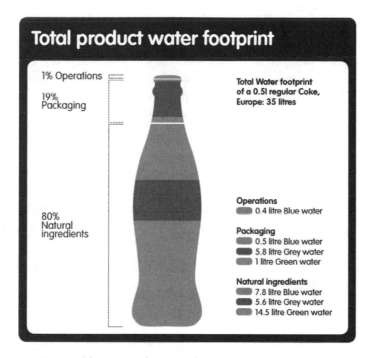

FIGURE 22.2 Coca-Cola's version of its water footprint. According to Coca-Cola and the Nature Conservancy, the total water footprint for Coca-Cola sweetened with beet sugar and produced in the Netherlands is 35 liters per half liter or 70 liters water per liter of soda. This industry-sponsored result comes to about one-fifth the 340-liter-per-liter footprint calculated by independent investigators. Source: Coca-Cola Europe, 2011.

percent. As shown in Figure 22.2, Coca-Cola and the Nature Conservancy estimated that each half-liter bottle required 15 liters of green water, 8 of blue, and 12 of gray. This comes to a total of 35 liters per half-liter bottle. Doubling that yields a 70-liter water footprint for one liter of Coca-Cola produced under conditions considered most optimal.[10]

The difference between the Nature Conservancy's water footprint of 70 liters per liter and the University of Twente's 340 for soda produced under the most conservative conditions must surely explain why Coca-Cola wanted to do its own study and why it recruited the Nature Conservancy as a partner. Accounting for the fivefold discrepancy requires a close examination of each of the assumptions underlying the various calculations, but the company-funded report does not provide enough detail to permit such scrutiny, nor does it provide references. Instead, the report admits, "Because we don't have all the data at our fingertips, we have to work with a lot of assumptions, some of which are questionable." Coca-Cola has a vested interest in wanting its water footprint to be as low as possible, and we can only assume that the consultants, consciously or unconsciously, made assumptions that minimized apparent water use. The Nature Conservancy's participation neutralizes suspicion of the company's motives and makes the results seem as though they come from a highly credible source.

The Nature Conservancy explains this partnership as deriving from common interests in water conservation:

> In 2007, Coca-Cola announced a sustainability effort to "replenish water equivalent to what is used in finished beverages" by the year 2020. Understanding their dependence and impact on water resources around the world, The Coca-Cola Company enlisted the expertise of The Nature Conservancy to help quantify the "replenishment credits" that the company could claim as a result of their investment in hundreds of local community watershed projects around the world. . . . The replenishment credits gained from these watershed projects are counted against the volume of water consumed in the company's bottling plants. This analysis revealed that the company will have achieved 42 percent of its replenishment goal by the end of 2013.[11]

Coca-Cola's press release pointed out that "the Company and the Conservancy found that the largest portion of the product water footprints assessed in the pilot studies comes from the field, not the factory." Translation: "It's not us, it's those sloppy sugar producers who use all the water." The discrepancy in these results casts doubt on the integrity of the sponsored Nature Conservancy study. Neither the Conservancy nor Coca-Cola makes it easy to find out how much money is involved in their partnership, but it must run to many millions.[12] Regardless of the size of its contributions, Coca-Cola gains invaluable reputational benefits from this partnership.

HOW DO SODA COMPANIES DEAL WITH WATER RISKS?

How soft drink companies deal with water issues is a topic for business case studies. As one such study explained, "The food and beverage sectors face water risk in both direct and indirect (supply chain) aspects of their business. These sectors also face the broadest types of potential risk (physical, reputational and regulatory) across their entire value chain."[13] Soda companies recognize these risks and deal with them in multiple ways. Over the years, they have assembled teams to deal with water risks, entered into partnerships with international agencies and nongovernmental environmental organizations such as the Nature Conservancy and the World Wildlife Fund, and created system-wide programs to back up commitments to reduce, recycle, and replenish. The companies say their goals are to return to communities and nature an amount of water equivalent to what they use (Coca-Cola) and to conserve water in operations and work with other organizations to bring safe water to developing countries (PepsiCo).

Coca-Cola, for example, has developed a "beverage process water recovery system" to reclaim wastewater using a combination of biological controls, ultrafiltration, reverse osmosis, ozone, and ultraviolet irradiation. The recovered water, although it meets or exceeds quality standards for drinking water, is to be used only for cleaning and bottle washing. Water conservation, says the company, is essential for the sustainability of its business and the communities it serves. By 2020, it will "safely return to communities and nature an amount of water equivalent to what we use in our finished beverages and their production." The company requires every bottling plant to develop a water-sustainability program to preserve community supplies. It works with U.S. growers of corn—the source of high-fructose corn syrup—to reduce their water footprints.[14] Coca-Cola's 2013 water stewardship report and 2013/2014 Sustainability Report sum up its global progress:

- Total liters used: 239 billion
- Water use ratio: 2.08 (direct)
- Plants in compliance: 96 percent
- Water replenished: 35 percent

PepsiCo says much the same. Its CEO was one of the first to sign the United Nations CEO Water Mandate in 2007. This committed companies to adhere to water management in six areas: direct operations, supply chain and watershed management, collective action, public policy, community engagement and transparency. PepsiCo reports considerable progress in these areas.[15]

PepsiCo's public policy commitments are particularly noteworthy. In 2009, it published guidelines in support of water as a fundamental human right, thereby endorsing the United Nations' goal of granting all people the right to safe, sufficient, acceptable, physically accessible, and affordable water for personal and domestic use. PepsiCo says it also consistently advocates for ethical engagement in water-related policy. Water stewardship, the company states, is good for society, but also good for business.[16] The business objectives explain why both soda companies so actively engage in community partnerships focused on water conservation.

THE DUAL BENEFITS OF COMMUNITY WATER PARTNERSHIPS

If you are a soda company and want to head off complaints about your appropriation of water, you fund reclamation projects in vulnerable communities and areas that earn you applause and honors. Here are a few examples.

PepsiCo and the Nature Conservancy

PepsiCo, as I noted earlier, also partners with the Nature Conservancy. Part of the partnership is the Recycle for Nature program, which links recycling to the Conservancy's water restoration projects. PepsiCo commits up to a million dollars a year to Conservancy projects to save and restore river water in nine states. The Conservancy "is drawn to this partnership with PepsiCo because we want to work with companies that can help us bend the trajectory of our common water future toward a more positive outcome by promoting widespread adoption of sustainable water practices." PepsiCo also supports the Nature Conservancy's Green Swamp Preserve in North Carolina, a haven for the endangered Venus flytrap and other carnivorous plants.[17]

Through its foundation, PepsiCo partners with groups working to provide access to safe water in developing countries, particularly in Ghana, Kenya, Brazil, China, and India, countries among Pepsi's most actively expanding markets. These projects install village water and irrigation systems, build harvesting cisterns, establish water health centers, improve sanitation programs, and recharge aquifers. In 2013, PepsiCo Jordan worked with the Jordan Valley Authority to construct a channel to collect surplus water and a new dam to collect rainwater to recharge underground water reserves.[18]

Coca-Cola Ekocenters

Coca-Cola's best-known partnerships are with groups that use advanced purification technology to provide clean water to children, health clinics, and rural communities in Africa and Latin America. The company says it will place nearly two thousand "Ekocenters"—kiosks providing water purification systems and other services—in twenty countries by the end of 2015.[19] Ekocenters use Slingshot (a reference to the story of David and Goliath) water distillers, developed by Dean Kamen, the American entrepreneur and inventor of the Segway, among many other patentable items. Ekocenters are capable of turning any source of impure water into 850 liters of safe drinking water a day. Coke's CEO, Muhtar Kent, says of the company's water partnership with Mr. Kamen:

> This is a really big deal. We believe that through our wide network of distribution and logistics, we can actually get these units to the last mile, where people don't have a source of electricity, where people don't have a source of clean drinking water, where people are dying.... Why are we doing all of this? Because when there's healthy communities, we have a healthy, sustainable business...In a very large geography in the world, that choice does not exist. Therefore, in my view, we are providing a huge service to humanity.[20]

Mr. Kamen also appreciates the partnership: "Coca-Cola is the largest, most efficient logistics operation ever put on this planet.... Coca-Cola can take their product and cost-effectively get it anywhere—and the poorest people in the world get access to it." The test-market Ekocenters dispense Slingshot water and provide solar-powered Wi-Fi. Not by coincidence, they also sell snacks and other Coca-Cola products. As one unimpressed critic puts it, "Fresh water and solar power are very nice of Coke to provide, in addition to marketing their products. But let's just call this EKOCENTER what it is: A glorified concession stand." Coca-Cola's CEO may promote them as a "big deal," but much about the Ekocenters remains theoretical. The units cost at least $100,000 each to build, and financing for them has remained elusive.[21]

Coca-Cola and WaterHealth International

Coca-Cola also holds a minority equity ownership in the for-profit WaterHealth International (WHI), which installs and operates water purification systems. Through its Child with Water program, WHI says it aims to deliver 500 million liters of safe drinking water per year to a million schoolchildren in developing countries by the end of 2015.[22] Perhaps it does, but I would like to know more about who bears the costs of this enterprise, whether the schools carry other Coke products, and what Coke gets out of the deal. But this is one way Coca-Cola wins enthusiastic support from such partners, who can be expected to overlook and remain silent about the health and environmental effects of soda production and consumption.

Other Community Water Projects

Overall, Coca-Cola is heavily invested in water projects. By its count:

- 386 community water partnership projects
- 94 countries
- 532 external partners
- $247 million invested
- 1.6 million beneficiaries[23]

Its most ambitious program is the Replenish Africa Initiative (RAIN), with a goal of improving access to safe water for two million Africans. Coca-Cola and its 140 partner organizations back RAIN with a $65 million commitment. By 2020, the company's Africa Foundation expects to "improve safe water access for 6 million Africans; economically empower up to 250,000 women and youth; promote health and hygiene in thousands of communities, schools, and health centers; and return up to 18.5 billion liters of water to nature and communities."[24]

PepsiCo also lists community access to clean water as one of its top CSR priorities, and it funds water projects run by the Earth Institute at Columbia University, Water.Org, the Safe Water Network, the Energy Resources Institute, the China Women's Development Foundation, WaterHope, WaterCredit, and PepsiCorps. Because Coca-Cola provides specific funding information about its international water projects, I list a few in Table 22.1.[25]

Soda company water partnerships cover all bases—private nongovernmental organizations, academic research enterprises, and government agencies, domestic and international. As is evident from Coca-Cola's partnership with the Nature Conservancy, these provide substantial benefits to soda companies as well as to recipients. Partnerships like these deflect at-

TABLE 22.1 Selected examples of Coca-Cola's water partnerships, programs, and initiatives, 2013

COUNTRY	DONATION	WATER PARTNER, PROJECT
Australia	$500,000	World Wildlife Fund, Inc.: Project Catalyst: Great Barrier Reef
Ecuador	$25,000	The Nature Conservancy: The Chongon-Colonche and Cerro Blanco ecological corridor: an initiative to conserve and restore key water sources and biodiversity
Indonesia	$74,887	Atma Jaya: rainwater harvesting system to support a healthy active school
Pakistan	$99,998	World Wide Fund for Nature: improving sub-watershed management and environmental awareness around Ayubia National Park (western Himalayas)
Spain	$199,212	University of Cordoba: reducing the hydrological impact of imported strawberries, Huelva region
Taiwan	$30,000	Environmental Quality Protection Foundation: green water school series: water adaptation school project
Thailand	$120,000	Population and Community Development Association: clean water for communities: solar-powered water systems
Vietnam	$180,000	World Wildlife Fund, Inc.: strengthening biodiversity conservation and improving dependent local livelihoods

tention to the companies' water use, build allies across the private and public sectors, and make regulation seem heavy-handed and unnecessary. And because the partnerships really do clean up water supplies and reduce water use, they provide unassailable public relations opportunities.

In 2012, for example, Coca-Cola gave grants to American Rivers, the National Fish and Wildlife Foundation, and the U.S. Forest Service to restore the Indian Valley meadow in Sierra Crest at the headwaters of the Mokelumne River in California. The river supports the water supplies of Contra Costa and Alameda counties along the East Bay across from San Francisco. Unsurprisingly, the river also supplies water for the region's Coca-Cola bottling plant. The public relations benefit of this particular project is evident from a video about the project from USDA's Forest Service that features Coca-Cola's involvement in this project.[26]

More recently, the USDA announced a public-private partnership with Coca-Cola to return more than a billion liters of water to the National Forest System. The company said it "supports more than 100 water projects throughout the United States in an effort to balance the water we use and help to ensure clean water supplies for communities," all of them, also not coincidentally, locations of Coke bottling plants.[27]

ACQUISITION OF WATER RIGHTS: CONSEQUENCES

Roughly 90 percent of the world's fresh water is under public control, but current trends are toward increasing privatization. Once corporations own water supplies, they charge more for water use and sometimes cut corners on water quality standards. The giant food corporation Nestlé (no relation) has leased or owns at least fifty spring sites throughout the United States. In some of these places, Nestlé is alleged to have inappropriately taken water from aquifers, raised prices, and polarized communities. Soda companies have not, to my knowledge, engaged in such practices in the United States. Instead, they typically buy brands of bottled water—Dasani (Coca-Cola) and Aquafina (PepsiCo)—and fill those bottles with water from taxpayer-supported municipal supplies or community springs. Soda companies buy municipal water at household rates. Customers pay for soda-company water twice: in city taxes and in the higher price of the water in bottles or in soda.[28]

Counterintuitive as it may seem, sodas are more profitable than bottled water. People choose sodas by brand but buy bottled water by price. Price competition means that soda companies do not make much money on their bottled water brands. For both Coke and Pepsi, bottled water represents less than 10 percent of total sales in the United States. This explains why both companies care so much about soda sales and why they look to countries such as China and India for sales growth.[29] Such places, however, have water problems of their own. To bottle sodas in India, for example, the companies must make deals for water rights that sometimes conflict with the water needs of local communities, as discussed below.

In the late 1990s, advocates for poor communities in India organized demonstrations against Coca-Cola to complain that its bottling plants were depleting village water supplies. The company recognized that it needed to protect its international business interests and asked for advice. Its consultant reported that 39 percent of Coca-Cola's worldwide bottling plants were located in water-stressed areas, precisely in the countries targeted for sales expansion. Developing markets are the riskiest for water scarcity and poor quality, and produce the world's highest water footprints for bottled water and soda. Both Coke and Pepsi want to reduce water use from local sources and protect their water supplies, and both win prizes for doing so. But they also want to head off community protests and environmental regulations.[30]

Coca-Cola's Water Problems in India

Coca-Cola's ongoing problems in India may be a sign of what is to come in other developing regions. In 1999, Hindustan Coca-Cola Beverages established a plant in Plachimada in Kerala state, in the south of India, and the village council licensed the company to begin production in 2000. Although Coca-Cola said that it would draw around 510,000 liters of water each day from boreholes and open wells, advocates claimed that it also pumped an additional 1.5 million liters a day from local reserves. They said the direct water-use ratio at that plant was 3.75 liters per liter. The bottling plant also produced a great deal of undrinkable wastewater. Within two years, local residents protested a drop in the water table so severe that farmers could no longer irrigate their crops. They complained that wastewater had polluted their land and wells to such an extent that residents were forced to walk miles to obtain clean water for drinking and irrigation.[31]

The protests grew into a movement—with the rallying cry "When you drink Coke you drink the blood of the people." When Coca-Cola gave up and closed the plant in 2004, its withdrawal inspired other such campaigns.[32] The Plachimada movement introduced two new terms into discussions of water access: "water mining" and "water democracy." The Indian environmental advocate Vandana Shiva, in an account of how women in Kerala had forced closure of the Coca-Cola plant, noted that their victory resulted from creation of broad alliances and use of multiple strategies, and led to widespread recognition of communities' rights to water. Her account of their successful advocacy reproduces the "Plachimada Declaration," which contains statements such as these:

- Water is not private property. It is a common resource for the sustenance of all.
- Water is a fundamental human right. It has to be conserved, protected, and managed.
- Water is not a commodity. We should resist all criminal attempts to marketize, privatize, and corporatize water.
- The production and marketing of the poisonous products of the Coca-Cola and Pepsi Cola corporations lead to total destruction and pollution and also endanger the very existence of local communities.

- We exhort the people all over the world to boycott the products of Coca-Cola and Pepsi Cola.[33]

To water advocates in India, the issue is clear: soda companies' mining of local water supplies is *preposterous*. Amit Srivastava, a director of Global Resistance, a group providing support to movements against corporate globalization in India, points out that the amount of water used by Coca-Cola in one year could meet the entire needs of people who lack access to clean drinking water for forty-seven days. "In a world where one of 5 people do not have access to potable water, it is indeed preposterous that any company could extract such large amounts of life sustaining water, and convert the vast majority of the freshwater into wastewater."[34]

Both Coke and Pepsi are committed to investing billions of dollars in the Indian market without having solved their water-sourcing problems. A Coca-Cola plant in Mehdiganj near Varanesi, which opened in 1999, has been under protest since 2003 over depletion of water supplies and polluted wastewater. In 2014, community protesters claimed a "colossal victory." Coca-Cola wanted to expand the plant, but the courts said that the company was violating its license, and the Central Ground Water Authority denied the expansion. Coca-Cola cancelled its plans on the grounds of "inordinate delays" in environmental clearances. It also stopped, or was forced to stop, plans for a bottling plant in Tamil Nadu. The company is facing similar problems in Indonesia.[35]

Such protests should be expected elsewhere as soda companies expand their marketing into the developing world. As University of Michigan business professor Aneel Karnani explains, water stewardship is not sufficient to overcome the "tragedy of the commons"—the overuse of common resources on which a business depends. "Asking companies to voluntarily act in the public interest will not be enough to solve these problems. It is essential to develop regulatory regimes with appropriate incentives and ability to enforce sanctions." Since a major purpose of CSR is to stave off regulation, it seems unlikely that soda companies will take his advice. Instead, the Coca-Cola Foundation's latest initiative is to partner with TERI University in New Delhi to create a department of regional water studies.[36]

Coca-Cola's Water Problems in the United States

Unlike India, the United States still has plenty of tap water available, at least in the East. But Coca-Cola's strategy is to encourage Americans to drink its bottled water or sodas instead. In the early 2000s, Coke developed a restaurant campaign called H2NO designed to discourage customers from drinking free tap water when they could be ordering soft drinks. In 2013, anti-soda advocates learned about a similar Coca-Cola program, Cap the Tap. The company had initiated the program in 2001 in partnership with Olive Garden restaurants as a means to increase revenues from sales of bottled waters and other branded drinks. The program's stated purpose is to capture revenue lost to tap water: "Every time your business fills a cup or glass with tap water, it pours potential profits down the drain. The good news: Cap the Tap—a program available through your Coca-Cola representative—changes these dynamics by teaching crew members or wait staff suggestive selling techniques to convert requests for tap water into orders for revenue-generating beverages."[37]

A program guide for Coca-Cola staff explains how managers can obtain a toolbox with posters and other information about how to avoid giving tap water to customers.[38] Cap the Tap comes with its own logo, shown in Figure 22.3.

Despite removal of the information from online sites, advocates suspect that such programs still exist. A 2014 advertisement for Pepsi's Gatorade, for example, called water "the enemy of performance," an announcement that induced advocates to file a complaint with the New York State attorney general. Health advocates are concerned about the implication of "turn off the tap" for First Lady Michelle Obama's Let's Move! campaign and its relationship to its private-sector collaborating group, the Partnership for a Healthier America (PHA). The PHA describes itself as devoted to working with the private sector to solve the childhood obesity crisis. Coca-Cola—directly through its Dasani brand of bottled water and indirectly through the ABA—supports the PHA's Drink Up campaign to encourage water consumption. The campaign actively promotes consumption of bottled water

Increase profits by selling
revenue-generating beverages
instead of tap water

FIGURE 22.3. Coca-Cola's Cap the Tap program logo, 2009. Information about the program was available online in 2013 but disappeared soon after the publication of critical blog posts.

but occasionally mentions that tap water is also acceptable.[39] Cap the Tap reveals the contradictions and potential conflicts of interest inherent in public health partnerships with food and beverage companies. From the soda industry's point of view, drinking tap water is bad for business. It can hardly be a coincidence that the featured speaker at PHA's 2015 summit meeting was Pepsi's CEO, Indra Nooyi.

THE DEBATE: A DILEMMA FOR ADVOCATES?

In 2014, as discussed in Chapter 21, Oxfam, along with an international coalition of anti-poverty advocacy groups, issued its annual assessment scorecard on the performance of global brands on a range of issues: land use, treatment of women, treatment of farmers and workers, effects on climate, transparency, and—relevant to this chapter—water conservation. Oxfam gave both Coca-Cola and PepsiCo scores of 5 out of 10 for their water conservation efforts, viewing both as having achieved some progress in this area.[40]

Let's agree that soda companies are indeed succeeding in using less water and producing less wastewater. Let's also grant that they are funding

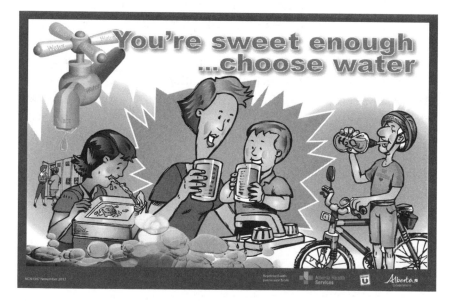

FIGURE 22.4 Poster promoting consumption of water, not sodas. Canada's Alberta Health Services produced this poster to encourage adults and children to drink water rather than sugary drinks. Courtesy Government of Alberta.

hundreds of community clean water and conservation initiatives. But if they win prizes for doing so, the awards are for fixing problems they caused in the first place. Soda companies' water stewardship efforts, effective as they may be, distract us from the fundamental issue: the extraction, use, waste, and pollution of hundreds of billions of liters of water every year to make products that promote obesity, tooth decay, and other human disease.

TAKE ACTION

Short of putting companies out of business, advocates are left with few options related to water issues.

- Monitor and hold soda companies accountable for their promises to reduce water footprints and to appropriately manage water resources, particularly in water-stressed areas.
- Discourage governments from approving bottling plants in water-stressed areas.
- Charge soda companies higher prices for use of taxpayer-supported community water supplies.
- Take legal action against soda company violations of rules for appropriate water use and waste disposal.
- Encourage consumption of water rather than sodas through education and policy options (see example in Figure 22.4).
- Support local water systems and public access to safe drinking water.
- Promote programs that make safe drinking water available in schools, parks, and workplaces.

"Hardball" Tactics: Defending Turf, Attacking Critics

23

Lobbying, the Revolving Door, Campaign Contributions, and Lawsuits

From its inception, the U.S. government has attempted to control, but has also responded to, what the founding fathers called "factions"—now known as special-interest groups. Then and now, such groups invest time and money in getting Congress and federal agencies to act on their behalf. Soda companies are prototypes of groups spending enormous sums to protect their ability to conduct business. For decades, the soda trade group now known as the American Beverage Association (ABA) has lobbied against any government action—no matter how beneficial to the public or seemingly trivial—that might raise the cost of soda production and marketing or discourage consumption. The ABA takes great pride in its successes, and the list of its lobbying issues is breathtakingly comprehensive. It has lobbied against nutrition labeling, packaging standards, fair labor standards, the exclusion of sodas from food assistance programs and school meals, limitations on franchises, quotas on sugar, container deposit laws, and restrictions on television advertising to children, among many other issues.[1]

In these next chapters, I deal with the ways soda companies work behind the scenes to pressure governments and government agencies to act on their behalf. This chapter examines soda industry lobbying, participation of lobbyists in the "revolving door," contributions to political campaigns, and use of lawsuits. Chapter 24 looks at soda company use of less transparent tactics such as third-party front groups to attack critics and gain popular support. Chapters 25 to 27 show how soda companies apply these tactics in real-world situations involving attempts to cap soda sizes and impose taxes.

This present chapter gets us into matters of money in politics and how all three branches of government foster Court promote a political system that permits wealthy corporations and individuals to exert extraordinary political power. Big Soda uses this system to its advantage. A system skewed to favor corporate interests involves rules and regulations so complicated, detailed, arcane, and obscure as to be beyond the comprehension of anyone who is not paid to understand them. Companies hire lobbyists to understand and use the rules on their behalf. To counter the influence of money in politics, advocates also must learn how this system works. Soda lobbying is a good place to start.

SODA LOBBYING AND LOBBYISTS

Lobbyists, by definition, are individuals paid by a company or organization to promote their clients' interest to the federal government—members of Congress, the president, or officials or staff of federal agencies. Lobbying in the United States is governed by the wonderfully named Honest Leadership and Open Government Act of 2007, an update of the Lobbying Disclosure Act of 1995. This act requires lobbyists to publicly disclose who pays them, how much they are paid, and which government entity they lobby, and to identify the issues they are discussing with federal officials. The law is vague about many of these requirements and leaves plenty of room for loopholes and evasions. Congress is not especially interested in enforcing the rules that do exist. It is no surprise that compliance with regulations is inconsistent, and many of the best-paid lobbyists do not even bother to register with the government. Furthermore, Congress does not require lobbyists to reveal either their position on issues or the amounts of time and money they spend lobbying on specific matters.[2]

The quarterly reports filed by individual corporations as well as the lobbying firms and lobbyists they hire are lengthy and tedious to read. Although the U.S. Senate compiles information about lobbying and lobbyists in a searchable database, the site is complicated and its use requires patience and practice. The Center for Responsive Politics performs an outstanding public service by compiling this information in an easier format at OpenSecrets.org. Its compilations reveal that in 2013 the sixty leading food and beverage companies spent $30,350,645 to support the work of 329 lobbyists. Coca-Cola, PepsiCo, and the ABA ranked first, second, and eighth, respectively, on the list of amounts spent on lobbying.[3]

TABLE 23.1 Soda lobbying activities, 2013: summary

LOBBYING ACTIVITIES	COCA-COLA	PEPSICO	AMERICAN BEVERAGE ASSOCIATION (ABA)	TOTAL
Expenditure for lobbyists	$5,981,527	$3,720,000	$1,240,000	$10,941,527
Number of in-house lobbyists	9	6	6	21
Number of outsourced lobbying firms	6	6	4	16
Number of outsourced lobbyists	32	21	17	70
Total number of lobbyists	41	27	23	91
Revolving door: lobbyists previously employed by government, number (percent)	32 (78%)	19 (70%)	15 (65%)	~70%

SOURCE: OpenSecrets.com, 2013.

Table 23.1 summarizes data obtained from Open Secrets on Big Soda lobbying activities in 2013. Together, Coca-Cola, PepsiCo, and the ABA reported spending nearly $11 million on lobbying, an amount that represents 37 percent of total lobbying expenditures by the sixty companies. The soda industry takes lobbying seriously. The three groups pay a remarkable number of individuals—ninety-one are listed—to lobby on their behalf. They either employ these lobbyists directly (in-house) or pay lobbying firms to recruit others to promote soda interests to federal or state governments.

The amount of money that food and beverage companies devote to lobbying depends on the issues Congress is considering. For example, soda lobbying expenditures rose sharply from 2008 to 2009. Whereas the ABA spent less than $700,000 on lobbying in 2008, the amount jumped to $19 million in 2009. Coca-Cola's lobbying expenses went from $2.5 million to $9.4 million, and Pepsi's from $1.1 million to $9.2 million that year. Altogether, Big Soda spent nearly $38 million in lobbying in 2009. Why the sharp increase? Congress was considering a tax on sodas. The lobbying funds were well spent: Congress soon gave up on that idea.[4]

In 2013, even with no such tax under consideration, soda lobbyists reported meeting with officials and staff of the House and Senate; the White House; the USDA, FDA, and EPA; the Departments of State, Treasury, and Homeland Security; the Commodity Futures Trading Commission; and the Securities and Exchange Commission, among others. It is difficult to think of a single issue relevant to soda companies that lobbyists did not discuss.

Although lobbyists for the ABA report issues mainly as "monitored," and PepsiCo's lobbyists say their discussions involve no specific legislation, Coca-Cola's lobbyists are sometimes more explicit about what they list as matters of concern. Table 23.2 gives some examples of Coca-Cola lobbying disclosures related to issues discussed in this book.

Even this short list of examples should be enough to demonstrate that any initiative that might affect soda production, transportation, sales, or

TABLE 23.2   Issues reported as discussed with federal officials in 2013 by lobbyists for Coca-Cola

ISSUE REPORTED	MY TRANSLATION
Promote active healthy lifestyles, obesity prevention, and additional funding for physical education programs	Physical activity is more important than soda intake as a causative factor in obesity
Oppose programs and legislation that discriminate against specific foods and beverages	Don't pass laws that single out sodas for taxes or size restriction
Educate policy makers on companies' voluntary efforts to reduce calories from beverages in schools	Do not pass or enforce rules that restrict soda sales in schools
Oppose proposals that restrict or ban the sale of certain sizes of beverage containers	Do not allow New York City—or any other state or municipal government—to limit the size of sodas that can be sold (Chapter 25)
Promote choice and fairness in the guidelines of the Supplemental Nutrition Assistance Program (SNAP); oppose policies that single out certain food and beverage items available to purchase under SNAP	Do not allow the USDA to make sodas ineligible for purchase with SNAP benefits (Chapter 16)
Oppose legislation that would tax bottled and canned beverages to pay for wastewater treatment and water infrastructure upgrades	Do not tax sodas (Chapters 26 and 27)
Support regulatory reform in commodity market for aluminum	Allow us to buy aluminum for our cans at lower prices
Support international and domestic tax reform for American-headquartered companies that compete globally	Reduce our corporate taxes
Seek assistance to urge the governments of Chile and Peru to include industry in discussions on proposed labeling regimes in those countries	Make sure that Chile and Peru do not require front-of-package food labels that might discourage soda purchases
Seek assistance to urge the Mexican government to work with industry to implement meaningful solutions to obesity	Ensure that Mexico does not impose a soda tax (Chapter 27)

SOURCE: OpenSecrets.com, 2014.

profitability—no matter how apparently obscure—is fair game for soda-company lobbying. The job of soda lobbyists is to make sure that government officials are well aware of the companies' interests in every issue that might affect business operations.

Although meetings of government officials with lobbyists take place behind closed doors, details occasionally surface. The White House Office of Management and Budget, for example, sometimes publishes lists of meeting attendees. In mid-2012, five of its regulatory affairs staff met with seven representatives of Coke, Pepsi, the ABA, and Dr Pepper Snapple. Of these, four were listed as registered lobbyists in the Open Secrets database. The USDA had recently released nutrition standards for school meals and snacks that would restrict the calories in beverages with added sugar to 25 per 8 ounces, well below the amounts in regular sodas. It is not far-fetched to guess that soda industry lobbyists hoped to convince the White House to ease the standards.[5] As discussed in Chapter 12, USDA later set 40 calories per 8 ounces as the cutoff point for drinks sold in high schools, more than its initial proposal but still below levels in full-calorie sodas and those in sports drinks such as Pepsi's Gatorade.

THE REVOLVING DOOR

The Open Secrets database reveals that 65 to 78 percent of soda industry lobbyists formerly held positions in government, a situation known as the "revolving door" (Table 23.1). The term is used to describe any industry's recruitment of former government officials as employees, as well as government's recruitment of people who formerly worked for industry. Lobbying laws put some restrictions on how quickly government officials taking jobs in industry can act on behalf of their new private-sector employers to influence legislation—usually not within one or two years. Even so, the potential for conflict of interest is high when former government officials employ their knowledge of how to work the system in the interests of the very industries they used to regulate.

Big Soda lobbyists report having held jobs as legislative aides and advisors, research directors, staff assistants, and advisors to members of the House and Senate, the president, and senior staff at the White House, as well as key positions in any number of federal agencies. To cite just a few examples from Open Secrets:

- Before he joined the C2 firm, which lobbies for PepsiCo, Nelson Litterst had a ten-year career as a legislative assistant to former House members Robert Michel (R-Ill.) and Gary Frank (R-Conn.), as a liaison to the George W. Bush presidential transition team, and as a legislative aide to the White House.
- Julia Sessoms, a lobbyist for PepsiCo who attended the White House Office of Management and Budget meeting I referred to earlier, formerly worked as a legislative aide to the late Senator Edward M. Kennedy (D-Mass.).
- Kirsten Chadwick, a partner in Fierce, Isakowitz & Blalock, a lobbying firm used by Coca-Cola, worked as a legislative aide to the White House under Presidents George H. W. Bush and George W. Bush, and as deputy assistant convention manager for the Republican National Committee.
- Kathleen Quint Black, a lobbyist for Coca-Cola, held positions as a tax and finance policy advisor to a current representative, Sam Johnson (R-Tex.), and a former senator, Olympia Snowe (R-Me.).
- The president of the ABA in 2014, Susan Neely, is also a registered lobbyist. She formerly held jobs as assistant secretary for public affairs at the Department of Homeland Security and as special assistant for Homeland Security at the White House under President George W. Bush.

Former government officials bring to their work as lobbyists an intimate knowledge of how the system operates, connections to leaders and staff of both political parties, and a vast address book of personal contacts accumulated on their jobs. Soda companies value Washington-insider information and attract former insiders with salaries that typically exceed those of government employees.[6]

ELECTION CAMPAIGNS: DISCLOSED CONTRIBUTIONS

Corporations as well as individuals are somewhat constrained by federal election laws in the amounts of money they are permitted to contribute to candidates. They are also somewhat constrained by how much they can give to political party committees or to political action committees (PACs), groups that raise and spend money to support or oppose political candidates. Prior to the Supreme Court's 2014 ruling in *McCutcheon v. Federal Election Commission*, individuals and corporations were limited to an aggregate total of $123,000 per election for the amounts they could give to candidates, national party committees, and state or local party committees.[7] These limitations explain why corporate campaign contributions appear lower than lobbying expenditures.

The Supreme Court's *McCutcheon* decision got rid of these restrictions. The Court ruled that because aggregate limits on campaign contributions "do not further the government's interest in preventing quid pro quo corruption or the appearance of such corruption, while at the same time seriously restricting participation in the democratic process, they are invalid under the First Amendment." In effect, this decision allowed corporate and individual election contributions to be virtually unlimited, especially when funneled through PACs or party committees.[8]

Table 23.3 summarizes information from Open Secrets about the contributions of Coca-Cola, PepsiCo, and the ABA in the 2012 election cycle, when the pre-*McCutcheon* restrictions still applied.[9] Such amounts were expected to increase greatly in subsequent election cycles.

TABLE 23.3   Big Soda campaign contributions, 2012 (pre-*McCutcheon*) election cycle*

CONTRIBUTIONS	COCA-COLA	PEPSICO	AMERICAN BEVERAGE ASSOCIATION (ABA)
Total campaign contributions	$2,900,000	$1,100,000	$1,500,000
To political parties	$150,000	$220,000	$16,000
To candidates	$830,000	$535,000	$200,000
To leadership PACs	$77,000	$51,000	$14,000
To 527 committees	$1,300,000	$220,000	$1,300,000
To the Republican Governors Association	$750,000	$50,000	$640,000
To the Democratic Governors Association	$410,000	$61,000	$310,000
Highest contribution to a single candidate	$54,000 (Barack Obama, D)	$50,000 (Mitt Romney, R)	$10,000 Tommy Thompson (R-Wisc.)
Contributions from individuals	$240,000	$220,000	$19,000
Contributions from PACs	$590,000	$320,000	$180,000

* Amounts rounded off for easier reading.

SOURCE: Center for Responsive Politics, Open Secrets, 2013. The Supreme Court's removal of restrictions on campaign contributions in *McCutcheon v. Federal Election Commission* did not apply until the 2014 election cycle.

Although not listed in Table 23.3, the Dr Pepper Snapple Group also contributes to political campaigns, but in relatively small amounts—$42,200 in 2012, mostly distributed in amounts of about $1,000.[10] In contrast, Coca-Cola, PepsiCo, and the ABA each reported contributing more than $5 million to candidates and their political parties. For Coca-Cola, the stated amount underestimates this company's investment in influencing Congress, as it only reflects the parent company's donations. Open Secrets also reports additional contributions, some quite substantial, from Coca-Cola Bottling United, Coca-Cola Enterprises, Coca-Cola Puerto Rico Bottlers, Coca-Cola Bottlers' Association, Coca-Cola Bottling Co., and Ozarks Coca-Cola Bottling.

Soda company contributions to political parties appear relatively modest, in line with the old legal restrictions, but the companies are equal-opportunity donors. The Open Secrets database indicates that the ABA, Coke, and Pepsi donate about equally to Democratic and Republican parties and candidates. Coke and Pepsi's largest contributions to individual candidates went to those running for president.

Soda company contributions to leadership PACs help current and former members of Congress and other prominent politicians raise funds for travel, office expenses, consultants, and other expenses. The soda industry contributes especially generously to 527 committees. These are tax-exempt political groups organized under section 527 of the tax code. In what may seem a subtle distinction, 527 groups are not permitted to "expressly advocate" for a candidate or party, meaning that as long as they avoid using phrases such as "elect," "defeat," or "Smith for Congress," they can say what they like about candidates' opinions and records to mobilize voters. They are allowed to raise as much money as they can get but must disclose their donors.

The Republican and Democratic Governors Associations, listed in Table 23.3, are state 527s. The ABA and Coca-Cola donate generously to both, but much more so to the Republican committees. Pepsi's much smaller contribution slightly favors the Democratic 527s. As political reporter Jim Hightower points out, shareholders rarely know that their soda company investments are funneled into the vaults of the Republican Governors Association, which "channels the political cash into the campaigns of assorted right-wing governors."[11]

The contributions summarized in the table come from individuals working for Coke, Pepsi, or the ABA, or their families, but Big Soda also contributes through PACs. One way or another, the laws permit many opportunities for attempting to influence elections to ensure that soda-friendly legislators are in place at the state and federal levels.

One additional point about disclosed influence: Open Secrets reports that forty-one members of the U.S. Congress owned stock in Coca-Cola, and forty-two owned stock in PepsiCo in 2013. Without knowing more about the extent of these holdings, or even of legislators' knowledge of them, you cannot assume that stock ownership influences voting decisions. But such ownership gives the appearance of conflict of interest. It suggests that legislators have a vested interest in making sure that no congressional action interferes with upward trends in company share prices.[12]

ELECTION CAMPAIGNS: UNDISCLOSED "DARK MONEY" CONTRIBUTIONS

In the methods for funding candidates discussed so far, the donors and the size of their donations are matters of public record. In 2010, however, the Supreme Court changed that requirement. In *Citizens United v. Federal Election Commission*, the Court permitted not only unlimited spending on election campaigns but also secrecy about its donors. It effectively granted everyone, including corporations, the right to give unlimited funds funneled through super PACs—on First Amendment grounds. Super PACs collect funds that can be used to support or oppose candidates through "independent expenditures," defined as money that is not donated directly to candidates or political parties. Super PACs must report donors but can accept anonymous contributions from nonprofit groups with some kind of stated social mission. By this route, corporate or private donors can donate anonymously to a nonprofit group set up for this express purpose. The group donates the funds to a super PAC, which uses the funds to run advertisements supporting or opposing candidates, reports the funds it gets from the nonprofit group, and allows the donors to that group to remain anonymous. This introduction of even more money into politics—and anonymous at that—seems like nothing less than corporate capture of the Supreme Court, as Figure 23.1 suggests.[13]

By July 2012, the anonymous "dark money" spent through this new loophole totaled an estimated $172 million, more than 90 percent of it donated by conservative, Republican-leaning groups. By 2014, business journals were reporting impressive growth in dark money spending outside of the

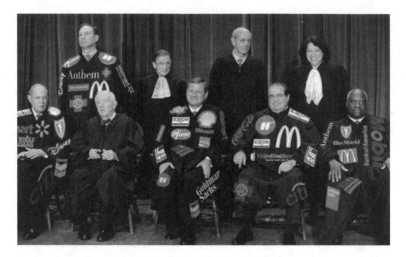

FIGURE 23.1 The Supreme Court's NASCAR sponsors. The Supreme Court's 2010 decision in *Citizens United v. Federal Election Commission* permitted unlimited, anonymous contributions to political campaigns. Only the four justices wearing robes free of corporate logos including Coca-Cola's voted against this decision. The court's decision in this case seems explicable only as the result of corporate capture of even this supposedly independent and nonpartisan branch of government. The image appeared at TucsonCitizen.com as "Wordless Editorial," February 2, 2010.

once standard campaign channels. The amounts were three times higher than those in the 2012 presidential campaign and seventeen times higher than elections before *Citizens United*, and were expected to total a billion dollars or more by the end of that year.[14] The *McCutcheon* decision should allow even higher spending.

Dark money makes it more difficult to track who influences policy. It also reinforces the power of lobbying. Legislators at the federal, state, and local levels must pay attention to what might happen the next time they run for office. Corporations offended by candidates' positions on issues will freely invest in negative advertising campaigns. Corporations favoring the candidates' stance will donate greater sums to their campaigns. The threat of unlimited expenditures on negative advertising should make any legislator think carefully about voting decisions that might affect donors' interests.

Do soda companies participate in dark money campaigns? Yes, they do. This became evident as a result of a court case in 2013 during the political fight over a Washington State proposition—Initiative 522—to label genetically modified foods (usually with "GMO," the abbreviation for "genetically modified organisms"). The Grocery Manufacturers Association (GMA) donated more than $11 million to the No on I-522 campaign—fully half of the $22 million total contributed to defeat that initiative. The attorney general in Washington State took the GMA to court on the grounds that it was violating state election laws by levying an assessment on its members and assuring them that their contributions would remain anonymous. In response to that lawsuit, GMA formed a PAC, Grocery Manufacturers Association Against I-522, and provided the attorney general with a list of its donors. The list, which makes fascinating reading, reveals that PepsiCo contributed precisely $2,352,965.71 to the GMA campaign and Coca-Cola donated $1,047,332.00.[15]

Why would soda companies care about a state initiative to label GMOs? Both Coke and Pepsi use high-fructose corn syrup (HFCS), undoubtedly made from genetically modified corn, and GMO corn is also undoubtedly used to make Pepsi's Frito-Lay snack foods. U.S. sugar beets are also mostly GMO. The biotechnology and food industry money that poured into Washington State succeeded in defeating I-522, but by a small margin: 51 percent to 49 percent.[16]

This was not the first time that soda companies had contributed to anti-GMO labeling campaigns. Both Coke and Pepsi donated to the ultimately successful campaign to defeat California's version of a GMO labeling initiative, Proposition 37. Pepsi contributed $2.5 million to that campaign, and Coke contributed $1.7 million. It also was not the last: both companies contributed generously to defeat GMO labeling initiatives in Colorado and Oregon in 2014. Ironically, both companies own organic brands. Their anti-labeling contributions led the Organic Consumers Association to call for a boycott of organic brands owned by soda companies: PepsiCo's Naked Juice, Tostitos Organic, and Tropicana Organic, and Coke's Honest Tea and Odwalla.[17]

Unsurprisingly, soda companies spend generously to defeat tax initiatives. Big Soda reportedly spent $12.8 million to defeat a proposed soda tax initiative in New York State, and greatly outspent proponents in California community tax initiatives, as detailed in Chapters 26 and 27.

DOES MONEY INFLUENCE VOTING DECISIONS?

The amounts spent on lobbying and election campaigns raise an obvious question: does soda money influence policy? Although it may seem self-evident that it does—why else would corporations spend so generously?—the question turns out to be difficult to answer. Research studies are few in number, yield contradictory results, and mostly focus on industries other than food. With respect to lobbying on a particular tax issue, for example, one analysis of audited corporate tax disclosures suggests that for every dollar spent on lobbying, the return to the corporation was $220—an excellent return on investment.[18] If true and applicable to other situations, the money is well used.

But researchers often find little correlation between corporate lobbying and voting behavior. Instead, they observe that the richest and best-performing corporations spend the most money in attempts to influence government. As for campaign contributions, one recent study of the telecommunications industry found a clear correlation between spending and outcome.[19]

A book devoted to this very question explains why the results of studies of lobbying effects on voting behavior are so difficult to interpret. Its author, Lynda Powell, a professor of political science at the University of Rochester, finds that although campaign donations do not seem clearly connected to voting patterns, they most definitely do influence what happens to bills and regulations *before* coming to a vote. Campaign contributions, she observes, clearly buy access to legislators, affect how bills are drafted, influence whether earmarks get into bills, and determine whether bills ever get to the floor for a vote. As Professor Powell explains, "The wording of just a sentence or two or the addition of an earmark makes all the difference to a special interest group. For other contributors, the goal may be to preserve the status quo and prevent a bill from coming to a vote at all."[20] These benefits are likely to be much the same for soda industry lobbying and contributions.

WHEN ALL ELSE FAILS: USE THE LAW

The chapters on soda size caps and taxes that follow describe how soda companies file lawsuits or try to get laws passed to protect their interests when they cannot achieve their goals by any other means. To cite one more example: in 2013, the North Carolina legislature passed the Commonsense Consumption Act, which blocks local jurisdictions from passing laws that might ban or restrict the sale of foods or beverages. The ABA celebrated the law:

> We're glad to see lawmakers are standing up for their constituents' freedom of choice by leaving the decision of what to eat or drink to

the people. It's not the government's responsibility to decide what we eat or drink—it's ours. And as we've said before, education will always be more impactful than trying to restrict what people can or can't eat or drink. That's why our industry is doing its part to provide more beverage options, as well as clear and useful information, for consumers.[21]

The ABA understandably prefers educational approaches to laws and regulations. Its officials know perfectly well that against massive soda marketing campaigns, education doesn't stand a chance.

CHALLENGE TO ADVOCATES

Public health advocates, with far fewer financial resources to spend on lobbying and election campaigns, are always at a disadvantage in this kind of political system. Corporations always can be counted on to outspend. The challenge for advocates is to find ways to bring corporate profit motives to public attention and to work with other public interest groups to help level the playing field.

This is the strategy behind the Boycott Coca-Cola campaign conducted by two advocacy groups, the Food Revolution Network and the Center for Food Safety. Their goal is to induce Coca-Cola to end its opposition to GMO labeling and to stop putting money into anti-labeling campaigns: "We have a unique opportunity to boycott the Coca-Cola brands being marketed as healthier alternatives until they pledge to cease any and all financial contributions to anti-GMO labeling efforts."[22]

In considering soda industry lobbying, I can never get over the extent of the effort these companies are willing to undertake to market a nutritionally empty sugary drink that contributes to poor health. The amounts of money spent on such efforts testify to the enormous profits generated by sales of such products. Although such issues may seem remote from immediate concerns about sodas, health advocates could do well to form alliances with groups devoted to overturning *Citizens United*, requiring lobbying to be more transparent, and funding election campaigns in ways that are less corrupting.[23]

24

Using Public Relations and Front Groups

Soda companies have ways of influencing policy that go beyond lobbying, campaign contributions, marketing, or support of worthy causes through corporate social responsibility (CSR). They also use some of the more hidden aspects of public relations to win allies, encourage favorable public opinion, and discredit anyone who suggests that consuming less soda might make people healthier. This chapter examines some of these behind-the-scenes "hardball" tactics.

FORGING BUSINESS AND PERSONAL CONNECTIONS

Early in 2013, the Stanford University physician-scientist Sanjay Basu assessed the soda industry's sphere of influence by identifying its ties to people and institutions. He used various sources of data to identify how soda company executives and board members are linked to prominent leaders in industry, government, and the private sector. He displayed the connections in circular maps too detailed and complicated to reproduce here.[1] The maps indicate that soda company executives or board members have corporate ties to former senators, cabinet secretaries, and ambassadors; foundations and international organizations dealing with global health policy; officials of governments in Latin America and Eastern Europe; owners of retail outlets and restaurants that serve Coke or Pepsi products; and executives in leading media companies. Many soda company board members are members of other boards, among them those of banks, oil companies, and major nonprofit art, environmental, health, and international development groups.

Of course they have such ties. All businesses have well-connected CEOs. But this industry seems unusually diligent in forging such connections and, thereby, raising questions about how business relationships might affect public policy. The map for Coca-Cola displays a link to Cathleen Black, for example, a member of the company's executive board who had just been nominated as chancellor of the New York City public school system. At the time, the city was engaged in a massive public health campaign to reduce soda drinking. Chancellor Black sat on the Coca-Cola board's policy committee, which dealt with its stance on obesity issues. If nothing else, such connections give the appearance of conflict of interest. To take the chancellor's job, Ms. Black was forced to give up her seat on the board, thereby forfeiting its substantial benefits. Since 1990, when she first joined the board, Coke had paid her more than $2 million in cash; she also held more than $3 million in Coca-Cola stock.[2] As noted in Chapter 19, at the time Dr. Victor Dzau was appointed head of the Institute of Medicine in 2014, he held a lucrative seat on the board of PepsiCo, raising similar questions about potential conflict of interest.

These maps, impressive as they are, understate the extent of such connections, as can be seen from the biographies of the companies' CEOs early in 2014. Indra Nooyi, the CEO of PepsiCo, was then a member of the board of directors for the Federal Reserve Bank of New York and Motorola, but also nonprofits such as the International Rescue Committee and the Lincoln Center for the Performing Arts. She was a Successor Fellow of the Yale Corporation, on the advisory board of the Yale School of Management, and on the boards of trustees for Eisenhower Fellowships and the Asia Society. She was also a member of the executive committee of the Trilateral Commission, which promotes cooperation between Japan, Europe, and North America. Through these affiliations, she had connections to 481 board members of twelve different organizations across eleven different industries. Such connections help Nooyi appear on lists of the world's best CEOs and most powerful women, and make her a frequent recipient of honorary degrees and many other awards.[3]

Muhtar Kent, the CEO of Coca-Cola since 2009, seems even more impressively connected. In 2014, he chaired the International Business Council of the World Economic Forum, co-chaired the Bipartisan Policy Center's CEO Council on Health and Innovation, and was a fellow of the Foreign Policy Association, a member of the Business Roundtable (a group of high-level business leaders), immediate past co-chair of the Consumer Goods Forum (a global food safety initiative), past chair of the U.S.-China Business

Council, and chair emeritus of the U.S. ASEAN (Association of Southeast Asian Nations) Business Council. He served on the boards of 3M (a company with $31 billion in revenues in 2013) and several nonprofits: Special Olympics International, Ronald McDonald House Charities, Catalyst, and Emory University. Through this service, Mr. Kent has the opportunity to form personal connections with many of the 342 other board members of nine different organizations representing eight different industries.[4]

To cite another example from the Coca-Cola board: Dr. Helene Gayle is the CEO of CARE (Cooperative for Assistance and Relief Everywhere, Inc.), a group devoted to fighting global poverty. She is linked to 133 other board members through Coca-Cola's and other board memberships. Dr. Gayle worked at the Centers for Disease Control and Prevention for twenty years, where she led HIV/AIDS initiatives and was deeply involved in minority health issues. Later, she led HIV/AIDS programs at the Gates Foundation. Coca-Cola benefits enormously from her participation on its board. Through her, Coca-Cola is personally connected to leaders of the nonprofit global health community who might otherwise be expected to oppose efforts to market sodas in developing countries or to minority groups in the United States.

Dr. Gayle's former employment with the Gates Foundation is also relevant. As Dr. Basu points out, the Gates Foundation owns more than fifteen million shares of Coca-Cola. This gives the foundation a vested interest in promoting Coca-Cola's growth and profitability. Writers who focus on the nonprofit world are troubled by the potential impropriety of this connection: "The question, of course, of whether Gates should be invested so heavily in Coca-Cola given its health focus is another very important matter that advocates should pursue. Investment is as much a declaration of mission intention and values as any other use of assets and there are serious questions about Coca Cola's contributions to the health of the world."[5]

Nevertheless, it is understandable how such business and personal connections flock to the wealthy heads of Coca-Cola and PepsiCo, who have the ability to spend generously on their fellow board members' favorite CSR causes. The people to whom soda company executives are connected through business—and often, therefore, personally—are likely to share soda company preferences for a corporate environment as free of government regulation as possible and to support the companies' positions on issues under debate. It is awkward to go on record against the views and policies of people with whom you have dinner or play golf or who encourage their companies to contribute to your favorite charities. "All in all," Dr. Basu concludes, "the picture is not very surprising, but the linkages at both the executive and political donor level appear to be unsubtle and tie the private sector to the public decision-making sector rather tightly as prominent decisions about soft drink regulation continue to be debated and voted on in the public sphere."

SPYING ON ADVOCACY GROUPS

Spying on citizens is common among world governments, as demonstrated in 2013 by Edward Snowden, the computer professional who leaked documents from the U.S. National Security Agency. Unless such leakages occur, spying remains a highly secret activity. Do soda companies engage in espionage? One leak suggests they do.

In 2012, WikiLeaks released a collection of emails revealing that the private intelligence firm Stratfor had been recruited by corporations to collect information about groups advocating for human rights, animal rights, and environmental sustainability. Coca-Cola was one such corporation. The company, a major sponsor of the Olympics, was worried that People for the Ethical Treatment of Animals (PETA) might organize protests at the 2010 Winter Games in Vancouver. It hired Stratfor to find out who was behind PETA's actions and what kind of methods PETA might use to plan and carry out its opposition. According to the leaked information, the Stratfor representative knew that the Federal Bureau of Investigation was running a classified investigation on PETA operatives and said, "I'll see what I can uncover." The emails did not reveal what Stratfor found or what it eventually reported to the company.[6] It seems plausible that soda companies are engaged in other such espionage, but it seems as though it will take further WikiLeaks or Snowdens to bring such information to public attention.

SUPPORTING THE ULTRA-RIGHT

In 2012, under pressure from public interest groups, both PepsiCo and Coca Cola withdrew their financial support of the ultraconservative American Legislative Exchange Council (ALEC). This organization drafts legislation

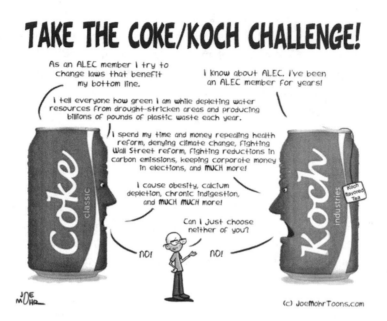

FIGURE 24.1 Take your pick: Coke vs. Koch. The cartoonist Joe Mohr explains why advocates called for Coca-Cola to stop funding ALEC, the ultraconservative American Legislative Exchange Council that is strongly supported by the wealthy, ultraconservative Koch Industries among other corporations. Coca-Cola and PepsiCo both withdrew funding in 2012. Courtesy of Joe Mohr.

and then lobbies for its adoption by state lawmakers. ALEC particularly promotes legislation to block gun control and restrict voting rights. Coca-Cola, along with representatives of Koch Industries, which prominently backs Tea Party Republicans, sat on ALEC's Private Enterprise Board. Figure 24.1 illustrates the linkage between Coke, Koch, and ALEC, which no doubt came about because ALEC "fully supports hardworking Americans, and opposes all efforts—federally and on the state level—to impose discriminatory taxes on food and/or beverages." In 2011, PR Watch organized a letter-writing campaign to induce Coca-Cola to withdraw from ALEC, arguing that it made no sense for a name-brand company to be associated with such far-right, consumer-unfriendly policies.[7]

Minority associations such as ColorOfChange were particularly unhappy about soda company support of an organization urging legal limitations on voter rights. They too organized a letter-writing campaign. In addition, they urged their members to boycott Coke and Pepsi. In 2012, PepsiCo quietly withdrew its membership in ALEC. A few months later, when Coca-Cola also severed its connection, it issued this statement: "The Coca-Cola Company has elected to discontinue its membership with the American Legislative Exchange Council. Our involvement with ALEC was focused on efforts to oppose discriminatory food and beverage taxes, not on issues that have no direct bearing on our business. We have a long-standing policy of only taking positions on issues that impact our Company and industry."[8]

Consider that the very reason ALEC attracted corporate supporters was its secrecy about its members, methods, and funding sources. According to *BusinessWeek*, ALEC "designed its entire structure to disguise industry-backed legislation as grassroots work from state legislators." Once the companies' connection to this strategy was publicly revealed, Coke and Pepsi no longer had any reason to remain with ALEC, and they withdrew—an action that elicited another call for a boycott, this time from Senator Charles "Chuck" Grassley (R-Iowa), who criticized Coca-Cola for yielding to leftist pressures.[9]

SUPPORTING FRONT GROUPS

Coca-Cola and PepsiCo are members of trade associations such as the American Beverage Association (ABA) and Grocery Manufacturers Association (GMA). Trade groups work on behalf of their members. They collect funds from their member companies, and use the funds for lobbying, campaign contributions, and public relations. For the most part, the financial connections between companies and trade associations are open and explicit.

Front groups, in contrast, operate covertly. They present themselves as populist and grassroots, and do everything they can get away with to cloak their industry funding. Their purpose is to gain popular support for positions on issues of concern, which they do through public relations, not lobbying. They are called front groups because they are out in front on the issues, while their funders remain hidden.

Front groups are important tools for soda companies. Coke and Pepsi put substantial public relations efforts into presenting their companies as exemplary corporate citizens. They do not want to be viewed as engaging in radical right-wing causes that might alienate their liberal customers, let alone in underhanded or aggressive tactics that might bring unfavorable publicity. Instead, they fund front groups to do the dirty work for them.

As Michele Simon explained in her cogent analysis of food industry front groups in 2013, the companies use "astroturf" (artificially "green" and grassroots) front groups to accomplish four goals:

- Appear as community-based representatives of the common people rather than big government and the elites
- Discredit critics through ridicule and terms such as "food police," "nannies," and "extremists"
- Create anxiety among consumers about loss of freedom of choice and Big Brother government
- Hire scientific and other experts to appear in the media, without disclosing who pays them
- Play to consumer anxieties, especially those related to higher food prices, job losses, or higher taxes[10]

Coca-Cola and the ABA use front groups frequently. PepsiCo apparently stays out of direct involvement but lets the ABA act on its behalf. Here are a few examples.

American Council on Science and Health (Coca-Cola, Dr Pepper Snapple)

The American Council on Science and Health (ACSH) presents itself as a national, nonprofit consumer health education and advocacy organization. ACSH was founded on the premise that "many important public policies related to health and the environment did not have a sound scientific basis." Its advisory board of 350 physicians, scientists, and policy advisors "add reason and balance to debates about public health issues and...bring common sense views to the public." It says its positions are strictly science-based and independent, but an investigative report in 2013 found that ACSH "depends heavily on funding from corporations that have a financial stake in the scientific debates it aims to shape." The ACSH does not disclose its donors, and it was only through leaked documents that reporters learned about Coca-Cola's $50,000 contribution and Dr Pepper Snapple's $5,000. The documents described Pepsi as an "ask," meaning that ACSH intended to solicit funds from PepsiCo (whether it actually did so is not recorded).

This organization gives soda companies what they pay for. The ACSH actively defends the safety of chemicals in the food supply, particularly of artificial sweeteners. It also strongly opposed New York City's attempt to limit the size of soft drink containers.[11]

Beverage Institute for Health and Wellness (Coca-Cola)

Although the Beverage Institute for Health and Wellness (BIHW) is fully disclosed as an enterprise of Coca-Cola, I consider it a front group because it purports to be about science and education, not marketing. Its Internet address (www.beverageinstitute.org) is separate from Coca-Cola's and suggests it is nonprofit. The institute's website explains that it is part of

> the Coca-Cola Company's ongoing commitment to use evidence-based science to advance knowledge and understanding of beverages, beverage ingredients, and the important role that active healthy lifestyles play in supporting health and wellbeing. It serves as a resource for health professionals, teachers, coaches and other professionals worldwide.... The BIHW also supports the educational needs of health professionals by sponsoring free continuing professional education (CE/CPE) programs led by recognized experts in fields such as nutrition, medicine, nursing, physical activity, behavior change, toxicology and various food science disciplines.... In addition, the BIHW regularly partners with credible third-party organizations and groups on programs that provide continuing education credit for physicians, nurses and other health professionals.[12]

As I discussed in Chapter 19, Coca-Cola uses this Institute to present its version of facts about nutrition and health to health professionals. Because the position statements come from BIHW, not Coca-Cola itself, they appear to be issued by a legitimate, unbiased source of scientific information.

"Astroturf" Groups Opposed to Soda Caps and Taxes (ABA)

When New York City mayor Michael Bloomberg suggested capping soda sizes at 16 ounces in 2012, the soda industry went into action (Chapter 25).

It quickly organized small and large businesses that sell sodas into a front group named for an issue likely to resonate well with the public: New Yorkers for Beverage Choices. The group advertised itself as a grassroots "coalition of citizens, businesses, and community organizations who believe that consumers have the right to purchase beverages in whatever size they choose." An investigation by the *Republic Report*, however, revealed the group's true origin. The ABA had contracted with Goddard Claussen Public Affairs (now Goddard Gunster) to organize the campaign. Goddard is anything but a group of concerned citizens in New York City. It is the Washington, D.C.-based public relations firm that ran the infamous "Harry and Louise" campaign responsible for derailing President Clinton's health care reform efforts in the early 1990s. The firm's slogan is "Get used to winning." Its website explains, "We drive the debate. Through facts and research, we define the parameters of the public debate and align consumer, corporate, and government interests."[13]

As discussed in Chapters 25–27, Goddard was the public relations agency responsible for the "grassroots" campaigns against New York City's soda cap initiative, as well as the campaigns against New York State governor David Paterson's proposed soda tax in 2010. The front group in the anti-Paterson campaign was called New Yorkers Against Unfair Taxes. Goddard also was behind the national group Americans Against Food Taxes and the California group Community Coalition Against Beverage Taxes, formed to oppose soda taxes in Richmond and El Monte, as well as the groups opposing tax initiatives in San Francisco and Berkeley (Chapter 27). The ABA funds the Goddard campaigns. Its president, Susan Neely, one of the lobbyists mentioned in Chapter 23, has a long history with the Goddard firm, and she managed its "Harry and Louise" campaign.

The many soda tax initiatives emerging in the United States keep Goddard busy with front-group organizing. The food blogger and advocate Nancy Huehnergarth compiled a list of ABA-funded "astroturf" anti-tax groups, which I adapt in Table 24.1.[14] Although the ABA website lists its corporate members, the front groups working through Goddard Gunster reveal their connection to the ABA in very small print, if at all. The ABA-created front group No Hawaii Beverage Tax, for example, does not mention the ABA anyplace on its website that I can find. Instead, it says it is "a coalition of individuals, families, businesses and community organizations in our state who are opposed to singling out certain beverages, like soft drinks, for a new tax."

TABLE 24.1 "Astroturf" American Beverage Association-funded city and state front groups organized to oppose soda taxes, 2012–2014

CITY OR STATE	ABA-FUNDED COALITION
Baltimore	Stop the Baltimore City Beverage Tax
Berkeley	No Berkeley Beverage Tax
California	Community Coalition Against Beverage Taxes
Chicago	Chicago Coalition Against Beverage Taxes
Hawaii	No Hawaii Beverage Tax
Illinois	Illinois Coalition Against Beverage Taxes
Kansas	Kansans Against Food and Beverage Taxes
New York	New Yorkers Against Unfair Taxes
Oregon	Oregon Coalition Against Beverage Taxes
Philadelphia	Philly Jobs. Not Taxes.
Pittsburgh	No Pittsburgh Beverage Tax
Rhode Island	Rhode Islanders Against the Beverage Tax
San Francisco	Coalition for an Affordable City
Texas	No Texas Beverage Tax
Vermont	Stop the Vermont Beverage Tax
Washington, D.C.	No DC Beverage Tax
Washington State	Washingtonians Against the Beverage Tax

THE CENTER FOR CONSUMER FREEDOM (COCA-COLA)

In 2014, the Center for Consumer Freedom (CCF) was subsumed into an umbrella "educational and charitable" organization called the Center for Organizational Research and Education (CORE, an abbreviation that conveniently if confusingly mimics that of the venerable civil rights group Congress of Racial Equality). This CORE website, however, explains that the organization is a "nonprofit dedicated to research and education about a wide variety of activist groups, exposing their funding, agendas, and tactics." CORE includes two other entities in addition to CCF: ActivistCash.com and a new front group, the Environmental Policy Alliance, abbreviated EPA. This abbreviation is also no coincidence. This EPA is "devoted to uncovering the funding and hidden agendas behind environmental activist groups and exploring the intersection between activists and government agencies"; by government agencies, it means the Environmental Protection Agency—the other EPA.[15]

CCF is the principal front group for food and beverage issues. Its website says CCF is a "nonprofit organization devoted to promoting personal responsibility and promoting consumer choices." The website explains the rationale for its formation:

A growing cabal of activists has meddled in Americans' lives in recent years. They include self-anointed "food police," health campaigners, trial lawyers, personal-finance do-gooders, animal-rights misanthropes, and meddling bureaucrats.... They all claim to know "what's best for you." In reality, they're eroding our basic freedoms—the freedom to buy what we want, eat what we want, drink what we want, and raise our children as we see fit.... We're here to push back.[16]

I must immediately disclose my involuntary membership in CCF's "cabal of activists." CORE's ActivistCash.com identifies me as a prominent member of the "food police" and says that I am "one of the country's most hysterical anti-food-industry fanatics" with "radical goals." Character assassination has long been typical of ActivistCash.com and CCF. They and their umbrella organization, CORE, were created and are headed by Richard Berman, a Washington, D.C.-based political consultant so controversial that an entire website is devoted to exposing his background and operating tactics.[17]

Rather than bothering to deal with issues, Berman explains, "our offensive strategy is to shoot the messenger.... We've got to attack [activists'] credibility as spokespersons." He adds, "We always have a knife in our teeth."[18]

As these statements might indicate, CORE is distinguished from other industry-funded front groups by its deliberately aggressive tactics. CORE's entities use no-holds-barred methods to attack and intimidate targets. For example, in response to President Barack Obama's announcement in 2014 of a plan to control carbon emissions, Berman's EPA placed a full-page ad in *USA Today* (June 3, 2014): "What would you call a radical organization that threatens to shut down 25% of our electric grid? ~~Anarchist. Militia. Terrorist.~~ Obama's EPA ... With radicals like this in power, who needs enemies?"[19]

Berman's groups are also distinguished by their secrecy. Companies and trade associations that would never dream of attacking health leaders or their campaigns in public can secretly fund CORE and hide behind what it does. Berman explains that he is not required to disclose his funders because he established CORE as a privately held nonprofit that ostensibly has no connection to his decidedly for-profit lobbying firm: "We run all of this stuff through nonprofit organizations that are insulated from having to disclose donors. There is total anonymity. People don't know who supports us."[20] But CORE entities, including CCF, pay handsome fees to his lobbying firm, a practice that has elicited lawsuits on the grounds of violation of nonprofit tax laws or regulations.

About the nondisclosure of donors, CCF says it "is supported by restaurants, food companies and thousands of individual consumers...businesses, their employees, and their customers. Many of the companies and individuals who support the Center financially have indicated that they want anonymity as contributors." Of course CCF's clients want anonymity. CCF is the public face—the attack dog—of the food and beverage industry in its attempts to block criticism, regulation, and legal challenges.

Coca-Cola, for example, has publicly supported campaigns by Mothers Against Drunk Driving (MADD) since the mid-1990s. But one of CCF's subsidiaries, the American Beverage Institute, a group created to support the alcoholic beverage industry, lobbies forcefully against more stringent drunk driving laws.[21] By supporting CCF, Coca-Cola has it both ways. It can oppose drunk driving in public while secretly supporting opposition to regulation of driving under the influence.

CCF has been the force behind tasteless campaigns against anti-obesity initiatives such as the full-page "nanny" ad ridiculing New York City Mayor Michael Bloomberg for his soda size-cap proposal (shown in Figure 25.4). CCF also operates internationally, as became evident in 2013 when the Mexican government was considering a tax on sodas (Chapter 27). CCF placed ads on school buses in Mexico City: "Can obesity be stopped by taxes? Yes or no to the tax on 'fatties.'"

Such actions strongly suggest that soda companies must be among CCF's most generous funders. According to a 2005 account in the *New York Times*, Berman admits that most of his funding comes from food and restaurant companies, some of them also clients of his lobbying firm. At the time, Coca-Cola admitted that it sponsored CCF, calling the group invaluable as "another voice in the debate." Pepsi, however, denied working with CCF because of discomfort with its arguments and approach.[22] In 2013, a former official of PepsiCo told me that the company did not fund CCF, but Coca-Cola does. Despite much suspicion and inquiry, I have been unable to find out if the ABA also supports the CCF or its parent organization.

USING PUBLIC RELATIONS

Throughout this book, I talk about soda companies' use of public relations in the context of specific advocacy initiatives. Here I will simply mention that the ABA runs a website, Let's Clear It Up, for the purpose of presenting the soda industry's views of current issues. It uses the website to give Big Soda's interpretation of the science linking sodas to diabetes and obesity and to counter "myths" about the health effects of caffeine, sugar, and the marketing of sodas to children.

Business analysts observing this and the other soda industry public relations campaigns are impressed by parallels to the campaigns run by the tobacco industry when its products came under scrutiny. These too involved "astroturf" organizations, full-page ads in newspapers, and assurances that the companies' main concern is and always will be the health of the public. These assurances, however, led to no fundamental change in the usual business model. Soda company goals are much the same—to get "more people to drink more sugar, regardless of the health consequences."[23] The real agenda, analysts observe, is to stave off regulations, particularly soda taxes that might raise the price of sodas and discourage consumption.

CHALLENGE FOR ADVOCATES

Secret connections, public relations, and front groups are by their very nature difficult to counter because their true purpose is hidden. The first line of advocacy, therefore, is to expose the soda industry's funding of public relations efforts and front groups and make sure that they are fully identified on campaign materials and by the media. The conflicts of interest raised by Big Soda's public relations and front groups are best observed in action when cities attempt to impose caps on soda sizes or soda taxes, as discussed in Chapters 25–27.

Advocacy: Soda Caps, Taxes, and More

25

Advocacy

Capping Soda Portion Sizes

In December 2011, New York City mayor Michael Bloomberg announced some excellent news. After years of city interventions to improve diet and physical activity patterns, the prevalence of obesity among New York children had started to decline. With this evidence that the city's public health measures were having the desired effect, Bloomberg appointed a task force to recommend further actions.

The task force released its report in May 2012. One of its twenty-six recommendations was to "establish a maximum size for sugary drinks in food service establishments." The task force noted that "sugary drink portion sizes have exploded over recent years.... Setting a maximum size for sugary drinks offered and sold in restaurants and other Food Service Establishments is a way we can change the default and help reacquaint New Yorkers with 'human size' portions to reduce excessive consumption of sugary drinks."[1]

On this basis, the mayor proposed what he—and advocates—formally named the "Sugary Drink Portion Cap Rule," a 16-ounce limit on the size of sugary drinks that can be offered in restaurants or retail stores overseen by the city. Opponents of the measure, however, immediately called it a "soda ban," a framing term far more likely to evoke public dismay, if not outrage.[2] The term "ban" took hold so quickly that even city officials sometimes slipped and used it. In this chapter, I review the rationale for public health initiatives to control portion sizes, and recount the fate of New York City's Portion Cap Rule, here abbreviated as "portion cap" or "rule."

THE SODA SIZE PROBLEM

Sodas were not always served in supersized containers. Coca-Cola's original 1916 contour bottle contained 6.5 ounces. Pepsi, as noted earlier, introduced the 12-ounce bottle in the 1930s. As late as 1954, 61 percent of bottled sodas contained less than 7 ounces and only 8 percent were larger than 20 ounces. Coca-Cola did not introduce sizes larger than 6.5 ounces until 1955.[3] Today's soda bottles range from 7.5 ounces to 2 liters (64 ounces), and the standard size in vending machines is 20 ounces—three times larger than the original.

Fountain drinks followed a similar trend. In the 1950s, McDonald's served 7-ounce drinks, but it added larger sizes throughout the 1960s and 1970s. As Lisa Young describes in her book *The Portion Teller*, Burger King's sodas in the 1950s contained 12 or 16 ounces, but by the early 2000s, the chain offered 12-ounce kiddie, 16-ounce small, 22-ounce medium, 32-ounce large, and 42-ounce king sizes. McDonald's did the same but called them child, small, medium, large, and supersize, respectively.[4] The 6.5-ounce soda, the industry standard for decades, is roughly half the size of a portion now considered suitable for a child.

Soda manufacturers encourage big sizes; the cost of the drink ingredients is trivial in comparison to that of the bottles, advertising, labor, and service. Restaurants and fast-food chains also encourage large portions. Customers like bargains, have come to expect large containers, and in places like Texas complain when they are not available.[5] Most of all, as I explained in Chapter 9, large sodas are wonderfully profitable for their makers and sellers.

PRICING STRATEGIES: EFFECT ON CALORIES

Soda companies have long marketed larger sizes as bargains. Pepsi's 1939 "twice as much for a nickel" demonstrably encouraged sales.[6] Soda companies continue to use this strategy. Doing the math at Walmart in 2013, for example, I could buy a 64-ounce bottle of Pepsi for 2 cents per ounce, but a 24-ounce bottle cost 3 cents per ounce. A 7.5-ounce can cost 6 cents per ounce, and I was obliged to buy more than one, as they only came in packs of eight, twelve, or twenty-four. As a supermarket retailer once explained to me, if customers want smaller portions, they ought to be willing to pay for them. This pricing strategy encourages everyone, and especially those who do not have much money, to buy sodas in larger sizes.

The higher price for a smaller amount would just be an amusing marketing technique except for its effect: larger portions have more calories. If an 8-ounce soda provides 100 calories, then a 16-ounce drink has 200 and a 64-ounce drink has 800 calories. On the basis of calories alone, larger portions are a sufficient explanation for rising rates of obesity. As noted earlier, the relationship of portion size to calories may seem self-evident but is not. Larger portions induce people to eat more and also to be fooled into underestimating how much they have eaten.[7] Most people cannot imagine that a soda of any size could contain 800 calories. Sugars in liquid form do not make people feel full, and food labels in 2015 still referred to the 100 calories in an 8-ounce serving.

THE DEFAULT ISSUE

The effects of larger servings are reasons to be concerned about the default—the automatic food choice when no easier alternative is available. People tend to eat what they buy or are served regardless of whether food comes in a container or is presented at the table. If a Happy Meal comes with a soda, kids drink soda; if it comes with milk, they drink milk. With milk or juice as the default, parents can always order a soda, but many will not. Changing the default to foods and drinks that are smaller and less sugary is the most effective way to promote healthier choices. Setting a 16-ounce cap on soda sizes does some of that. Customers can still drink as much soda as they want; they just have to ask for additional 16-ounce servings.[8] Hence cap rule, not ban.

CALLS TO REDUCE PORTION SIZES

I can think of at least six reasons why sodas are best consumed in small amounts. Because larger food portions (1) have more calories, (2) induce people to consume more calories, and (3) fool people into underestimating the calories they are consuming, reducing portion sizes ought to be a prime goal of obesity intervention. But sodas provide three additional reasons for avoiding large sizes: (4) their calories are empty, (5) their sugars are in liquid form, and (6) larger sizes are usually less expensive per volume than smaller sizes. And, I might add, sodas are heavily advertised to everyone, but especially to those most vulnerable—youth and minorities.

In 2001, the U.S. surgeon general issued a "call to action" to prevent obesity. This, among other recommendations, urged the food industry to produce foods and drinks in smaller portions. Aimed at changing the behavior of food companies rather than individuals, this message was largely ignored by federal agencies. Instead, government dietary advice continued to focus on improving personal food choices. The 2005 Dietary Guidelines said, "Special attention should be given to portion sizes which have increased significantly over the past two decades." The 2010 guidelines included a similar personal-choice message: "When eating out, choose smaller portions.... Prepare, serve, and consume smaller portions of foods and beverages." The My-Plate food guide in 2011 advised, "Avoid oversized portions."[9]

Inducing the food industry to reduce portion sizes, however, is far more controversial. In 2010, to provide an evidence base for the First Lady's Let's Move! campaign, President Obama appointed a task force to review evidence and make recommendations. With respect to portion sizes, the task force made two: "Restaurants should *consider* their portion sizes" and "Restaurants should be...*attentive to* the effects of plate and portion size" (my emphasis). The 2010 Dietary Guidelines were similarly tentative: "Initiate partnerships with food producers, suppliers, and retailers to promote the development and availability of appropriate portions." The Partnership for a Healthier America, the food industry group that works with Let's Move!, says nothing about its member companies' responsibility to reduce portion sizes as a means to address childhood obesity. While the cap rule was under consideration, Coca-Cola was lobbying Congress to "oppose policies that restrict the sale of certain beverages in packages larger than 16 fluid ounces."[10] Neither the federal government nor Congress seemed likely to take on portion sizes as a means to prevent obesity.

To the food industry, portion size is a matter of simple economics. If large portions cost little to produce and increase sales, companies need them. No wonder fast-food companies have done little to respond to "reduce portion size" messages. If anything, they have increased their serving sizes. McDonald's, for example, dropped the term "supersize" but continues to sell such portions in special promotions. European fast-food outlets, however, manage to sell smaller portions and stay in business. In 2012, the largest Coca-Cola served in the British Burger King was 12 ounces smaller (and provided nearly 150 fewer calories) than the largest U.S. size, and that in the

British McDonald's was 8 ounces smaller (100 fewer calories) than its American counterpart.[11] But because Americans expect to be served large amounts of food and drink when eating out, restaurants and food producers are reluctant to do anything to risk alienating customers. Given these observations, it is easy to understand why New York City's sensible proposal to cap the sizes of sugary drinks at 16 ounces elicited a firestorm of protest.

ADVOCACY: NEW YORK CITY'S "SUGARY DRINK PORTION CAP RULE"

On May 30, 2012, Mayor Michael Bloomberg called a press conference to announce a limit on the sale of sugary drinks larger than 16 ounces in restaurants, movie theaters, street carts, bodegas, and all other retail locations over which the city holds jurisdiction. The portion rule would apply to sugar-added drinks containing more than 25 calories in 8 ounces.[12]

Bloomberg is a billionaire who paid for his own election campaigns, took no city salary, and appeared impervious to public criticism. Under his administration, health commissioner Dr. Thomas Friedan and his successor, Dr. Thomas Farley—both deeply committed to improving the health of city residents—led the nation by developing a series of interventions to improve the environment of food choice. The city banned the use of trans fats in restaurants in 2006, and required calorie labeling on restaurant menus in 2007. Although some critics complained, the trans fat ban was quickly adopted by city restaurants.[13] Congress passed national menu labeling in 2010.

Several of the campaigns specifically aimed to reduce soda consumption. These began with subway posters illustrating the amount of sugar in sodas, how those sugars are converted to fat in the body, and the number of miles needed to walk off soda calories (Figure 17.1). The campaign used slogans such as "NYC! Go Sugary Drink Free." A 2012 poster campaign illustrated the link between large soda portions and amputations resulting from type 2 diabetes (Figure 25.1).[14] As noted in Chapter 16, the city also tried—but failed—to obtain permission from USDA to block sales of sodas to those receiving SNAP benefits (food stamps).

To public health advocates, the portion cap rule was another such intervention, this time aimed at changing the default soda size. A 16-ounce sugary drink is not exactly abstemious. It contains two of the old standard 8-ounce servings and provides nearly 50 grams of sugars and 200 empty, liquid calories. During the press conference, city officials displayed an

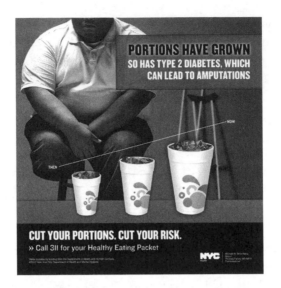

FIGURE 25.1 In 2012, the New York City Department of Health and Mental Hygiene placed this poster in subways. It illustrates the connection between larger soda sizes and amputations that result from type 2 diabetes. This campaign elicited particular criticism when the "amputee" turned out to be Photoshopped from a stock photo.

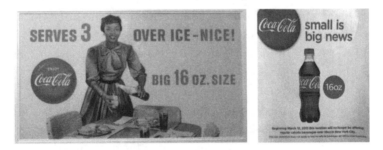

FIGURE 25.2 The change in views of 16-ounce sodas since the 1950s. In the 1950s, Coca-Cola advertised a 16-ounce bottle as "big" and capable of serving three. In 2013, shortly before the soda portion cap rule was to go into effect, the company advertised the same size as "small." The 1950s ad is an early example of soda marketing targeted to African Americans. The more recent sign says, "Beginning March 12, 2013 this location will no longer be offering regular calorie beverages over 16 oz in New York City. The size restriction does not apply to low/no-calorie beverages served by crew members." On March 11, however, a judge blocked the portion rule from going into effect.

advertisement from the 1950s when Coca-Cola viewed a 16-ounce bottle as big—enough to serve three over ice. The city's idea was to return sodas to reasonable sizes.[15] "Reasonable," of course, is a matter of perception. Shortly before the cap was to go into effect, retailers posted signs referring to the 16-ounce size as *small*. Figure 25.2 illustrates this comparison.

THE SODA "BAN": ABA-ORGANIZED OPPOSITION

The American Beverage Association (ABA) mounted an enormous public relations campaign to convince New Yorkers that the "ban" on large soda sizes infringed on freedom of choice.[16] It began by attacking the science in a full-page ad in the *New York Times* (June 1, 2012): "Are soda and sugar-sweetened beverages driving obesity? Not according to the facts." The ABA explained: "The facts make it clear—beverage calories and added sugars have decreased for more than a decade, while the CDC reports obesity rates

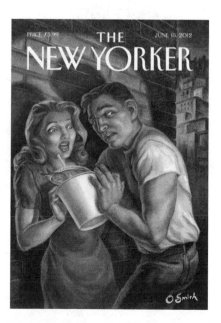

FIGURE 25.3 The *New Yorker* cover of June 18, 2012. Owen Smith's illustration depicted the common but misleading interpretation of the portion cap rule as a "ban" that would force innocent consumers of oversize sodas into hiding from the food police. Owen Smith/*The New Yorker*/©Condé Nast.

continue to climb." The ad did not mention the overall leveling off of obesity in parallel with the decline in soda sales (see Figure 5.1).

The ABA and its allies complained that the "ban" was a "nanny-state" move that would force people to sneak off to drink large sodas in secret, as Figure 25.3 suggests. Even the *New York Times* misinterpreted the cap as a ban: "Mr. Bloomberg, however, is overreaching with his new plan.... The administration should be focusing its energies on programs that educate and encourage people to make sound choices.... [T]oo much nannying with a ban might well cause people to tune out."[17]

The soda and restaurant industries bought help from the Center for Consumer Freedom (CCF). Its full-page advertisement, shown in Figure 25.4,

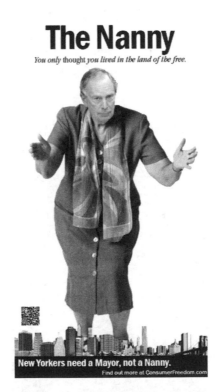

FIGURE 25.4 The infamous "Bloomberg nanny" ad, *New York Times*, June 2, 2012. The ad was placed by the Center for Consumer Freedom, the industry-funded public relations firm discussed in the previous chapter. "Bye Bye Venti. Nanny Bloomberg has taken his strange obsession with what you eat one step further. He now wants to make it illegal to serve "sugary drinks" bigger than 16 oz. What's next? Limits on the width of a pizza slice, size of a hamburger or amount of cream cheese on your bagel?"

depicted Mayor Bloomberg wearing a dowdy blue dress: "The Nanny. You only thought you lived in the land of the free. Nanny Bloomberg has taken his strange obsession with what you eat one step further....New Yorkers need a mayor, not a nanny." Bloomberg, fortunately, has a sense of humor: when asked about the ad at a press conference, he said, "Would I wear a dress like that? No! It was one of the more unflattering dresses."[18]

As I explained in Chapter 24, the CCF does not reveal its funding sources, but both Coca-Cola and the National Restaurant Association have been identified as clients. The Restaurant Association's interest is easily explained. According to *Advertising Age,* soft drinks account for about 10 percent of sales in fast-food and casual restaurants, and come with a profit margin of 90 percent.[19]

The ABA created a new astroturf organization, Let's Clear It Up, and a website to "clarify myths" and give the industry's spin on the science of sodas and health.[20] Coca-Cola used a different strategy: divert attention from sugars and calories. Its *New York Times* advertisement on June 10 said, "Everything in moderation. Except fun, try to have lots of that...By promoting balanced diets and active lifestyles, we can make a positive difference." Coca-Cola's president of sparkling beverages in North America, Katie Bayne, explained the company's opposition to the cap rule to a reporter from *USA Today*:

Q: Is there any merit to limits being placed on the size of sugary drinks folks can buy?

A: Sugary drinks can be a part of any diet as long as your calories in balance with the calories out. Our responsibility is to provide drink in all the sizes that consumers might need....

Q: But critics call soft drinks "empty" calories.

A: A calorie is a calorie. What our drinks offer is hydration. That's essential to the human body. We offer great taste and benefits whether it's an uplift or carbohydrates or energy. We don't believe in empty calories. We believe in hydration.[21]

The campaign against the cap rule appeared to be well orchestrated and lavishly funded, and it consistently invoked nanny states, intrusion on personal choice, and lack of patriotism. Groups of young people gathered at farmers' markets and other crowded places to collect signatures on petitions to block

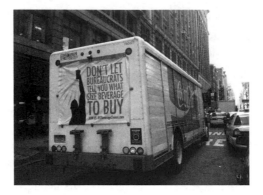

FIGURE 25.5 Coca-Cola delivery truck, New York City, 2012. During the debates about the portion cap, Pepsi and Coca-Cola delivery trucks carried signs telling customers, "Don't let bureaucrats tell you what size beverage to buy." The signs remained on the trucks well into 2014. Photo courtesy of Daniel Bowman Simon.

the cap. Paid $30 an hour (or so they said) by another ABA-sponsored front group, New Yorkers for Beverage Choice, they wore T-shirts saying "I picked out my beverage all by myself" and handed out cards: "Don't let bureaucrats tell you what size beverage to buy." Soda delivery trucks were emblazoned with such slogans (Figure 25.5). Ads appeared on television, in movie theaters, and on airplane banners. As a resident of New York City, I received a home mailing from the ABA with instructions on how to protest the "ban."[22]

It is impossible to know how much of the protest was spontaneous, as opposed to deliberately organized by the soda and restaurant industries, but the website of New Yorkers for Beverage Choice revealed that it was maintained by Goddard Clausen, the public relations firm recruited by the ABA to defeat soda tax initiatives. It is also difficult to know the extent to which these industries were behind federal and state initiatives to block similar attempts. Senator Ted Cruz (R-Tex.), for example, introduced an amendment to the congressional budget resolution intended to prevent federal regulation of the size of foods and beverages. The amendment failed to pass. But Mississippi, where nearly 35 percent of the population is obese and overall health ranks last among the fifty states, passed a bill preventing local communities from setting limits on soda size as well as on salt content, toys in fast-food children's meals, calorie counts on menus, and genetically modified foods. By 2014, such bills had been introduced in at least eight other states.[23]

I wish I could tell you how much money the soda industry spent to defeat the cap rule, but this was not an election and expenditures did not have to be disclosed. The amounts must have run into the millions in advertising, home mailings, payment of astroturf "volunteers," and the not inconsiderable costs of the subsequent legal challenges.

THE ABA'S LEGAL CHALLENGE

The city argued that for reasons of history and necessity, the mayor had the authority to propose the cap rule if the Board of Health agreed.[24] That the board would agree was never in question—the mayor appoints its members—and it approved the rule on September 13, 2012. Because the portion cap would not go into effect until March 2013, the soda industry had six months to try to block it. The ABA quickly organized a coalition of community organizations to join in petitioning the state supreme court to stop the rule or declare it unconstitutional.[25]

On March 11, 2013, the day before the portion cap was to go into effect, New York State Supreme Court justice Milton Tingling issued an injunction against it. The rule, he said, was:

> fraught with arbitrary and capricious consequences...uneven enforcement even within a particular City block, much less the City as a whole...It is arbitrary and capricious because it applies to some but not all food establishments in the City, it excludes other beverages that have significantly higher concentrations of sugar sweeteners and/or calories on suspect grounds, and...no limitations on re-fills...The Portion Cap Rule, if upheld, would create an administrative Leviathan...The Rule would not only violate the separation of powers doctrine, it would eviscerate it. Such an evisceration has the potential to be more troubling than sugar sweetened beverages.[26]

Justice Tingling was referring to some of the complications faced by the city in developing the cap rule, particularly that of jurisdiction. As his decision explained, the city health code applies to food service places such as fast-food restaurants and supermarkets, but because of an agreement between the city and the New York State Department of Agriculture and Markets, it does not apply to grocery stores, bodegas, or convenience stores like "7-Eleven market chains and their famous, or infamous, Big Gulp containers."

Tingling's decision caused the ABA to react with a "sigh of relief." The mayor, however, said the city would appeal: "Being the first to do something is never easy.... Anytime you adopt a groundbreaking policy, special interests will sue. That's America. But we strongly believe that, in the end, the courts will recognize the Board of Health's authority to regulate the sale of beverages ... leading to disease and death for thousands of people every year."[27]

In July 2013, the appellate court confirmed the injunction. Only the City Council, it said, had the authority to pass such rules. Mayor Bloomberg issued a ringing defense: "Since New York City's ground-breaking limit on the portion size of sugary beverages was prevented from going into effect on March 12th, more than 2,000 New Yorkers have died from the effects of diabetes.... Today's decision is a temporary setback, and we plan to appeal this decision as we continue the fight against the obesity epidemic."[28]

While the last appeal was under review, Dr. Tom Farley, who had been health commissioner in the Bloomberg administration, explained his surprise at the public reaction and the court rulings.

> The portion cap rule isn't a ban, and it isn't about restricting freedom or choice. It's simply a regulation on the size of containers, not on the amount people drink.... The case is about whether the New York City Board of Health has the authority to regulate restaurants in ways that protect the health of the City's residents, over the fierce objections of some of the world's biggest corporations, the soda companies. And, more important, whether the Board can protect New Yorkers from many other current and future health hazards, from unsafe conditions on the city's beaches to toxic chemicals in food or water.[29]

What started out as a legal challenge to the portion cap had become a test of a much larger issue: whether city health departments had the authority to pass rules to protect and promote the health of citizens. In June 2014, the State Appeals Court ruled that they did not: "We hold that the New York City Board of Health, in adopting the 'Sugary Drinks Portion Cap Rule,' exceeded the scope of its regulatory authority. By choosing among competing policy goals, without any legislative delegation or guidance, the Board engaged in law-making and thus infringed upon the legislative jurisdiction of the City Council of New York."[30] Because the timing of these events can be confusing, Table 25.1 provides a summary.

TABLE 25.1 New York City's Sugary Drink Portion Cap Rule: time line of events during the legal challenges

DATE	EVENTS IN THE LEGAL CHALLENGES
2012	
May	Obesity Task Force issues report recommending limits on the sizes of sugary drinks sold in New York City. Mayor Michael Bloomberg proposes Portion Size Rule to limit sales of sugary drinks (> 25 calories per 8 ounces) to containers of 16 ounces or less by retail establishments under city jurisdiction.
June	Fourteen of 51 New York City Council members write mayor insisting that the rule be put to the council for a vote. It is not.
July	Board of Health holds public hearing on the rule. Several City Council members testify against the rule.
September	Board of Health adopts rule to take effect March 12, 2013.
October	The ABA organizes coalition of groups (Hispanic Chambers of Commerce et al.) to jointly petition New York State Supreme Court (New York County) to block rule.
November	Five members of the City Council file an *amici* brief in support of the soda industry's petition.
December	The New York State Conference of the National Association for the Advancement of Colored People (NAACP) and the Hispanic Federation file brief supporting the soda industry's position.
2013	
January	State Supreme Court holds hearing, presided over by Justice Milton Tingling.
February	Mayor Bloomberg asks New York State governor Andrew Cuomo to extend rule to convenience stores regulated by state. Cuomo denies request.
March	Supreme Court issues injunction; blocks the "ban" as "arbitrary and capricious." Bloomberg administration appeals. National minority, community, public health, and medical groups file *amici* briefs supporting the rule. City officials (including then public advocate but soon to be mayor Bill de Blasio) and representatives of minority and health community groups speak out in favor of rule.
June	New York State Appellate Division (First Department) holds hearings.
July	Appellate Division upholds lower court ruling; says mayor lacks authority to adopt health policy without vote of City Council. Bloomberg administration appeals.
August	Polls say 60 percent of New Yorkers oppose the rule.
October	New York State Court of Appeals agrees to review case.
November	Public advocate Bill de Blasio, who favors rule, is elected mayor. City Council member Letitia James, who opposes rule, is elected public advocate.
2014	
January	Bill de Blasio replaces Bloomberg as mayor; appoints Dr. Mary Bassett, who supports rule, as health commissioner. City Council member Melissa Mark-Viverito, who opposes rule, is elected its Speaker.
April	National Alliance for Hispanic Health and other prominent minority groups file *amici* brief in support of rule.

(continued)

TABLE 25.1 Continued

DATE	EVENTS IN THE LEGAL CHALLENGES
May	The majority (32 of 51) of members of the New York City Council, along with the public advocate, file *amici* brief opposing the rule.
June	Appeals Court holds hearing. National public health leaders issue statements in support of rule. Appeals Court decides that the rule exceeded the authority of the New York City Board of Health and infringed on power reserved for the New York City Council.
October	Mayor de Blasio says his administration is meeting with health advocates and lobbyists to consider alternative ways to cap the size of sugary drinks.

The ABA's Strange Bedfellows

It is understandable why groups whose sales might be threatened by the soda "ban," such as the National Restaurant Association and the New York State Association of Theater Owners, would oppose it. The soda industry's allies also included unions representing workers in bottling plants and those who transport sodas, such as the International Brotherhood of Teamsters and the Soft Drink and Brewery Workers Union Local 812, along with minority business associations such as the Hispanic Chambers of Commerce and the New York Korean-American Grocers Association.[31]

But the New York City Council also weighed in: five members signed an *amicus curiae* brief arguing that they, not the Board of Health, had the authority to set such a policy. And to the surprise of many city officials and public health advocates, the New York State chapter of the National Association for the Advancement of Colored People (NAACP) and the Hispanic Federation also filed a brief opposing the cap rule. Their concern: damage to small and minority-owned businesses by "discriminatorily preventing them from selling large 'sugary beverages' while allowing their large competitors such as 7-Eleven and grocery stores to carry the banned sugary beverages."[32]

Why would minority groups, whose health would most benefit from drinking less soda, support the industry's opposition to the rule? The NAACP and the Hispanic Federation argued from principle that it was discriminatory, paternalistic, and damaging to minority-owned small businesses. But they shared one other relevant characteristic: for years, Coca-Cola and PepsiCo have generously supported their programs.[33]

The same question must be asked of the City Council, many of whose members represent communities where obesity and type 2 diabetes are rampant. City Council member Dan Halloran, for example, who took the lead in City Council protests against the rule, viewed it as challenging "nothing less than the principles on which our country was founded." He was the recipient of a $2,000 contribution from PepsiCo's Concerned Citizens Fund. Executives of Coca-Cola and PepsiCo contributed to other council candidates as well as those running for public advocate, borough president, and mayor. For the most part, soda company employees' donations to candidates were tiny, ranging from $25 to $1,500; most were under $200. Among the City Council members who accepted donations from soda company officials, some spoke out against the rule, but others did not. This was also true of elected officials who accepted such donations.[34]

But even such small donations or less direct ties to soda companies raise questions, not least because the larger donations track closely with viewpoint. For example, Coca-Cola executives gave about $10,000 to Christine Quinn, the Speaker of the City Council, who was then the leading candidate for mayor. Quinn said the "ban" was punitive, unlikely to be effective, and something that should be reconsidered once Bloomberg was out of office.[35] Some of the members who spoke out against the rule—Melissa Mark-Viverito and Letitia James, for example—received higher campaign contributions and were also most active in seeking grants from the Coca-Cola Foundation to community groups in their districts. But at least one beneficiary of such grants, the Children's Aid Society, joined a brief in support of the rule. Although such financial connections invariably appear as conflicts of interest—and track closely with outcome—exceptions do exist. But in this instance, soda companies' donations to City Council members' campaigns and districts, no matter how small, paid off: the majority of council members opposed the rule.

Late in 2014, I attended a lecture on the cap rule given by Dr. Andrew Goodman, who had recently retired from the City Health Department. He talked about the extensive soda industry lobbying that had occurred while the rule was under consideration. Executives of soda companies and the ABA wrote the mayor and met with health officials. Coca-Cola even offered to fund a city-wide physical education program (the city turned it down). Former health commissioner Tom Farley also talked about the lobbying. He told the *Wall Street Journal*, "The soda companies hated [the cap rule]. They lobbied hard against it, and they reached a lot of council members. So, it would not be an easy thing to pass."[36] Soda lobbyists visited every City Council member. Health Department officials doubted they could get the rule through the City Council and thought it would have a better chance of passing if they worked through the Board of Health.

SUPPORT FOR THE CAP RULE: BETTER LATE THAN NEVER

Perhaps surprised by the breadth and intensity of the opposition, the city was late in organizing support. Public health advocates only learned about the cap rule when it was announced publicly; they had to scramble to catch up. Some Health Department staff members told me they too heard about it at the last minute. Although Dr. Goodman said that health officials had spent a year discussing how best to develop the cap rule before releasing it, the announcement appeared spontaneous and unplanned. Perhaps they and the mayor assumed that most people would agree that their public health initiatives had done a great deal of good. If so, they were wrong. Early polls found the majority of residents to be opposed to the rule, often to the point of ridicule. On this basis, *The Onion* observed satirically that the portion size issue had achieved a miracle: it had roused Americans out of political apathy.[37]

If the city was doing anything to organize support for the cap rule, its efforts did not become visible until February 2013. In response to complaints about the 7-Eleven exemption, Bloomberg appealed to Governor Andrew Cuomo to extend coverage to places operating under state jurisdiction. According to press accounts, the governor denied the appeal, saying, "It is not something we are considering at this time.... Haven't really studied it."[38]

In March—at long last—an impressive collection of medical, public health, and minority community groups filed *amici* briefs in support of the cap. The National Alliance for Hispanic Health led one group of *amici*. It was joined by groups such as the Harlem Health Promotion Center, National Congress of Black Women, Inc., the New York Chapter of the National Association of Hispanic Nurses, the Association of Black Cardiologists, and the United Puerto Rican Organization of Sunset Park, along with an equally impressive coalition of medical centers, physicians' organizations, and public health institutes. Another brief came from the Association of Local Boards of Healthcare, public health advocacy organizations, and university legal groups.[39]

A year later, the National Alliance for Hispanic Health filed a second brief in support of the rule, joined by additional minority community groups. The brief said: "For the one of every three children born in 2000 who will develop type 2 diabetes, and for the one of every two African-American and Hispanic girls who will get the disease, the question is not whether the Rule was justified but rather 'What else is being done?' It is for their sake that the Rule was adopted....It is for their sake that *amici* urge this Court to uphold the Rule." In a statement, the alliance's president, Dr. Jane L. Delgado, succinctly summarized the underlying issue: "The beverage industry has pursued a strategy of legal obstruction and put profits over the health of its customers." Soon after, many other proponents of the rule came forward with supporting statements.[40]

Would the portion cap have encountered less public opposition if the city had engaged in coalition building right from the start? I think so. In his lecture, Dr. Goodman agreed. Health Department officials did not try to get support for the initiative because they did not want to tip their hand to the soda industry. But organizing support before taking action is essential to effective advocacy. Ben Jealous, the president of the NAACP chapter responsible for the *amici* brief opposing the "ban," emphasized this point when he later commented that his organization

> would support the idea of a ban but you have to do it well... it's not the details about the policy. This is about organizing. This is about come talk to us, right? Let's figure out how to do this together.... Rather than pitting each other against each other, let's just be good organizers and do it the right way.... [The Mayor's] got to come clean and actually humble himself to listen to his constituents and say let's solve this together. Our folks at the NAACP here in New York want to help him push through a comprehensive policy.[41]

Like Mr. Jealous, others criticized Mayor Bloomberg for proposing the soda cap with so little consultation, and for not understanding that such measures are likely to be received more favorably "within the context of a more consistent and compassionate message about the city's commitment to the underserved."[42]

This interpretation is borne out by public polls. Although a Gallup poll found that only 30 percent of Americans said they were for soda cap regulations, the percentage was *higher* among low-income and minority respondents. A Pew Research poll found that 67 percent of African and Hispanic American respondents agreed that government has a role in public health, as compared to just 33 percent of whites. Results like these suggest that the very groups most at risk of obesity and type 2 diabetes would be willing to support such interventions if approached with greater sensitivity to issues that concern them.[43]

The Hispanic Institute wants its constituency to understand the issues at stake. It compares the tactics of the soda industry to those of the tobacco industry.

In the case of tobacco companies, minority community organizations walked away when they found themselves condemned by their constituents and were able to find other sources of revenue to replace the lost donations. It is critical, therefore, for the Hispanic organizations that are not tied by financial strings to big sugary drinks to speak out.... The Hispanic organizations that have thrown in their lot with big sugary drinks can make a choice to break the ties and to support the health needs of their constituents.... In doing so, they will also serve the health needs of the entire country.[44]

In June 2014, the appeals court handed down its verdict. The portion size rule, it said, infringed on power reserved for the New York City Council. If the city wanted to cap soda sizes, it would have to obtain approval from a majority of City Council members. Regardless of this disappointing decision, advocacy for size caps is unlikely to disappear. Even the European president of Coca-Cola, James Quincey, conceded that "serving sizes had to be reduced." Coca-Cola's CEO, Muhtar Kent, informed investors that the "romance of the smaller package" had become the most important driver of soda sales in North America. Health-conscious consumers were flocking to the 7.5-ounce cans, the very ones that cost more and provide higher profit margins to the company and retailers.[45]

Eventually, we will learn whether people who choose the 7.5-ounce cans drink less soda and gain less weight, or whether they follow generally healthier diets to begin with. But for now, it's worth pondering whether the portion cap initiative failed in part because the 16-ounce limit was set too high.

ADVOCATE: CAP SODA SERVING SIZES

Understand the Issue

Larger soda portions:

- Provide more calories
- Provide more sugars
- Induce greater consumption of sugars and calories
- Induce underestimation of sugar and calorie intake
- Cost less per ounce
- Are heavily promoted

Engage in the Debate

TABLE 25.2 Topic for debate: soda sizes should be capped at 16 ounces*

THE SODA INDUSTRY AND ITS SUPPORTERS SAY	ADVOCATES SAY
Cities have no right to impose size limits on foods.	Cities have a responsibility to ensure the health of their residents.
Soda caps are an infringement of personal freedom.	Large sodas limit parents' freedom to raise healthy children.
The cap rule is a ban on soda consumption.	The cap rule sets a maximum size per serving.
The cap rule restricts customers' choice.	The cap rule restricts the soda industry's choice.
People have the right to drink as much soda as they wish.	People may order as many drinks as they wish; free refills are also permitted.
Caps on soda sizes unfairly affect the poor.	Soda-related obesity and type 2 diabetes unfairly affect the poor.
The ban discriminates against minorities.	Minorities bear the discriminatory burden of higher levels of obesity and type 2 diabetes.
The ban will not improve health.	The default size affects consumption; soda consumption is strongly linked to obesity, type 2 diabetes, and other health conditions.
Soda caps are unfair to small businesses.	The health care burden from obesity and type 2 diabetes is unfair to small businesses.
Only the New York City Council has the authority to set a cap on soda sizes.	The New York City Board of Health has the responsibility to ensure the health of residents.

* Adapted in part from New York City Department of Health and Mental Hygiene, "Sugary Drink Portion Cap Rule: Fact vs. Fiction."

Take Action

- Build coalitions to support portion size limits.
- Frame caps on portion sizes as part of a broad commitment to address the health and economic needs of the underserved.
- Ask city councils to set maximum limits on soda sizes.
- Ask city agencies to stop selling and serving sodas on city property or to set maximum limits on their sizes.
- Be prepared to address concerns about nanny-state infringement on personal choice.
- Pressure soda companies to reduce the price differential between large and small serving sizes.
- Ask the FDA to require the full number of calories in a container—not just calories per serving—on the front of soda cans or bottles of all sizes.

26

Advocacy

Taxing Sugary Drinks—Early Attempts

Taxing sodas is not a new idea. Any unnecessary, non-nutritious, but widely consumed comestible is a sitting target for taxation. Had sodas existed in 1776, Adam Smith undoubtedly would have listed them along with sugar, rum, and tobacco as "extremely proper subjects of taxation." What the soda industry prefers to call the "threat" of taxes first emerged in the United States in 1898 during the Spanish-American War, but Congress did not actually impose such taxes until the Revenue Act of 1918. That act included a 10 percent tax on sodas, an affront the industry considered so objectionable that it organized a trade association, the American Bottlers of Carbonated Beverages, later renamed the American Beverage Association (ABA), to lobby for repeal. Taxes raise prices and, when they go high enough, demonstrably reduce purchases. As revenue generators, soda taxes may appear attractive, but they create a dilemma for government: if the tax rate is too high, federal revenues decline along with sales.[1]

The soda industry and retailers always oppose taxation, even at rates too low to affect purchase patterns. Their rationale: once taxes exist, they can always be raised. In 1919, while New York officials were predicting that soda taxes would enrich state coffers by $6 million a year, drugstore owners formed the Soda Fountain Association to whip up public sentiment and collect signatures on petitions to end the tax. By 1920 New York City reported that soda taxes were generating a quarter of a million dollars a month from fountain sales, just within the boroughs of Manhattan and the Bronx. Although Congress repealed the 1918 wartime tax three years later, nearly every state was considering such taxes as a way to raise revenues. As

Mark Pendergrast explains, "lawmakers (with 'upturned palm') saw the wealthy bottlers and The Coca-Cola Company as a convenient source of special sin taxes."[2]

The industry fought state tax initiatives such as Pennsylvania's attempt to impose a 20 percent soda tax in the 1940s. By the 1950s, only two states had soda taxes: South Carolina's 1-cent-per-bottle tax, passed in 1925, and West Virginia's 1951 sales tax. All other attempts lasted only a few years or failed. From then until now, all segments of the soda industry vigilantly opposed such attempts. States continued to consider and occasionally pass soda taxes, but most were small—in the range of 1 cent per 12 ounces—and did not affect buying habits. In Puerto Rico, however, a tax of 5 cents per 12-ounce drink did seem to reduce sales. Although the industry did all it could to fight them, the smaller taxes did not elicit much opposition from the public, especially when revenues were earmarked for social purposes such as drug education, medical education, or public parks.[3]

TAXES FOR A CAUSE: OBESITY PREVENTION

Throughout this history, soda taxes had only one purpose: to generate revenue. But in 1994, Kelly Brownell, a professor of psychology who then directed a center for eating and weight disorders at Yale University, came up with a new strategy. He suggested that funds collected from taxes on junk foods should be used to support physical activity or nutrition education in order to counter rising rates of obesity. He did not single out soft drinks for special consideration in that article or in a later one written in 2000 with Michael Jacobson of the Center for Science in the Public Interest (CSPI). He and Jacobson simply pointed out that a penny-a-can tax on soft drinks, too small to affect consumption, could generate $1.5 billion annually to fund health programs. Over the next several years, both authors continued to document the growing body of evidence linking soft drink consumption to poor diets and obesity, the historical justification for soda taxes, and the value of small taxes as a way to raise funds for programs to discourage consumption.[4]

By 2008, twenty-eight states were taxing soft drinks at rates too low to affect sales and putting all of the revenues into general funds. The turning point came in 2009. That year, Brownell and colleagues proposed a different strategy: taxing soft drinks at levels high enough to discourage consumption. In two articles in the *New England Journal of Medicine*, they called for a national excise tax of 1 cent per ounce. Unlike sales taxes, excise taxes—those levied on the production of specific items—appear as part of the purchase price and are not paid separately by consumers. Brownell and his co-authors estimated that an excise tax at this level would increase the price of a 20-ounce soft drink by up to 20 percent. This, they suggested, not only would generate $15 billion in annual revenue, serious money that could be used to fund health programs, but also would reduce consumption by about 10 percent. This difference, they suggested, could over time lead to significant weight loss and a reduction in health care costs over time. Although one study showed that even a 12 percent price increase led to significantly fewer soda purchases, models developed by economists and others predicted better results from taxes at 20 percent.[5]

Beginning in 2009 and thereafter, many states considered the introduction of soda taxes as an obesity control measure as well as a revenue generator. Although no state measures had passed by 2014, their introduction suggested a growing interest in this approach at a time of severe budget restrictions. That year, as discussed in Chapter 27, tax initiatives in two cities in California, San Francisco and Berkeley, won majority votes. At the federal level, Representative Rosa DeLauro (D-Conn.) introduced legislation to tax sugars at 1 cent per teaspoon, with the revenues going to disease prevention programs. Survey results indicated that although voters generally oppose taxes on sugars and sodas, many people would be willing to approve them if they were linked to desirable social and health programs.[6]

This brief history holds lessons for soda tax initiatives aimed at addressing obesity and its health consequences.[7] It reveals that any proposed tax on soda has a good chance of addressing obesity if it is constructed as an excise tax levied per ounce, raises the purchase price by at least 20 percent, and is earmarked explicitly for public health or social service programs.

ARGUMENTS AND ACTIONS AGAINST SODA TAXES

Opponents of soft drink taxes argue that taxation is neither a good nor an effective way to prevent obesity. They say it hurts small businesses, causes job losses, and—horrors—represents nanny-state government policy.[8] These arguments, of course, ignore the effects of soda marketing on food choices and the high costs of obesity and its consequences to individuals and to society.

The soda industry lobbies Congress on "issues pertaining to beverage taxes" and wants legislators to "monitor potential initiatives to impose a tax on sugar-sweetened beverages."[9] The industry also uses its considerably financial resources to influence community and health groups that might otherwise favor soda taxes.

Let me give two particularly blatant examples. In 2009, the U.S. advocacy group Save the Children (STC) campaigned for soft drink taxes in four states and Washington, D.C. But then STC accepted $5 million in grants from PepsiCo for international work in India and Bangladesh, and negotiated with Coca-Cola for additional support. Late in 2010, STC announced that it would no longer be working on soda tax issues. A second example: when Philadelphia mayor Michael Nutter asked his city council to pass a 2-cent-per-ounce soda tax as an anti-obesity measure, the ABA promised to deliver a $10 million donation to Children's Hospital of Philadelphia (CHOP) for obesity prevention programs. The City Council promptly withdrew Philadelphia's soda tax measure.[10]

As I explained in Chapter 24, the soda industry generously funds astroturf groups to organize petition and public relations campaigns.[11] The largest of these groups, Americans Against Food Taxes, is a coalition of "57,000 concerned individuals" and a great many food and beverage business groups. The coalition sponsors a website that encourages visitors to take action against soda taxes:

> The food and beverage industry is doing its part to reduce childhood obesity through innovation, nutrition education, and encouraging physical activity.... Discriminatory and punitive taxes on soda and juice drinks do not teach our children to have a healthy lifestyle and have no meaningful impact on child obesity or public health.... American families and small businesses are struggling to survive in the current economy. CLICK HERE to learn more about the devastating economic impact of raising more taxes on the food and beverage industry... and on the millions of Americans who eat and drink every day.[12]

As noted in Chapter 23, Coca-Cola and PepsiCo spent more than $9 million each, and the ABA another $19 million, on lobbying against state soda taxes in 2009.[13] The industry uses its funds and its funded front groups to great advantage in turning public opinion against such measures. In this chapter, I present three examples of national and international soda tax initiatives that resulted in a variety of outcomes, all unsuccessful: New York State (withdrawn), two cities in California (voted down), and Denmark (passed but later rescinded). In Chapter 27, I explain how the lessons learned from these experiences led to more successful soda tax advocacy in Mexico, other California cities, and the Navajo Nation in New Mexico.

NEW YORK STATE

Late in 2008, New York State governor David Paterson proposed an 18 percent sales tax on soft drinks along with other measures aimed at reducing a budget shortfall. He expected his "obesity tax" to generate more than $400 million a year to be used for public health programs. The tax was meant to be high enough to affect consumption—and to be used for social purposes—but it was not designed as an excise tax.[14]

As the *New York Times* understated the matter, Paterson's proposal caused a "spirited debate." The ABA argued that taxes such as these hurt the middle class and would cause job losses. It promised a major lobbying effort, which it delivered. After experiencing relentless lobbying for a month or two, and recognizing that the legislature was unlikely to pass the bill, Governor Paterson retreated. His explanation: he was merely trying to create a conversation: "The tax on soda was really a public policy argument.... In other words, it's not something that we necessarily thought we would get. But we just wanted the population to know some issues about childhood obesity."[15]

Paterson observed that the soda industry bought off lawmakers with nearly $13 million in donations and advertising, even spending large sums in districts where 40 percent of minority children were overweight or obese. He told reporters, "We ran into the machine the way anti-smoking activists did in the early '60s.... It's not a fight you're going to win right away."[16]

In 2010, Paterson tried again, this time with a carrot-and-stick tactic: pairing the soda tax (stick) with state tax exemptions for diet sodas and bottled water (carrots). This approach fared no better. During the first four months of 2010, the ABA spent $9.4 million on lobbying against the tax. Reportedly, all but $120,000 of that amount went to Goddard Claussen, the public relations firm well experienced in countering such initiatives—and evidently well paid. Goddard Claussen's astroturf group, New Yorkers Against Unfair Taxes ("a name calculated to make the blood boil"), signed on more than 10,000 individuals and 158 businesses.[17] Soda companies mounted their own campaigns, as Figure 26.1 illustrates.

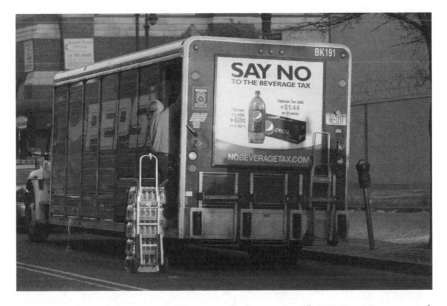

FIGURE 26.1 Pepsi delivery truck, "Say no to the beverage tax," 2010. PepsiCo converted its delivery trucks in New York City to billboards arguing against soda taxes. This photo illustrated an article on soda industry anti-tax spending in the *New York Times*, July 2, 2010. Photo: Earl Wilson/*New York Times*/Redux. Used with permission.

Where was the public on all this? A Quinnipiac University poll released in April 2010 found that nearly 70 percent of New Yorkers opposed "fat taxes" (the polltakers' term) on sugary drinks but that the percentage dropped substantially when respondents were told that the revenues would be used to fund health care.[18]

Although the New York State soda tax never came to a vote, at least thirty other states had introduced similar bills or were doing so. Coca-Cola, PepsiCo, and the ABA collectively spent at least $70 million to defeat soda tax initiatives from 2009 to 2012.[19] They must view that amount as minor in comparison to the losses in sales expected if state soda taxes actually passed.

RICHMOND AND EL MONTE, CALIFORNIA

California towns such as Richmond and El Monte would seem unlikely places to break new ground on soda taxes. In 2012, both had populations of about 100,000, largely African and Hispanic American, and unemployment rates of about 15 percent. In El Monte, per capita average annual income was less than $15,000; in Richmond, it was just over $23,000. In both, more than half of elementary school children were overweight or obese, and soft drink consumption was high, especially among teenagers. City health officials viewed soda taxes as a good way to address such problems.[20]

At the instigation of Dr. Jeff Ritterman, a member of the Richmond City Council, the council voted to place a soda tax of 1 cent per ounce on the November ballot—Measure N. The impetus for the measure came from a report prepared by the Contra Costa County Department of Health Services. The county report found levels of soda consumption, obesity, and obesity-related diseases to be higher among Richmond residents than those in other Contra Costa cities, and costly to local and state government. It included a map locating the abundant retail stores selling sodas within city limits, many of them close to schools. Among its suggestions for City Council action was a "sugar-sweetened beverage regulatory fee"—in other words, a tax.[21]

Based on this report, the council designed the ballot initiative to tax soda sales at a rate expected to raise more than $2 million a year. The council wanted to apply these funds to obesity programs, school gardens, and playing fields. But California's Proposition 13, passed in 1978, requires any local tax measure earmarked for special purposes to be passed by a two-thirds majority, a percentage guaranteed to be difficult to achieve. Instead, the council proposed a separate ballot initiative—Measure O—to specify where the funds would go.[22] El Monte's initiative also involved two distinct ballot measures. Voters would need to understand that Measures N and O were linked, a challenge in itself.

The ABA went into action in both communities. In Richmond, its astroturf group, the Community Coalition Against Beverage Taxes, registered by the Goddard Claussen public relations firm, funded street teams wearing T-shirts and holding signs with anti-tax slogans. Its "No on N" materials focused on the higher cost of sports drinks, baby formulas, and horchata and agua fresca (the latter two consumed largely by Hispanic residents). Campaign materials said: "Richmond needs real solutions like more jobs, better schools and safer streets. Not more taxes on working people!" And it exploited the division between the two measures: "No on N: millions in new taxes and not one dime guaranteed for our kids."[23]

An after-the-fact investigative report found that much of the anti-tax advertising deliberately invoked race and discrimination to generate minority opposition to the measure. The ABA recruited African and Hispanic American community members to canvass against the tax. It also used issues of race and class to divide health advocates working to reduce obesity from anti-poverty advocates. Another investigative report, this one examining news coverage of ballot measures from late 2011 to early 2013 in Richmond, El Monte, and Telluride, Colorado (which also ran a failed tax initiative), documented substantial "infiltration" of news accounts by the soda industry. Without identifying its role, the ABA-funded public relations agency recruited—and paid—community members to speak out against soda taxes. As Dr. Wendel Brunner, then director of public health for Contra Costa County, once told me, "Everybody was bought off." This strategy permitted soda companies to appear as though they had nothing to do with promoting opposition to the tax and that actions against it instead arose spontaneously from the community.[24]

Election campaign laws, full of holes as they are, still require spending disclosure. That is how we know that the ABA spent $2.2 million to fight the Richmond initiative, nearly ninety times the measly $25,000 spent by pro-tax advocates.[25] It used the funding to produce billboards such as the one shown in Figure 26.2, mailings, and television advertisements portraying

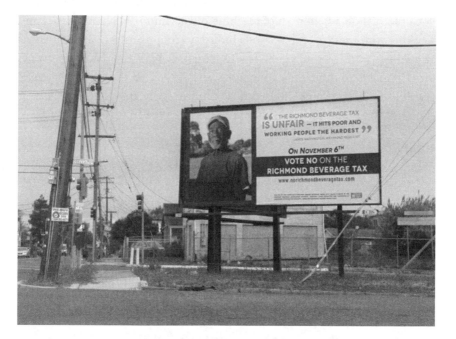

FIGURE 26.2 Billboard, Richmond, California, 2013. The ad framed the soda tax as unfair to poor and working people, especially those of color. It illustrated an article, "Race-Baiting in Richmond," in the *East Bay Express*, January 23, 2013. Photo by Rachel De Leon, courtesy of Robert Gannon, editor, East Bay Express.

proponents of the tax as white elitists who were seeking to impose unfair taxes on minorities and the working poor. In El Monte, it spent $1.3 million for similar purposes.

Against this kind of opposition, the pro-tax initiatives did not stand much of a chance, and the measures were overwhelmingly defeated. In both cities, 67 percent of voters cast ballots against the taxes. But at the same time, at least 60 percent of these voters approved the additional measures—now moot—that would have authorized soda tax revenues to fund parks, recreation, and wellness programs. All in all, the ABA spent an estimated $115 for every single vote cast in its favor, most of it funneled through Goddard Claussen. Given this level of spending, the California Endowment asked an obvious question: how could soda companies have used that money to help these low-income communities? By its 2012 estimation, the soda industry's anti-tax spending could have paid for 41 playgrounds, 82 miles of bike lanes, 1,100 water fountains, and 318,000 jump ropes (see Figure 27.1 for the 2014 update).[26]

The Richmond and El Monte examples taught important lessons. Advocates must do a better job of reaching out to minority communities and working with them to stop the soda industry from using race and elitism as strategies to undermine public health efforts.[27] Advocates must do everything possible to force soda companies, the ABA, and the Goddard public relations firm to disclose the amounts of money they are spending to defeat such initiatives, and the ways they are deploying the funds.

THE DANISH "FAT TAX"

In 2009, the Danish government announced a major tax overhaul aimed at cushioning the shock of the recent global economic crisis, promoting renewable energy, protecting the environment, discouraging climate change, and improving health—all while maintaining current revenue levels. The tax reforms made it more expensive to produce products likely to harm the environment and to consume products likely to harm health, such as sugar-sweetened beverages. Because the targeted foods included a new category—those containing at least 2.3 percent saturated fat—the tax was quickly framed as a "fat tax."[28]

Denmark has taxed candy for nearly ninety years, and it was the first country to ban trans fats, in 2003. Because its income disparity is relatively small, the effects of such taxes are less regressive than in many other places. Although the Danes are already fairly healthy as a population, they could be healthier. Thus, the tax policies aimed to increase life expectancy as well as to reduce the burden and cost of illness from diet-related diseases in a country where health care is universal and funded by taxpayers. The new "health taxes" were supposed to raise nearly $500 million annually, with the tax on saturated fat expected to account for more than one-third of that amount. Overall, the taxes were set at relatively low levels, and no one knew how they might affect consumption.

The experiment ended in 2012 with a change in government. Under intense pressure from the food industry in an already weakened economy, the new government repealed the tax. It explained the repeal as responding to complaints from consumers who resented having to pay more for an ingredient intrinsic to many foods, but the real reason was to appease business interests. A coalition of Danish food businesses had begun a national campaign to undo the taxes, insisting that they would lead to a loss of 1,300 jobs, generate high administrative expenses, and increase cross-border shopping. In ending the taxes, the government used precisely those arguments: higher food prices raised the costs of doing business, put Danish jobs at risk, and drove customers to travel to Sweden and Germany to buy food.[29]

In its short lifetime, the tax did raise revenue. As for consumption, University of Copenhagen economists observed up to a 20 percent drop in purchases of taxed foods during the first three months, but they could not say whether the decrease occurred because of the tax or the depression in the Danish economy.[30] Overall, Danish food prices increased up to 9 percent—enough to generate a political firestorm but not to make a measurable difference in health within the short period of observation.

As for lessons learned, it seemed evident that goals for taxation must be more clearly defined, and taxing a natural ingredient such as saturated fat is not a good strategy. The lesson for Europeans is that a small country with open borders cannot get away with raising food prices unless its neighboring countries do so as well.

These examples describe tax advocacies that failed. But advocates observed these cases carefully, and learned from them, as Chapter 27 demonstrates.

27

Advocacy

Taxing Sugary Drinks—Lessons Learned

Taxes do reduce consumption. In 2012, France instituted a 7-cent-per-liter tax on sodas as part of a fiscal measure aimed at reducing the cost of social security to farm workers and, perhaps, reducing obesity as well. Since the early 2000s, Coca-Cola had considered France a "growth engine," but the tax led to a sharp drop in sales. In 2014, soda companies responded with a promise to reduce the sugars by 5 percent in their drink portfolios in France by 2015.[1] The tax had this effect as well.

Advocates, therefore, had no reason to be discouraged by the failure of other soda tax initiatives. They could learn from those failures and try again in strategically chosen California communities such as San Francisco and Berkeley. They were inspired by the surprising adoption of a tax on sodas and junk foods in Mexico, a country with especially high soda consumption, obesity, and type 2 diabetes. The Mexico example demonstrated that soda tax advocacy has a good chance of succeeding when it is done skillfully, generates public support—and is well funded.

THE MEXICAN "BLOOMBERG" TAX

Late in October 2013, Mexico's president, Enrique Peña Nieto, signed into law an excise tax on sodas of 1 peso (about 8 cents) per liter. The tax was part of a fiscal reform program, which also included an 8 percent tax on snacks and candies. The government designed these taxes for two explicit purposes: to reduce obesity and to raise revenues. Obesity and its consequences are acute problems in Mexico, as nearly 70 percent of Mexicans are overweight or obese and 15 percent are known to have type 2 diabetes.[2] Another law a few months later specified that 80 percent of the revenues were to be earmarked for public health programs to combat malnutrition, to prevent obesity, and—most critical for popular support—to improve access to clean water in rural areas, schools, and public spaces. Table 27.1 summarizes the details of the Mexican soda tax law.

Mexican health authorities viewed the need to address obesity as an urgent priority. Although Mexico was still a relatively poor country, its economy was improving. Its population was becoming increasingly obese, a transition widely attributed to the introduction of processed foods and beverages. Health officials suspected that their efforts to deal with poverty were promoting obesity, and they wanted to make sure that measures aimed at raising revenues would also deal with obesity prevention. Mexicans were spending more than $14 billion a year on soft drinks, about 163 liters of sodas a year per capita, amounting to more than one 12-ounce serving per day.[3] Raising the price of sugary drinks also might help counter the ways these beverages were so deeply entrenched in Mexican culture.

The origins of this entrenchment date back to the 1950s, when Coca-Cola began intense marketing campaigns in Mexico. By the 1970s, sodas were well established as components of daily cultural life. In the early 2000s, the company embarked on more aggressive sales strategies. It commissioned people to deliver bottles, campaigned against local colas, threatened store owners selling competing drinks, contracted with schools, and sold sodas at prices below that of water in rural communities. For such practices, some of which pushed legal limits, the company was fined $13 million in 2003.[4]

TABLE 27.1 The Mexican soda tax law: summary

ISSUE	DETAILS
The tax	Passed by Congress, October 31, 2013; went into effect January 1, 2014
Type of tax	Excise
Amount of tax	1 peso per liter (about 8 cents U.S.)
Price increase	About 10 percent
Taxable items	All drinks with added sugar, except milks and yogurts
Anticipated reduction in consumption	10 percent to 13 percent
Anticipated revenues	12 billion pesos per year ($900 million U.S.)
Earmark	Passed May 2014: public health measures to address obesity and diabetes, beginning with installation of potable water fountains or dispensers in all schools throughout the country

The marketing campaign succeeded in promoting an increase in soda intake, in part because of the widespread unavailability of potable water. Large segments of the Mexican population live in areas without clean running water. Sodas, however, are sold everywhere and quickly became integrated into the cultural fabric of Mexican society, particularly in rural areas. Sodas are served to guests, mark social status, are given as bridal dowries, and replace wine in religious rituals.[5] Mexico's president from 2000 to 2006, Vicente Fox, had been president of Coca-Cola Mexico before he took office. Today, places selling sodas are ubiquitous, and bottles come in 3-liter sizes. These often sell for less than bottled water, in part because the price of Mexican sugar is so low. Mexico grows its own cane sugar and sells it at market prices unaffected by U.S. tariffs and quotas. In 2013, I saw buses in Mexico City covered with ads for sugar: "It's natural. A little happiness each day. Only 15 calories per spoon."

The Soda Industry's View of the Tax

Mexican advocates tell me that the soda industry's pushback against the tax was ferocious, using all the usual tactics and then some. The soda and sugar industries used job losses as the main talking point. Their advertisements argued that the tax would put 3.5 million people out of work. I saw ads from sugarcane producers in major newspapers saying that higher soda prices would burden workers and the poorest families: "This tax will not solve the obesity problem. It will generate unemployment, and discourage productivity and investment." One ad from the Mexican Beverage Association must surely be unique to Mexico. It not only attacked the science linking sodas to obesity but also extolled the nutritional benefits of drinking sodas: "Sugar is nutritious; it's a carbohydrate. Carbohydrates are essential for life. Sugar is indispensable for the brain. Soft drinks hydrate and bring energy."

The soda industry even brought in the Center for Consumer Freedom (Centro para la Libertád del Consumo) to help with the anti-tax campaign. The CCF placed ads on school buses: "Can obesity be stopped by taxes? Yes or no to the tax on 'fatties.'" The Mexican branch of the Coca-Cola Foundation tried a softer approach. It spent $131,000 to install drinking fountains that purify tap water in forty-two schools, and said it would soon put the devices in another seven hundred schools at a cost of $2 million. These "Centros de Hydratación" are marked clearly with the Coca-Cola logo, ensuring that children remain familiar with the brand.[6]

How Did Mexico Pass the Soda Tax?

It is worth asking how the Mexican government succeeded in promoting public health against the opposition of some of its most important industries—cane sugar, sodas, candy, and snack foods. Evidence suggests that the answer lies in unusually effective pro-tax advocacy from members of the Alianza por la Salud Alimentaria (Alliance for Healthy Food), a coalition of twenty-two nongovernmental organizations and networks representing some 650 nonprofit and grassroots organizations. These groups worked closely with government officials and research scientists from the National Public Health Institute. The most prominent of the groups, El Poder del Consumidor (Consumer Power), is led by Alejandro Calvillo, a former Greenpeace organizer.

Together, these groups did advocacy by the book. They thoroughly researched the facts, reached out to potential allies, and built a strong and united coalition. They forged alliances with Mexico's president, the tax authorities, and members of opposition parties. They explicitly linked the tax to an issue of major popular concern: providing clean water to schools.

But beyond its careful planning, the alliance had one other, critically important asset: it was unusually well funded. Bloomberg Philanthropies provided three-year grants eventually adding up to $16.5 million to three groups in the alliance, including El Poder and the collaborating public health research institute. The funds were to be used to advocate for banning the marketing of unhealthy foods to kids, improving front-of-package food labels, and improving guidelines for the sale and preparation of food in schools. But their immediate purpose was to promote the soda tax. As Bloomberg Philanthropies explains on its website: "In the Fall of 2013, our partners helped Mexico's President Enrique Peña Nieto propose a new tax on sugar-sweetened beverages. We acted quickly to fund aggressive media campaigns in support of the tax."[7]

With this kind of funding, advocates could recruit allies, among them the World Health Organization, and engage support of the tax. They could bring international journalists and anti-soda advocates, such as Dr. Jeff Ritterman of California's Richmond campaign, to Mexico to meet with them and government officials.[8]

They also could invest in media. They produced a powerful film emphasizing linkages between soda consumption and type 2 diabetes. They produced two videos translating the real meaning of Coca-Cola's television

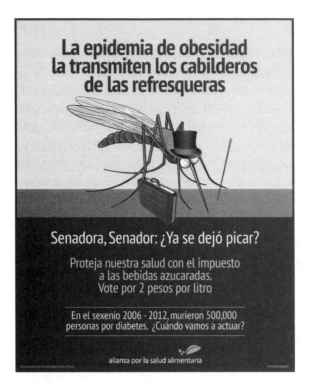

FIGURE 27.1 Advertisement for the Mexican soda tax, 2013. The Alianza por la Salud Alimentaria (Alliance for Healthy Food) placed this ad in *Reforma*, October 24, 2013. My translation: "The obesity epidemic is transmitted by soft drink lobbyists. Senators: did you let them bite you already? Protect our health with a tax on sweetened beverages. Vote for 2 pesos per liter." The Mexican government passed the soda tax the following week, but at 1 peso per liter. Courtesy of Alianza por la Salud Alimentaria/El Poder del Consumidor.

ads and depicting Santa Claus apologizing for his version of the "karmic debt" he owed for having worked for Coca-Cola since 1931. Throughout the campaign, they placed pro-tax advertisements in subway stations, on television, and in newspapers. Figure 27.1 shows one such advertisement.[9]

Advocates in Mexico had other advantages. They could frame their campaign as countering the cost of obesity and type 2 diabetes to the economy and to the universal, single-payer health care system instituted the previous year. The political situation also helped. The three major political parties in Mexico had agreed that they would not actively try to undermine measures supported by the majority.[10] And the earmarking of tax funds for clean water greatly helped to recruit allies.

In addition, advocates could take advantage of strategic mistakes made by the soda industry. Advertisements framing the tax as something imposed by the United States—"No to the Bloomberg tax...don't let a gringo tell you what to drink"—struck Mexicans as xenophobic, overly aggressive, antagonistic to other food and beverage producers, and "out of step with the rest of the Mexican political system." People were offended when the soda industry forced major media, which typically ran soda commercials, to block the alliance's pro-tax advertisements in major magazines and radio and television stations. They also did not appreciate the industry's personal attacks on Alejandro Calvillo.[11]

The soda tax went into effect in January 2014, and results were observed immediately—a drop in sales of up to 10 percent, despite soda companies' efforts to maintain demand by reducing prices in rural areas. This percentage was half that expected if the tax had been 2 pesos per liter, but advocates thought it would still have useful effects. Mexican bottlers said the price increase would force them to substitute less expensive high-fructose corn syrup for cane sugar, but the parent Coca-Cola Company denied it was changing its sweetener. Instead, it promised to invest $8.2 billion in Mexico from 2014 to 2020. PepsiCo also said the tax would have no effect on its expansion plans in Mexico. By October 2014, it was evident that Mexicans were drinking less soda, so much less that Coca-Cola FEMSA, Mexico's largest bottler, said it was forced to close production lines and cut 1,300 jobs. Business analysts observing these events predicted that the market would shift to increased consumption of water, juice, and milk, and less of soft drinks—just what the tax intended.[12]

At a Soda Summit meeting in Washington, D.C., in June 2014, Alejandro Calvillo summarized what advocates for the Mexican soda tax had done right.[13] To win such campaigns, he suggested, advocates should:

- Begin with the public health problem, in this case rampant type 2 diabetes and the amputations that result.
- Identify the enemy—here, the soda industry—and position the tax as a solution.
- Link tax revenues to a cause, in this case drinking water in schools.
- Form alliances with academics, public interest groups, and government officials.
- Develop a strong research basis.
- Obtain adequate funding.

- Use the funds to engage public debate, call on experts, bring diverse voices in support, model the effects of the tax, reinforce economic and financial analyses, and use the media.

Amen.

SAN FRANCISCO: CHOOSE HEALTH SF

Back in the United States, two neighboring cities in Northern California, San Francisco and Berkeley, put soda tax initiatives on the 2014 November ballot. Health advocates framed San Francisco's Proposition E as "Choose Health SF: Our Community's Health Matters. Let's Fight for It." The public health community strongly supported the measure, as did the *San Francisco Chronicle*: "A statewide approach would be preferable, but there is no way the politicians in Sacramento—let alone Washington—are going to stand up to the beverage industry. It's time once again for San Francisco to lead the way on a critical matter of public health. Vote yes on Proposition E."[14]

Proposition E called for a tax of 2 cents per ounce on sugary beverages, and specified that the revenues were to go for physical education and nutrition programs for children. The city's economists estimated that the tax would raise the price of soda by 23 to 36 percent, reduce consumption by 31 percent, and bring in $35 million to $54 million annually for the targeted purposes.[15] Recall that for ballot measures specifying how revenues are to be spent, California law requires approval by two-thirds of city voters rather than a simple majority. Thus, although Proposition E won 56 percent of the vote, the measure did not pass. In contrast, as I soon explain, Berkeley's measure required only a majority vote and passed easily.

The differences between the situations and outcomes in the two cities have been subjected to endless analysis.[16] In the following sections I summarize the main reasons for the loss in San Francisco.

The Two-Thirds Plurality Requirement

Proponents of the soda tax would have preferred to try for a simple majority vote but did not trust the city government to use the revenues for health purposes. A poll sponsored by the California Endowment showed that two-thirds of voters would back a soda tax if the revenues were earmarked for programs for children and not just funneled into the city's general spending account. But neither the San Francisco Board of Supervisors nor the mayor's office fully supported the tax, and proponents did not think the city government could be held accountable for spending the funds for social purposes.[17] They chose to try for a two-thirds vote.

Community Demographics

The grassroots campaign, which worked well in higher-income, white neighborhoods, did not start early enough or work hard enough in low-income communities. San Francisco is a more ethnically and economically diverse city than Berkeley, and proponents of Proposition E were unable to do sufficient outreach into Chinese, African American, and immigrant neighborhoods.[18]

Soda Industry Opposition

As might be expected, the No on E campaign was especially well funded and comprehensive. The soda industry did not want San Francisco to set a tax precedent. The American Beverage Association (ABA) framed the soda tax as a burden on the poor that would make living in San Francisco even less affordable. Its website, www.affordableSF.com, made that clear as did the name of its Astroturf group, Coalition for an Affordable City, and its slogan: "Stop unfair beverage taxes." The website acknowledged who paid for it in small type: "With major funding by American Beverage Association California PAC."

The ABA spent lavishly—nearly $10 million—to defeat Proposition E, much of it on TV and radio advertising, billboards, home mailings, polls, and political consultants. Reportedly, it paid the Goddard Gunster firm nearly $950,000 to run the campaign, which among other tactics used billboards featuring local business owners declaring that they planned to vote no. But a brilliant exposé by ABC News' *Nightline* investigators revealed how the ABA had recruited and paid people $13 per hour to "spontaneously" demonstrate against the tax, and how some business owners cited in the ads actually planned to vote yes.[19]

The ABA also gave generously to local political clubs, including the Harvey Milk LGBT Democratic Club, the Affordable Housing Alliance, the

Black Young Democrats of San Francisco, the Chinese American Democratic Club, and the San Francisco Black Leadership Forum. In contrast, Yes on E was only able to raise less than $300,000. Although Bloomberg Philanthropies initially expressed interest in supporting Yes on E, its polls suggested that a measure requiring a two-thirds vote was a lost cause and not worth the investment.[20]

From the Advocacy Perspective, a Success, Not a Loss

Although Proposition E lost, San Francisco advocates count some lasting gains. The campaign brought the health effects of sugary drinks to wide public attention. It gained the support of a broad coalition of nonprofit organizations, Democratic clubs, parent-teacher associations, the school board, more than half the board of supervisors, and the *San Francisco Chronicle*. It exposed the underhanded methods and crass commercial goals of Big Soda. It induced companies to change their policies about sugary drinks in the workplace. Three supportive members of San Francisco's board of supervisors summarized the positive effects:

> Despite over $10 million spent by Coke, Pepsi and Red Bull—the most ever spent on a campaign in San Francisco—the voters have spoken, and a majority support a soda tax.... The first domino has fallen, and more cities will be emboldened to follow, because we now know that taxing soda reduces consumption, just as tobacco taxes reduced smoking, and as Mexico's consumption of soda and sugary beverages has dropped 10 percent since they instituted their soda tax this year. We were able to accomplish an incredible amount over 10 months with 1/30th of the funds the No side had.... This isn't about one soda tax. This is about a national movement that was kicked off tonight, and we are proud to have raised the conversation about the health impacts of soda and sugary beverages, and exposed the beverage industry's deceptive tactics.[21]

BERKELEY VS. BIG SODA

In the one spectacular victory for U.S. soda tax advocates, the citizens of Berkeley, California, passed Measure D, a 1-cent-per-ounce tax on sugary beverages, with a whopping 76 percent of the vote.[22] Dr. Xavier Morales, executive director of the Latino Coalition for a Healthy California and a member of the campaign steering committee, exulted:

> Berkeley's fight against industry money can be put into the same category as the Battle of Thermopylae in 480 BC—when a vastly under-resourced and outnumbered few defended and held off hordes of invaders. Yes, lots of hyperbole here, but this is what happens when you think you can buy an election in Berkeley. We believe our neighbors more than we believe industry's paid operatives who only have one goal: to protect the sales of sugary beverages.[23]

Morales was referring to the $2.4 million spent by the ABA to defeat Berkeley's Measure D, and to its usual buying of Astroturf "volunteers." But he also was referring to how well Berkeley voters recognized the ABA's tactics. University of California, Berkeley, professor Robert Reich, for example, produced a video exposing the ABA's actions. Voters did not appreciate the way the ABA had papered Berkeley BART (transit) stations with No on D advertisements. They also did not appreciate the lawsuit filed against the measure by two Berkeley "residents," both associated with public relations firms working for the ABA. One had registered as a new Berkeley voter on August 4 and sued the city ten days later.[24]

Berkeley, of course, was an obvious choice for a soda tax challenge. It is a small university town with a proud tradition of national leadership in civil rights, free speech, nonsmoking sections in restaurants, access for the handicapped, curbside recycling, and school food policies. If soda taxes could win anywhere, they could win in Berkeley. Alternatively, if Big Soda could defeat the tax in Berkeley, no tax measure would have a chance anyplace else.

When I was an undergraduate and graduate student at Berkeley, we fondly called it "Beserkeley" or the "People's Republic of Berkeley." Less fondly thinking of it this way, the ABA thought that if Berkeley voters passed the tax, no one would believe it meant anything. Roger Salazar, a spokesman for the No on D campaign, said "Berkeley is not necessarily the trendsetter that they claim to be.... They are a nuclear-free zone. They give free pot to low-income folks. Berkeley is Berkeley." Supporters, however, viewed the Berkeley win as "very much like tobacco... This is how it happens. It has to be encouraged for other cities. This is the beginning of a movement." CSPI's Michael Jacobson agreed: "Big Soda's PR machine can spin all it wants about Berkeley's being out of step with the rest of the country, but it's the industry that's out of step."[25]

What Berkeley Did Right

The Berkeley campaign avoided the mistakes made in Richmond and El Monte. Morales, who worked on the campaign with Dr. Vicki Alexander, a retired African American physician and public health official, noted the sharp change in the political climate since those campaigns: "In 2012, the soda industry skillfully navigated the racial dynamics of Richmond, portraying the measure there as a regressive tax backed by white elitists that would boost grocery bills of working-class people of color.... What's going right in Berkeley is that it's an inclusive effort with a very strong, diverse coalition that wants to do something about health disparities."[26]

Larry Tramutola, a political consultant for Berkeley's Yes on D campaign, observed that the measure had unprecedented local political support from all eight city council members, all five school board members, the mayor, and most of the political candidates. He observed how offended they and many other Berkeley residents were by the amount of money spent by the soda industry to defeat the measure.[27]

In contrast to the campaign in San Francisco, Bloomberg Philanthropies thought the Berkeley efforts were worth a $650,000 grant. This paid for canvassing and television advertising, and a commercial during the World Series (eventually won by the San Francisco Giants). The campaign also received smaller but still significant donations from the American Heart Association and CSPI.[28]

Lynn Silver, a veteran of the New York City Health Department's anti-obesity campaigns who was then on the West Coast at the Public Health Institute, explained the win as the result of Berkeley's supportive political leadership and the residents' confidence that the City Council would spend the money on nutrition and public health. "As it turned out the city's highly educated electorate, an Obama-style door-to-door grassroots campaign, getting pretty much every organization in town signed on, and the choice of the 50 percent threshold, created a 'this one's gonna win' energy that ended up getting us way over the top with 75 percent."[29]

Political consultant Larry Tramutola is even more specific about the winning strategies. In a summary that makes it clear that the Yes on D campaign had followed the rules of successful advocacy, he said that the campaign achieved the following:

- Built a broad coalition of health experts and community leaders who knew the research
- Proposed the measure as a general tax requiring a simple majority vote to pass
- Recruited volunteers to conduct an aggressive door-to-door campaign in every Berkeley neighborhood
- Recruited every elected official in Berkeley and every candidate for office, from school board to city council, to support the measure
- Obtained backing from the League of Women Voters and the Berkeley chapter of the NAACP, and focused on people likely to vote
- Made sure voters knew that the beverage industry was behind the No on D campaign[30]

WHAT'S NEXT FOR SODA TAXES?

Soon after the November 2014 elections, the Navajo Nation raised its taxes on sodas and junk foods, and linked the increase to an elimination of an existing tax on fresh fruits and vegetables. This nation includes the 300,000 people who live in 110 communities on and off its 27,000-square-mile reservation. One-third of Navajos are diabetic or pre-diabetic, and diabetes is the fourth-leading cause of death among tribal members. The revenues from the tax increase are to pay for farmer's markets, vegetable gardens, and exercise equipment.[31]

In Congress, Representative Rosa De Lauro (D-Conn.) introduced the Sugar-Sweetened Beverage Tax Act of 2014 (the SWEET Act) to raise $10 billion a year to help prevent and treat diseases caused by excess soda consumption. The act had little chance of passing, but it was a sign of the expanding popular support for taxing sodas.

Will the ABA continue to pour millions into defeating these initiatives? By the end of 2014, it had spent about $117 million to fight soda taxes since 2009, but to that must be added the $513,000 it spent to oppose a 2015 tax initiative in Vermont. The California Endowment considered how the millions spent to defeat the soda tax measures in San Francisco and Berkeley could have been used to improve the health and fitness of California's children.[32] Figure 27.2 illustrates its suggestions.

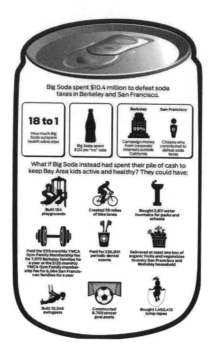

FIGURE 27.2 How the soda industry's anti-tax money could have been better spent. The California Endowment created this chart to illustrate how soda industry expenditures to fight the soda tax could have been used to promote children's health. The illustration appeared in the *San Francisco Chronicle*, November 14, 2014. Courtesy Anne Stuhldreher, California Endowment.

The endowment points out that the $122 spent by the ABA on every vote in those two cities could have paid for a bag of organic fruits and vegetables for every household, or 104 playgrounds, 78 miles of bike lanes, 2,611 water fountains for parks and schools, 6,705 soccer goal posts, or 1,492,413 jump ropes—among other health-promoting options.

ADVOCATE: TAX SODAS

Understand the Issues

In 2012, the Rudd Center's Roberta Friedman and Kelly Brownell summarized the arguments in favor of soda taxes:[33]

- Habitual consumption of sugar-sweetened beverages is linked to poor diets, obesity, and obesity-related chronic diseases.

- Sodas contain sugars but no nutrients; their calories are "empty."
- Liquid calories do not induce satiety as well as those in food.
- Sodas are not necessary for survival, but are widely consumed.
- Sodas are marketed extensively to children, adolescents, and low-income groups most at risk of overweight and its consequences.
- Soda consumption is highest among such groups.
- Taxes reduce soda consumption.
- When used to pay for health programs, taxes can help balance the societal cost of soda consumption in lost productivity and health care.

Engage in the Debate

Obviously, the soda tax issue generates fierce debate.[34] Friedman and Brownell laid out the principal anti-tax arguments and suggested ways that advocates could rebut them. Table 27.2 draws on their format to contrast the main debating points.

TABLE 27.2 Topic for debate: sugar-sweetened sodas should be subject to excise taxes

OPPONENTS SAY	ADVOCATES SAY
Taxes are a blunt instrument of government intervention.	Taxes can encourage healthier food choices while generating needed revenue.
No compelling evidence links sodas to obesity or other health problems.	Research sponsored by independent agencies, not soda companies, clearly links soda consumption to overweight and poor health.
Soda taxes are regressive. They disproportionately hurt poor people.	Diabetes is regressive. Obesity and diabetes disproportionately hurt poor people.
Governments should stay out of personal choice.	Governments should protect the health of citizens.
Soda choice is a matter of personal responsibility.	Taxpayers fund health care costs. Obesity and diabetes are matters of social responsibility.
Soda companies are already making healthful changes to their products.	Soda companies heavily market sugary beverages.
Soda sales have declined while obesity rates remain high; Sodas cannot be responsible for obesity.	Obesity rates are stabilizing as soda sales decline. Sales of some other sweetened beverages are increasing. All should be taxed.
Sodas are not cigarettes or alcohol. They do not cause the same level of harm.	The health effects of sodas increase health care costs for everyone.
Soda taxes lead to unintended consequences. Decreases in consumption will be offset by other sources of calories.	Cigarette taxes decreased smoking. Let's try taxing sodas and see whether it works.
Everyone opposes nanny-state soda taxes.	Soda taxes linked to health programs have strong bipartisan support from public health organizations, city officials, and policy centers.

Take Action

- Propose excise taxes.
- Work to have the taxes increase the price of soft drinks by at least 20 percent.
- Explicitly link revenues to support of health, activity, or school programs.
- Build a broad coalition of supporters that include health, university, and government organizations, including representatives of minority groups.
- Engage communities most likely to be affected by the taxes.
- Explain the tax as part of a broader commitment to address the needs of the underserved.
- Expect strong opposition from the soda and other industries and strategize accordingly.
- Counter that opposition with adequate funding.

Join the Campaigns

Several advocacy groups in the United States are actively engaged in supporting soda tax initiatives. Appendix 1 provides information about them.

28

Conclusion

Taking Action

In her opening address to the Eighth Global Conference on Health Promotion in 2013, Dr. Margaret Chan, director-general of the World Health Organization (WHO), concluded with a statement that touches on many of the themes of this book:

> Efforts to prevent noncommunicable diseases go against the business interests of powerful economic operators...it is not just Big Tobacco anymore. Public health must also contend with Big Food, Big Soda, and Big Alcohol. All of these industries fear regulation, and protect themselves by using the same tactics...front groups, lobbies, promises of self-regulation, lawsuits, and industry-funded research that confuses the evidence and keeps the public in doubt... gifts, grants, and contributions to worthy causes that cast these industries as respectable corporate citizens in the eyes of politicians and the public. They include arguments that place the responsibility for harm to health on individuals, and portray government actions as interference in personal liberties and free choice.... Few governments prioritize health over big business. As we learned from experience with the tobacco industry, a powerful corporation can sell the public just about anything.[1]

"Just about anything," in this context, means sugar-sweetened beverages—calorically empty, demonstrably unhealthful, environmentally polluting, and extravagantly marketed. Figure 28.1 illustrates some of these points.

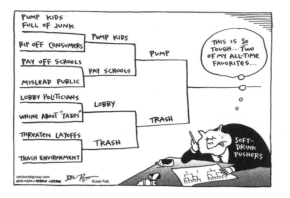

FIGURE 28.1 How soft-drink pushers think. Joel Pett suggests that the drive for corporate profit causes Big Soda to engage in marketing and lobbying efforts that pump kids full of junk and trash the environment. Such methods are no different from those used by Big Food, Big Alcohol, or Big Tobacco. Joel Pett editorial cartoon, with permission of Joel Pett and the Cartoonist Group. All rights reserved.

Dr. Chan continued by reminding the audience that no country to date has been able to reverse obesity. This, she said, is "not a failure of individual will-power. This is a failure of political will to take on big business.... When industry is involved in policy-making, rest assured that the most effective control measures will be downplayed or left out entirely." The influence of industry on health policy, she added, is "well documented, and dangerous," so much so that "in the view of WHO, the formulation of health policies must be protected from distortion by commercial or vested interests."

Her point is that the marketing strategies of Big Soda, Big Food, and Big Alcohol are much the same as those of Big Tobacco. Their profit goals are similar and conflict with those of public health. Singly and together, Big Food and Big Soda promote obesity and type 2 diabetes, a condition now understood to be a public health problem as prevalent and costly as those caused by alcohol and tobacco. This book focuses on Big Soda, but the lessons learned from this analysis apply just as well to any other ingested substance that leads to poor health.

In her speech, Dr. Chan did not suggest steps that governments must take to protect their health policies against corporate interests, nor did she say what advocates could do to encourage governments to take such steps. Others, however, have done so, drawing especially on parallels with Big Tobacco.[2] In this concluding chapter, I review some of the more prominent campaigns to limit the actions and impact of Big Soda, introduce several additional advocacy approaches currently under consideration, and sum- marize the principal strategies needed for effective advocacy for any inter- vention aimed at promoting healthier food choices.

Let me acknowledge immediately that advocacy to reduce soda intake faces special challenges that distinguish it from advocacy for reduction of al- cohol, tobacco, or junk foods. Like these other industries, the soda industry sells relatively inexpensive products that are available in almost every corner of the globe. Like them, this industry is extremely wealthy. Also like the others, health is the industry's Achilles' heel. But in sharp contrast to companies selling junk food, alcohol, or tobacco, Coca-Cola and PepsiCo consistently rank among the most admired, respected, and honored companies in the world.[3] Health and environmental advocates must recognize the power of this favorable public perception when encouraging others to resist it.

CURRENT ADVOCACY CAMPAIGNS

In the United States, many groups have developed health campaigns aimed at reducing soda consumption. Among them at the time of this writing, three had taken the lead. The California Center for Public Health Advocacy, based in Davis, California, is the organizing center for healthy beverage policies. It runs the Kick the Can campaign in collaboration with the Center for Science in the Public Interest (CSPI) in Washington, D.C., and the Rudd Center for Food Policy and Obesity, formerly at Yale and now at the University of Con- necticut. A fourth organization, the Berkeley Media Studies Group, provides technical assistance in advocacy methods, and a fifth, ChangeLab, provides models for legal challenges. Together and separately, these groups have devel- oped—and make publicly available—extensive materials for use by advocates: research summaries, training videos and slide shows, and model letters, peti- tions, and laws. These materials support advocacy for public education about the need to reduce soda consumption as well as for policies to establish a food environment that supports healthier choices of foods and beverages. Appendix 1 provides information about how to find and use these materials.

Government agencies concerned about the rising prevalence of obesity among their constituents also have developed education campaigns about sugary drinks. Appendix 2 presents examples of soda-reduction campaigns developed and run by U.S. government agencies at the national, state, county, and city levels.

One other organization deserves separate discussion: Killer Coke. This group, led by Ray Rogers, began the Campaign to Stop Killer Coke in 2003. Its purpose, in his words, is to hold "bottlers and subsidiaries accountable and to end the gruesome cycle of violence and collaboration with paramilitary thugs, particularly in Colombia." Despite the rhetoric—and Coca-Cola's insistent denials of responsibility—Rogers's claims deserve serious consideration. At least two well-researched books and the documentary film cited in Figure 15.3 offer details and eyewitness accounts of the otherwise alleged harassment and murders of union organizers at Coca-Cola bottling plants in Central America and elsewhere.[4]

The company says it has no responsibility for these problems and indeed has a stated policy on human rights: Coca-Cola "respects our employees' right to join, form or not to join a labor union without fear of reprisal, intimidation or harassment. Where employees are represented by a legally recognized union, we are committed to establishing a constructive dialogue with their freely chosen representatives."[5] As noted earlier, the parent Coca-Cola Company typically owns less than a majority share of its international franchise bottling operations. Whether it bears responsibility for labor relations in those franchises is debatable, I suppose, but Rogers's point is that a 49 percent stockholder could and should insist—forcefully—that its bottlers uphold the human rights of unionizing workers.

Rogers views Coca-Cola's denial of responsibility as disingenuous. His campaign challenges "the company's widespread labor, human rights and environmental abuses and aggressive marketing to children of unhealthy beverages that fuel the childhood obesity, high blood pressure and diabetes epidemics."[6] The Killer Coke website provides information about the Coca-Cola Company and its alleged criminal actions (by country), and much else about soda-related lawsuits, racial discrimination, campus activism, and health issues. Killer Coke's slogans include such messages as "The Drink That Represses," "Murder—It's the Real Thing," and "Unthinkable, Undrinkable." Figure 28.2 provides an example.

Ray Rogers is a formidable advocate. He owns a single share of stock in Coca-Cola. This entitles him to attend annual corporate meetings, where he can and does stage protests. The Securities and Exchange Commission (SEC) warned him that shareholders must abide by SEC rules and that he must delete portions of the Killer Coke website containing inflammatory statements about Coca-Cola. Rogers's reply: "The SEC plays patsy with the Wall Street banks and corporations and then they try to shut me up.... What's that about?"[7]

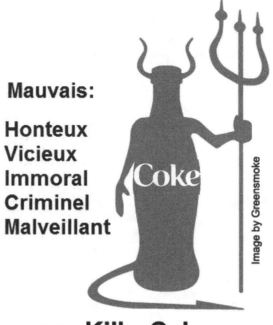

FIGURE 28.2 The Campaign to Stop Killer Coke equates Coca-Cola with the devil: bad, shameless, vicious, immoral, criminal, malevolent. This poster is also available in Spanish and Chinese. Courtesy of Ray Rogers and Killer Coke.

Killer Coke's activities in the United States aim to induce college campuses to ban Coca-Cola on the basis of the company's tacit tolerance of human rights violations. The campaign succeeded at the City University of New York, which replaced Coke with Pepsi in a $21 million deal (see Figure 12.1). It was less successful at New York University (NYU), where I teach. NYU banned Coke in 2005 but rescinded the ban a few years later.

In 2014, the Killer Coke Campaign announced a new ally. The 1.6-million-member American Federation of Teachers (AFT) passed a resolution to ban all Coca-Cola products from its facilities and events and to urge its affiliates to do the same. The ban, however, lasted only four months. Coca-Cola requested and got meetings with the AFT executive committee. The result: the AFT cancelled the resolution and instead announced a partnership with the company "in areas where we have a strong mutual interest, such as the elimination of hazardous child labor and advocating for increased educational opportunities for children." If contributions from Coca-Cola were involved, neither Coke nor the AFT mentioned them. But Ray Rogers, as always, came right to the point: "The most effective way for Coca-Cola to help end illegal child labor in places like the Philippines and El Salvador is...to pay sugar processors enough money to pay fair wages to sugar cane harvesters." He and others petitioned AFT to end the new partnership.[8] More such campaigns should be expected.

EMERGING TARGETS FOR SUGARY DRINKS ADVOCACY

Throughout this book, I have been talking about advocacy efforts to remove sodas from schools, stop soda marketing to children, cap soda sizes, and tax them. Let's now take a quick look at some additional strategies proposed or introduced by advocates.

Remove Sodas from Kids' Menus in Chain Restaurants

CSPI is campaigning to convince the twenty-three leading U.S. restaurant chains to remove all sugary drinks from meals aimed at children. More than 160 organizations and individuals have signed on to this campaign (including me). Although the National Restaurant Association has its own voluntary Kids LiveWell program for putting healthier items on kids' menus, and a few of the smaller restaurant chains already have adopted no-soda policies for kids' meals, CSPI wants the big ones to make this commitment. In 2013, McDonald's said it would phase out sodas; Wendy's did so early in 2015, as did Burger King.[9] If healthier drinks are the default in kids' meals, CSPI argues, it is easier for health-conscious parents to take their families to chain restaurants.

Eliminate Tax Deductions for Soda Marketing to Children

The U.S. tax code permits companies to deduct the costs of marketing—even to children—as business expenses. Because marketing is so powerful an influence on food choice, eliminating the deduction for soda and fast-food advertising directed at children should discourage companies from doing so. In 2014, advocates encouraged two senators to introduce the Stop Subsidizing Childhood Obesity Act, which would prevent companies from taking tax deductions on expenses for marketing junk foods to children under age fourteen. A similar bill was introduced in the House: "To amend the Internal Revenue Code of 1986 to deny any deduction for marketing directed at children to promote the consumption of food of poor nutritional quality." The bills got nowhere, but they brought the issue to congressional—and public—attention. Attention is useful, but real progress takes action.[10] The lack of congressional support for this and similar public health measures is a reason why advocacy is so urgently needed, and why advocates need to engage in the political process.

Put Warning Labels on Soda Packages

Warning labels for cigarettes, especially those with photographs of the consequences of smoking, have been effective in helping smokers to stop. Why not try them for sodas? In 2012, the Ontario Medical Association (OMA) examined tobacco-control policies to see how they might be applied to obesity prevention. Among other measures, the OMA recommended placing a warning label on sugar-sweetened beverages. Its proposal for such a label is shown in Figure 28.3.[11]

The California Center for Public Health Advocacy is equally concerned about how excessive soda consumption can lead to diabetes. It worked with the UCLA Center for Health Policy Research to survey Central Valley residents hospitalized in 2011. Among all hospitalized patients, 31 percent had type 2 diabetes, but the percentage was even higher—42.5 percent—among hospitalized Latinos. On this basis, the center lobbied the California legislature to introduce a Sugar-Sweetened Beverages Safety Warning Bill in 2014. The bill would have placed a warning message similar to that shown in Figure 28.3, but without the photograph, not just on Coke and Pepsi but also on hundreds of other sweetened drink products that contain more than 75 calories per 12 ounces.[12]

The bill gained remarkably strong public support from more than one hundred groups representing hospitals, medical associations, nurses, labor, clinics, and health advocates, among them the Latino Coalition for a Healthy California and the California Black Health Network, and polls showed that almost 75 percent of California voters supported the measure. Understandably, the soda industry did not. Although the state senate passed the measure, the health committee of the assembly rejected it. Because this committee is in charge of California's health, the no vote seemed an especially telling sign of soda industry influence. But the bill's widespread public support suggested that this strategy would be worth trying again. Indeed,

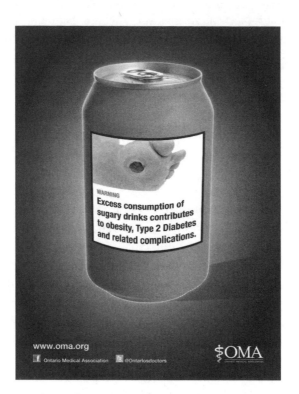

FIGURE 28.3 A proposed soda warning label. The Ontario Medical Association (OMA) wants to warn Canadians about how excessive consumption of sugary drinks can contribute to obesity and its health consequences. Like the photographs of lung cancers and other diseases shown on cigarette packages in Europe, the OMA label depicts foot ulcers that can result from type 2 diabetes. Courtesy of the Ontario Medical Association.

the New York State Assembly soon introduced a similar measure for a "SAFETY WARNING: Drinking beverages with added sugar contributes to obesity, diabetes and tooth decay." Members of the San Francisco Board of Supervisors introduced a similar measure in 2015, and other such attempts were sure to follow.[13]

Use the Legal System to Curb Soda Marketing

Public interest lawyers have scrutinized tobacco-control strategies for ways that could be applied to sodas. One idea is to ban the public sale of sugary drinks to minors on the basis that "the concurrent travesty underlying childhood obesity is the relative societal failure to slow and reverse its spread. If obesity were a highly infectious disease, then government would have declared states of public health emergency decades ago and used nearly every legally supported intervention possible to stymie its impacts."[14]

Lawyers are also looking for precedents to require food companies to pay for their contribution to obesity-related health care costs.[15] The Valorem Law Group in Chicago invoked a legal doctrine used in tobacco legislation, *parens patrie* (father of country), which refers to the government's responsibility to protect its citizens. In letters to the attorneys general in sixteen states, the firm pointed out the need for taxpayer relief from the skyrocketing state costs of obesity-related health care. However unlikely the immediate success of such approaches, they too raise awareness of the ways in which obesity poses problems for society as well as individuals. The Public Health Advocacy Institute at Northeastern University School of Law and the Public Health Law Center at the William Mitchell College of Law are two examples of a growing number of legal training sites that produce materials especially relevant to sugary beverage and other food legislation.

Change Institutional Beverage Procurement Practices

One way to create a healthier beverage environment is to set nutritional standards for drinks that can be offered or sold in government offices, child care facilities, hospitals, prisons, senior centers, and other such institutions. The U.S.-Canada Healthy Beverages Challenge, for example, calls on hospitals to begin increasing the proportion of healthy beverages they sell as a first step to becoming zones free of sugary drinks. For cash-strapped institutions, this approach presents challenges. A similar campaign, the Healthy Hospitals Initiative, surveyed participating hospitals in 2012 and found them to be in widely different stages of implementing healthy beverage programs. Only about half had made significant progress. Nevertheless, many hospitals are replacing sodas with water, low-fat or nonfat milk, unsweetened coffee and tea, and smaller sizes of fruit and vegetable juices. For hospitals and other institutions that are engaged in community health programs, getting rid of sugary beverages is a logical step. So is getting rid of McDonald's, especially from children's hospitals.[16]

Reach Out to Large Audiences

Although countless documentary films have shown how food marketing affects health, none has been distributed as widely as *Fed Up*, "the film the food industry doesn't want you to see," released in 2014 (I appear in it, briefly). The producers, Katie Couric and Laurie David, and director, Stephanie Soechtig, interviewed dozens of experts who take a hard, critical look at how food and beverage marketing promotes obesity.[17] Although the film focused mainly on the effects of sugars on obesity and type 2 diabetes, it had plenty to say about soft drinks as sugar delivery systems aimed at young children. One of the posters designed to promote the film picked up on this theme, as shown in Figure 28.4.

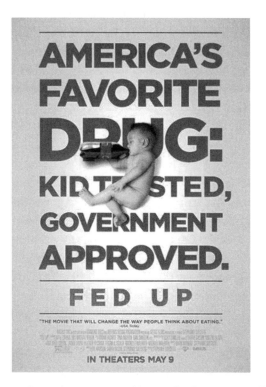

FIGURE 28.4 The award-winning poster to advertise the documentary film *Fed Up*, 2014. Although the producers used a different poster to market the film, this one conveys a powerful message about government's collusion with industry in selling sodas. Courtesy of RADIUS-TWC and the Weinstein Company.

Join the Do-It-Yourself Healthy Beverage Movement

Small machines for making carbonated water at home, such as those from SodaStream, have been cutting into soda sales and undermining soda marketing. These are fitted with rechargeable carbonation cartridges. You fill a compatible bottle with tap water, screw it into the machine, and press a lever that squirts carbon dioxide into the water. You can drink the soda water plain, add sugary syrups supplied by soda manufacturers, add fruit juices, or make your own concoctions. At least one book provides recipes for using these machines to produce healthier carbonated drinks at home. Late in 2014, PepsiCo began test-marketing some of its products in a partnership with SodaStream, an action expected to improve the fortunes of both companies.[18]

Jam the Culture

With little money to spend on public relations and organizing, community and public health advocates must seek other ways to educate and engage the public. Soda marketers have no problem using the frames of "happiness," "pause," and "refresh" to convince you that sugary drinks will make you feel good, all day long, especially if you consume them everywhere and in large amounts. Advocates are looking for ways to reframe those messages to counter the disproportionate resources and political power of food companies. "Jamming the culture" refers to the conversion of corporate advertising to advocacy purposes, as in creating satirical versions of Coca-Cola commercials or songs, or organizing "beautiful trouble"—artistic activism that brings issues to public attention and engages people in political action. The Occupy Big Food movement is one example of such activism.[19] These outside-the-mainstream methods are limited only by imagination. Expect to see more of them.

GUIDELINES FOR EFFECTIVE ADVOCACY

The history of social movements and personal accounts by community organizers and advocates for a wide range of causes suggest basic guidelines for conducting successful advocacy campaigns. The food policy analyst Corinna Hawkes, for example, extracted the take-home lessons from a review of international actions to improve food choices. Advocacy, she concludes, is likely to be most effective when it involves multiple components—a comprehensive policy approach—that includes education to change personal behavior along with interventions to make the food environment more supportive of healthier food choices. She points out that soda companies use multiple strategies when they back product reformulations with advertising campaigns. Governments do too when they link classroom instruction to new school nutrition standards. Her research argues that education works better with policy and program interventions, and that policies have a greater chance of succeeding when backed up by public education.[20]

The Berkeley Media Studies Group (BMSG) has distilled lessons learned from social movements into a succinct summary of the essential steps necessary for successful advocacy campaigns, and the methods for applying these steps to policy change.[21] Advocates working to improve the environment of food choice need to:

- Define the problem—health, social, economic, political—that demands a change in policy or program.
- Do the research and establish a thoroughly documented basis for concern about the problem.
- Choose a goal that represents the best—or the most practical or politically feasible—way to address the problem.
- Identify the person, agency, or institution with the authority or power to achieve that goal.
- Enlist allies who can help support and promote the goal.
- Work with allies to create messages ("frames") that describe the problem, the proposed solution, and why it is important to solve the problem.
- Use the media to educate the public and generate support.
- Work with allies to determine actions—letters, petitions, demonstrations, use of social media, lobbying, and others—to convey these messages to the target authority.
- Take these actions.

But advocacy does not end with the action or intervention. Advocates must do even more:

- Evaluate how well the actions worked to achieve the goal.
- Review, reconsider, and take further action.
- Persist.

To this list, I must add one other critically important step that emerges from the experience with soda tax initiatives:

- Obtain adequate funding.

What strikes me most about these steps is how straightforward they appear, yet how extraordinarily difficult they can be in actual practice. In my experience, it can be difficult for food advocates to define problems clearly, set specific goals, frame messages, or enlist allies. Many well-intentioned campaigns falter because they have not done the groundwork—especially the deep and sensitive community organizing needed to gain support for campaign goals. Effective advocacy requires knowledge, skills, and experience to put these steps into practice and to overcome the obstacles that inevitably crop up. The obstacles are not only political. Sometimes they are personal. Confrontational and culture-jamming methods, for example, may well take potential allies outside of their comfort zones.

Advocacy requires persistence, patience, and time—in seemingly infinite amounts. It requires a level of commitment—and the persistence, patience, and time that go with it—far beyond the capacity of most volunteers, especially if they are not paid. Money helps. Advocacy campaigns based on volunteers are difficult to sustain in the long run. It is not an accident that the two successful soda tax campaigns to date were funded by Bloomberg Philanthropies (Chapter 27). Most advocacy campaigns are not so fortunate and must compete for grants from the same few foundations. One explanation for CSPI's decades of longevity is its firm funding base. Nearly a million readers subscribe to its monthly publication, *Nutrition Action Healthletter*. The subscriptions pay for 90 percent or so of the center's expenses, and foundations cover the rest.

Although the funding and other challenges of effective advocacy cannot be underestimated, I see much cause for optimism. Advocacy has had a profound effect in reducing soda consumption in the United States, so profound that this book can be read as a case study of successful health advocacy.

ADVOCACY IS WINNING

In 2014, I attended CSPI's Soda Summit in Washington, D.C., a meeting that brought together hundreds of advocates engaged in a variety of projects to reduce soda consumption. One speaker after another began with what seemed like the meeting's overriding theme: "We are winning." Sales of sugar-sweetened sodas have been falling steadily in the United States for a decade, with no sign of reversal. And sales are falling faster in places with active "drink less soda" campaigns. In Great Britain, where 60 percent of drinks already contain no sugar, sales of sports drinks are also falling as public health campaigns such as Give Up Loving Pop (GULP) are having an effect. In 2015, the French parliament banned unlimited refills of soft drinks. Drink preferences are changing to the healthier—or to the perceived healthier—and not just as a result of economic recession or changing food prices. By far the most convincing explanation for this downward trend is the public's response to health advocacy.[22]

To the dismay of soda companies, diet drinks have also become the subject of health concerns, and their sales too are falling rapidly. In 2015, in an attempt to reverse this trend, Pepsi announced that it would no longer use aspartame to sweeten these drinks. Because customers singled out aspartame as the main reason why they stopped drinking Diet Pepsi, the company said it would replace aspartame with artificial sweeteners perceived as less harmful. But if these perceptions change, diet soda could be at even greater risk.[23]

Without question, advocacy has gained media attention, increased public awareness of the health effects of sodas, and engaged communities and young people. Nearly two-thirds of Americans now say they are avoiding sodas in their diet—an increase of 20 percent since 2002. It is no coincidence that along with the decline in consumption of sugary drinks, the prevalence of obesity is leveling off and even declining in some groups.[24]

Soda companies are responding to this "failure and disarray" in their business by lowering their revenue and growth targets, and by diversifying their product portfolios in ways that were unimaginable just a few years ago. In 2014, Coca-Cola paid more than $2 billion to acquire a significant stake in Monster Beverage, the maker of highly caffeinated energy drinks recently associated with the deaths of several young people (see Chapter 3). It also invested in Fairlife, a milk filtered and treated with lactase (the enzyme that splits lactose, the sugar in milk that some people cannot digest, into glucose and galactose) to produce a milk product with 50 percent more protein and 30 percent less sugar. This product will cost twice as much as regular milk, but the company expects it to "rain money."[25]

Also in 2014, in a move widely viewed as an admission that sugary drinks promote obesity, the Alliance for a Healthier Generation (founded by the American Heart Association and the Clinton Foundation) and the American Beverage Association (funded mainly by Coca-Cola and PepsiCo) jointly pledged to reduce the calories in such drinks by 20 percent by 2025. Although Risa Lavizzo-Mourey, president and CEO of the Robert Wood Johnson Foundation, was "especially pleased that this commitment will target communities with disproportionately high consumption rates of sugar-sweetened beverages," the move appeared more as public relations than as a genuine commitment to health. The industry was still pouring millions into fighting soda tax initiatives and warning labels and into promoting its products in African American and Hispanic American communities.[26]

Business analysts worry about the soda industry's response to health concerns. They think soda companies should be working harder to reduce the impact of their products on health and the environment. They are well aware that this industry is vulnerable to attacks by competitors such as Brita, the maker of devices that filter tap water; this company advertised its filters by displaying the number of sugar cubes soda drinkers consume in a year. The *Wall Street Journal* produced a video highly critical of Coca-Cola's seemingly desperate marketing response to declining sales. *Bloomberg BusinessWeek* displayed similar views, as illustrated in Figure 28.5.[27]

Business analysts also want soda companies to clean up some of their more unsustainable management practices. The billionaire Warren Buffett, a major investor in Coca-Cola, thinks the company's executives are paid too much. So does Calvert Investments, which notes that the compensation paid to Coke's CEO is "not well aligned with sustainable shareholder interests." Coca-Cola, Calvert says, should modernize its board of directors to deal with its members' age, entrenchment, and lack of independence, so as better to "address sustainability challenges and opportunities," especially in emerging markets. Another group, Wintergreen Advisers, runs a website (fixbigsoda.com) devoted to getting better value from the 2.5 million shares of Coca-Cola it manages for its clients. In 2015, the Gates Foundation liquidated its holdings in Coca-Cola, valued at $914 million, along with holdings in McDonald's and ExxonMobil. Analysts interpreted these actions as consistent with the foundation's policy not to invest in companies whose corporate activities it finds to be "egregious."[28]

But before celebrating, consider the work that still needs to be done. Soda companies are marketing sugary juice drinks, teas, coffees, waters, and sports drinks as healthier options. They have shifted their soda marketing to target the low-income populations of the developing world, particularly in Asia,

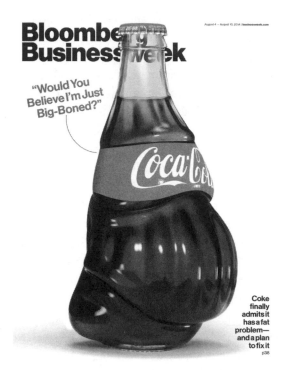

FIGURE 28.5 *Bloomberg BusinessWeek*, August 4–10, 2014. The cover story focused on the threat posed by obesity to Coca-Cola's sales and profits. The magazine took a dim view of Coca-Cola's announcement that it would be concentrating its marketing efforts on smaller cans and bottles. Used with permission of Bloomberg L.P. Copyright© 2014. All rights reserved.

Latin America, and Africa. These actions demand further advocacy. The actions of advocates for reduced soda intake may be less advanced in emerging markets, but they are increasing in scope and intensity as international governments confront the personal and economic costs of obesity and type 2 diabetes in their countries. The Mexican government's banning of soda and junk food advertisements on daytime television in 2014 may well signal the beginning of major international efforts to counter soda marketing.[29]

Also relevant is increasing public support for a new kind of corporate structure—benefit corporations—that link profit mandates to production of measurable societal benefits. By 2014, nearly half the states authorized such structures for incorporation of new businesses. These states require corporate directors to consider the interests of all stakeholders, not just owners of shares, when making business decisions.[30] Although it is unlikely that either Coca-Cola or PepsiCo will switch to this model, benefit corporations put pressure on other businesses to make their corporate social responsibility actions more genuinely socially responsible.

As I hope is evident, the purpose of this book has been to encourage everyone who cares about their own health and that of their children to engage in advocacy for healthier beverages, but also to advocate for healthier diets—and societies. The examples I discuss here aim to bring the relationship between sugary drinks and health to the forefront of public attention. But they also point to the need to advocate for the full range of food issues that affect health and the environment. This, of course, requires engagement with and use of the political system, no matter how distasteful that task might appear. Such engagement can be less frustrating and more effective at the local level, which is why city soda tax initiatives have a good chance of succeeding when advocacy is done right.

Like businesses in general, food businesses—even the most socially conscious—must put profits first. To be effective, advocates must understand that soda and other food corporations are willing to spend fortunes to influence political processes. Without anywhere near that kind of funding, it becomes necessary to find smarter methods for using the political process to counter soda industry marketing. At the very least, advocates should hold legislators and food companies accountable when they fail to support— or actively oppose—public health and environmental measures.

Enormous opportunities are available for advocacy work to counter pressures on corporations to grow at any cost, to push back on relentless marketing and lobbying, and to educate the public about the need to create systems and environments that support healthier food choices. My hope is that *Soda Politics* provides compelling evidence for the value of food advocacy work. I wrote it to inspire readers to action. Join the food movement. Work with others to make adequate, safe, accessible, affordable, healthy, and delicious food available for everyone, everywhere.

Afterword

Neal Baer, M.D.

Sodas are everywhere. Marion Nestle stings us with their ubiquity in *Soda Politics*, their seemingly banal presence in our lives suddenly taking on new, shocking meaning. Sodas are advertised on billboards, television, and the Internet, available in convenience and grocery stores, in movie theaters and fast-food restaurants. Anytime you desire a soda, you can get one—often at less expense than a bottle of water. And that's true virtually anywhere in the world, from small villages in Kenya to schools, sports events, and even hospitals. The availability of sodas anyplace at any time inures us to their harmful effects on our health. And just in case you start to question their nutritional value, Big Soda, as Nestle calls the corporate entities and their pals who produce and promote them, forcefully creates a different story through advertisements that feature the most prominent celebrities of our time or by tying sodas to philanthropic donations to deserving nonprofit organizations.

I approached Marion Nestle about writing *Soda Politics* because, as a pediatrician and a storyteller, I knew the real story of soda had to be told. I'd read academic articles in top medical journals demonstrating through compelling data that sodas are the number one contributor to childhood obesity. As Nestle presents in the book, a plethora of recent studies now show that sodas simply are not good for you. And yet soda companies still cling to tired claims that they are reducing calories in their products by offering smaller-sized bottles or cans, or tout connections between enjoyment of sodas and an active lifestyle (undoubtedly to burn up the empty calories they so doggedly push on consumers around the world).

Sodas are big business—a multibillion-dollar business, in fact. Big Soda has much to lose if people turn to healthier choices for hydration—namely, water. It's no accident that these businesses now own bottled water brands as well.

Sodas, as this insightful book shows, have a fascinating story of their own. How a product that is made for pennies from water, high-fructose corn syrup, and flavoring and which has absolutely no nutritional value can command such admiration and respect is a marvel of advertising. Add to that the legions of lobbyists who tirelessly promote soda at great expense to protect the product from taxes and to keep them in schools. The result—sodas are no longer just refreshment or a source of liquid "happiness," but a major corporate powerhouse that spares no expense to keep people drinking in all corners of the world.

After reading *Soda Politics*, you're probably angry, even outraged. How can companies knowingly promote a product that is deleterious to people's health? The answer is simple: money. Sodas make lots of money, just as cigarettes do. And when money collides with health, corporations turn to the mantras of "choice" and "individual responsibility." They insist that they are giving consumers what they want. Of course, they never acknowledge their role in manufacturing that desire with decades of advertisements, philanthropy, and other clever promotional gambits.

I view sodas as the hub of a corporate wheel, with spokes extending to all the areas in which sodas have an impact. First is health. There is no question that drinking sodas every day is harmful. Certainly, enjoying sodas as a treat once in a while is fine, but making them a habitual part of one's diet, as Nestle shows, contributes to obesity and other health problems.

Another spoke is government. Sodas are supported by subsidies that provide farmers with payments for raising corn, from which high-fructose corn syrup is derived.

Sodas reach into the philanthropic world, another spoke, where millions of dollars of consumer-generated profits are served up to deserving organizations, a salve on Big Soda's corporate conscience. Of course, logos everywhere proclaiming soda companies' largesse is another clever way to promote the product while receiving a tax break.

A fourth spoke is the environment. While sodas are cheap to the consumer, their cost, as Nestle shows, is profound. The amount of water needed to raise enough sugar beets to make one liter of soda is staggering. And soda companies have fought recycling programs and deposit charges on their containers for years.

Still another spoke emanating from the soda hub is youth. Sodas are targeted at children and adolescents in many ways, including through school vending machines, sports events, pouring rights at colleges and universities, and, of course, through ever-present advertisements. Soda companies will tell you that they voluntarily do not advertise to children. Technically that's true, but, for example, they do advertise extensively on television, and we all know that children watch much more than the shows directly aimed at them. And since sodas are the number one contributor to childhood obesity, which is arguably the greatest health problem facing our country, it's hard to ignore soda's astonishing impact on youth.

So what can we do to level the playing field? We can bring Nestle's story of soda to others. We can make our schools' lunch programs healthier. We can educate young people—as well as adults—about the health hazards of drinking soda on a regular basis. There are many steps individuals can take to change their diet or initiate a soda tax in their communities. Readers interested in taking action can turn to ActionLab.org/Soda, my new social action platform, which will provide a plethora of things you can do, from learning how to read labels to a practical guide for taking soda vending machines out of your children's schools. *Soda Politics* has the power to inspire, to open our eyes to the harm these products are causing to ourselves and our families. Now it's up to you to draw on what's inspired *you* and put it into action in your own community. And ActionLab.org/Soda, is here to help you do that.

Appendix 1

THE PRINCIPAL U.S. GROUPS ADVOCATING FOR HEALTHIER BEVERAGE CHOICES

ADVOCACY GROUP	RESOURCES
Berkeley Media Studies Group http://bmsg.org	Technical assistance on the design, framing, implementation and evaluation of media advocacy campaigns. See especially: • Working Upstream: Skills for Social Change (Publications) • Layers of strategy (Training); Framing 101 (Resources)
California Center for Public Health Advocacy http://www.publichealthadvocacy.org	Kick the Can: Giving the Boot to Sugary Drinks http://www.kickthecan.info Fact sheets, research reports, advocacy tools, polling data, campaigns, state and local legislation and initiatives, videos, images, links to other sources
Center for Science in the Public Interest (CSPI) https://www.cspinet.org	Sugar drinks home page http://www.cspinet.org/liquidcandy/index.html Current events, reports, fact sheets, links, campaigns, petitions, summit materials • Global Dump Soft Drinks campaign http://www.dumpsoda.org/campaigns.html • National Alliance for Nutrition and Activity (NANA) https://www.cspinet.org/nutritionpolicy/nana.html • Food Marketing Workgroup http://www.foodmarketing.org

(*continued*)

Continued

ADVOCACY GROUP	RESOURCES
ChangeLab Solutions http://changelabsolutions.org	Childhood obesity home page http://changelabsolutions.org/childhood-obesity This site provides extensive toolkits and model legislation to promote: • Active, healthy communities • Healthier food environments • Limits on unhealthy foods • Junk food marketing • Healthier schools • Law & policy 101
Rudd Center for Food Policy and Obesity http://www.uconnruddcenter.org	What We Do home page http://www.uconnruddcenter.org/what-we-do Research, policy briefs, fact sheets, graphs, maps, videos, guides to advocacy in these policy areas: • Economics • Food Marketing to Youth • Schools, Families & Communities • Weight Bias & Stigma • Public Policy • Sugary Drinks/Taxes

Links were active at the time of publication.

Appendix 2

NATIONAL, STATE, AND LOCAL CAMPAIGNS TO REDUCE SODA CONSUMPTION: SELECTED U.S. EXAMPLES

LEVEL	SPONSOR	CAMPAIGN
National	CDC	Rethink Your Drink http://www.cdc.gov/healthyweight/healthy_eating/drinks.html Reducing sugary drink access to youth http://www.cdc.gov/features/healthybeverages
State	Illinois	Illinois Alliance to Prevent Obesity: Rethink Your Drink http://preventobesityil.org/?page_id=453
	Kentucky	Kentucky Department for Public Health: Zero Soda campaign http://chfs.ky.gov/dph/mch/hp/5210/default.htm
County	Howard, Maryland	Howard County, Unsweetened. Better Choices Coalition http://www.betterchoicescoalition.org
	Los Angeles, California	Los Angeles County Department of Public Health Choose Health LA http://www.choosehealthla.com/eat-healthy/sugar-loaded-beverages/
	King County, Washington	Seattle & King County Public Health Department: Nutrition and Health http://www.kingcounty.gov/healthservices/health/nutrition.aspx Search for Sugary Drinks. See: • 10 Things Parents Should Know About Sugary Drinks • 10 Things Families & Organizations Can Do to Cut Down on Sugary Drinks

(*continued*)

Continued

LEVEL	SPONSOR	CAMPAIGN
City	Boston, Massachusetts	Boston Public Health Commission: Sugar Smarts http://www.bphc.org/whatwedo/healthy-eating-active-living/ sugar-smarts/Pages/Sugar-Smarts.aspx
	New York, New York	New York City Department of Health and Mental Hygiene Sugary drinks home page http://www.nyc.gov/html/doh/ html/living/cdp_pan_pop.shtml

Links were active at the time of publication. If inactive, refer to the California Center for Public Health Advocacy's current list of educational and legislative campaigns about soda consumption at http://www.kickthecan.info (see Campaigns).

Appendix 3

A BIBLIOGRAPHIC NOTE ON SOURCES

In writing a book about advocacy to reduce consumption of Coke, Pepsi, and other sugary drinks, I had to confront a daunting reality. I am not the first person to write about these topics. Indeed, the existing published work on the soda industry could fill a small library on its own. From slogging through this material, I came to understand that no official of Coca-Cola—from the 1880s on—ever threw out a scrap of paper; every one of those scraps found its way into some company or university archive; and every one of those archives has already been mined to the hilt by an army of scholars and journalists. Even more sobering: many of those researchers had already produced works of remarkably distinguished scholarship.

Existing books about soda companies include histories, business analyses, biographies, personal accounts, political analyses, advertising ephemera, technical manuals, and company trade books. These cover the ground from the academic to hagiography, diatribe, and gossip. Most focus on Coca-Cola, and for good reason. The company's source materials are extensive and its history is rich with fascinating characters and domestic and international political intrigue. From this library, PepsiCo appears to be a far less interesting company, or perhaps it is just that its executives kept paper trails under lock and key. Below, I provide an annotated list of the books I found most useful for producing this particular addition to this genre.

Making sense of current events in soda advocacy required me to keep up not just with new research articles, which seemed to appear every day, but also with a Niagara Falls of online material. For most of the three years I worked on this book, I subscribed to a Google Scholar feed for Coca-Cola and PepsiCo. These typically listed twenty-five to fifty articles a day mentioning Coca-Cola, and half that number for Pepsi. Friends and colleagues, knowing that I was writing about the soda industry, sent items they had run across. I eventually figured out how to sort through and organize this avalanche of material, but doing so required daily diligence. The research review in this book is current through May 2015, but I firmly believe that the themes, history, and advocacy material should remain relevant for years to come.

BOOKS ABOUT THE SODA INDUSTRY: A HIGHLY SELECTIVE LIST

Among the library of books written about soda companies and their industry, I found some to be especially germane to advocacy. Any such list must start with the now classic history written by Mark Pendergrast, to whom all current writers, including me, are deeply indebted. I list the others by topic but otherwise in no particular order.

Histories of the Companies

Pendergrast, Mark. *For God, Country & Coca-Cola: The Definitive History of the Great American Soft Drink and the Company That Makes It,* **3rd ed. Basic Books, 2013.** Pendergrast produced the first edition of his book in 1993, and the second in 2000. Although this 3rd edition adds three new chapters to update events through 2012, it is 100 pages shorter than the 2nd because—and scholars like me are aghast—it omits endnotes. You can get the notes to the 2nd edition at *http://www.markpendergrast.com*, but you are on your own for the 3rd. Nevertheless, the writers of several books I mention here thank Mr. Pendergrast for his support, and I do too. He is extraordinarily generous with information and encouragement. When I was unable to find a discussion of something I was certain had to be in his book, Pendergrast sent me a searchable electronic file. He has made his research papers publicly available at Emory University—a gift to scholars. And he tells wonderful stories, backing each of them up with meticulous research. His (I hope) ironic bottom line: "And aside from controversies over nutrition, obesity, culture, advertising, politics, water depletion, labor issues, and death squads, The Coca-Cola Company has been a force for good in the world" (p. 483). Readers of what Pendergrast has to say about such issues, however, may come to quite different conclusions, as I most definitely did.

    Allen, Frederick L. *Secret Formula: How Brilliant Marketing and Relentless Salesmanship Made Coca-Cola the Best-Known Product in the World.* **Harper-Business, 1994.** Despite its flashy title, this is a work of serious historical scholarship up to the early 1990s. The author, a journalist, did just what Pendergrast did and at much the same time (Pendergrast tells me they met once at the Coca-Cola archives). Allen's book, which followed Pendergrast's first edition by a year, is also carefully researched—a detailed historical account of how a company selling a product based in patent medicine—nothing but flavored, colored, caffeinated sugar water—became an international symbol of America, admired more for its iconic brand than for its taste.

Hays, Constance L. *The Real Thing: Truth and Power at the Coca-Cola Company*. Random House, 2004. This history by a now deceased business writer for the *New York Times* homed in on the company's business aspects—leadership, acquisitions, and stock prices. Hays's book is especially useful for its discussion of race issues, both historical and recent. The company, she points out, is headquartered in the South, where issues related to slavery and the Civil War continue to be alive and well and highly contemporary.

Louis, J. C., and Harvey Z. Yazijian. *The Cola Wars: The Story of the Global Corporate Battle Between the Coca-Cola Company and PepsiCo, Inc.* Everest House, 1980. The subtitle does not do justice to the content of this book, a carefully researched account of both companies' involvement in the seamiest aspects of national and international politics. Beginning with the idea that soft drinks constitute the essence of American capitalism, the authors describe how Pepsi favored Republicans (especially President Richard Nixon) and Coca-Cola favored Democrats (especially President Jimmy Carter), and how both "siblings" were rewarded accordingly. On the international scene, the book documents how one or the other company was involved in such matters as heroin and opium trafficking in South Vietnam, the Bay of Pigs invasion of Cuba, the overthrow of democratic governments in Guatemala and Chile, and Teamster payoffs. They quote a president of Pepsi: "I think businessmen should take a very vital interest in politics and governmental affairs.... It's necessary to protect their own interest from punitive legislation" (p. 133). The authors conclude that

> Coke and Pepsi operate within overlapping political and corporate networks that seek to preserve the marketplace favorable to both companies. On a symbolic plane, both contribute to an advertising structure that reinforces the values favorable to soft drinks.... [T]he companies stand toe-to-toe in the center of a whole system merging economic and political organization with certain very basic patterns of social behavior—primarily consumption (p. 370).

Their point is that competition between the two companies in reality is a close collaboration that works to the benefit of both.

Riley, John J. *A History of the American Soft Drink Industry: Bottled Carbonated Beverages, 1807–1957*. American Bottlers of Carbonated Beverages, 1958. This is an authorized, uncritical, industry perspective on the origins of the soft drink industry and its commercial development, with an emphasis on the technical aspects—carbonation, bottles, bottling equipment, plants, trucks— and personalities. A useful appendix provides a detailed chronology of key events in this history, with preliminaries that begin in 1450 and events summarized by decade from 1800 to 1957.

Lofland, Cheryl Harris. *The National Soft Drink Association.* **NSDA, 1986.** Trade associations have histories too. Soda trade associations started out in 1882 and formally united as the American Bottlers of Carbonated Beverages in 1919. The name changed to the National Soft Drink Association in 1966 and to the American Beverage Association (ABA) in 2004. The book provides ample documentation of how this organization has from its earliest days deliberately, systematically—and with great pride—lobbied for tax breaks, favorable trade rules, and exemptions from labeling requirements, but against sugar quotas, bottle deposit laws, nutrition standards for school meals, restrictions on advertising to children, and soda taxes.

Stoddard, Bob. *Pepsi-Cola: 100 Years.* **General Publishing Group, 1997.** It's a pity that Pepsi lacks a Pendergrast. This is one of the few books with any real content about PepsiCo, as most books about the company stick to collectibles. Stoddard's is a coffee-table book, lavishly illustrated, with a detailed—but undocumented—account of the company's history. Unreferenced as it is, and beyond what Pepsi posts on its website, it's all we have. While the book comes with a disclaimer—"This book has neither been authorized nor approved by Pepsi-Cola Company"—it is introduced both by Roger Enrico, then CEO, and by one of its past CEOs, Donald Kendall. Kendall sets the tone:

> I'm convinced free enterprise has been good for our country and for the world too. Among the things I'm most proud of is the part Pepsi-Cola may have played in the downfall of Communism. I can't prove that Pepsi gave Eastern Bloc consumers their first taste of freedom, but I'd sure like to think so.

Stoddard provides an index, but no sources at all—no references and no footnotes. Although researchers interested in checking his facts have to go to the company's website or other histories that mention PepsiCo, or must dig for their own primary sources, this book is a good starting place—the only one, really—for understanding what this company is about.

Cultural and Political Histories

Kahn, E. J., Jr. *The Big Drink: The Story of Coca-Cola.* **Random House, 1960.** Kahn was a staff writer for the *New Yorker* when he produced this book based on articles he published in the magazine in the 1950s. It is not scholarly and lacks references, endnotes, and an index. Instead, it is a breezy, gossipy account of the role of soda companies in American and international culture of that era. Many of the anecdotes told here show up in later histories, so the lack of citations to original sources is especially unfortunate. But you will learn such tidbits here as how a Pepsi bottler visiting Egypt "returned with the uplifting report that the camel he was riding was named Coca-Cola" (p. 37) and that Coca-Cola was offered the chance to buy the nearly bankrupt Pepsi company in 1931 but declined.

Capparell, Stephanie. *The Real Pepsi Challenge: How One Pioneering Company Broke Color Barriers in 1940s American Business*. Wall Street Books, 2007. Pepsi's contribution to the civil rights movement began in 1940 when it hired its first African American salesman and, later, a team of a dozen, to expand the company's reach into the "Negro" or "special" market. These jobs were highly prized by young African American men eager to go into business but with few such opportunities in the deeply racially segregated society of that time. The book documents the hardships these men had to endure not only on the road (hotels and restaurants refused to serve them) but also in corporate headquarters, where slights and slurs were common. The book tells the stories of individual team members and explains why these jobs were so groundbreaking. It is illustrated with photographs of the team and of advertisements targeted to African American publications. An added bonus: the book comes with a thought-provoking study guide. For example, "Throughout the 1940s, African-American publishers and civic leaders pushed hard to get corporations to pursue the so-called Negro market. What were their motives? What did the lack of recognition of African-American spending clout have on individuals, companies, and society as a whole?" Here's another: "One of the salesmen said he would use 'the race bit' to sell Pepsi. What did he mean? How did the two biggest cola rivals use race in their campaigns in the 1940s and 1950s to sell their product?"

Foster, Robert J. *Coca-Globalization: Following Soft Drinks from New York to New Guinea*. Palgrave Macmillan, 2008. Foster is an anthropologist who uses sodas as an entry point into discussions of the cultural implications of globalization, particularly in Papua New Guinea. He also delves into shareholder activism and obesity advocacy. He is persuasive about the cultural and political power of soda companies. Shareholder activism, he points out, is not the same as shareholder democracy. "How could it, when one director, Warren Buffett, controls about 200 million shares of The Coca-Cola Company (and thus 200 million votes), and I own five?" (p. 209).

Thomas, Mark. *Belching out the Devil: Global Adventures with Coca-Cola*. Nation Books, 2009. Thomas, who describes himself as a human rights activist and recovering Coca-Cola addict, moves quickly from the "happiness factory" at the Coca-Cola museum in Atlanta to Coke's history of labor and other human rights abuses in Colombia, El Salvador, Turkey, and India, among other places—all firmly denied by the company. These are ugly stories, particularly because, as Thomas puts it, "you can talk of consumers inviting you into their lives and you can treasure secret formulas but all you are selling is essentially sugar and water: fizzy pop. No one actually needs Coca-Cola and no one would die if it disappeared off the planet tomorrow" (p. 324).

Blanding, Michael. *The Coke Machine: The Dirty Truth Behind the World's Favorite Soft Drink.* Avery, 2010. Blanding is not a fan of Coca-Cola. He begins with a tough look at the history of the company, an antidote to what the company says on its website. He hangs out all the dirty laundry: selling Coke by making portions bigger, getting products into schools, pushing bottled water, pushing sodas in developing countries, taking over water supplies in India, allegations of complicity in the murder of union organizers in Colombia, and fighting shareholders upset about Killer Coke.

Elmore, Bartow J. *Citizen Coke: The Making of Coca-Cola Capitalism.* Norton, 2015. Elmore is a historian at the University of Alabama who takes a fresh look at how soda companies manage to make fortunes selling cheap sugar water. Advertising, he says, is only a minor factor in generating soda profits. The real money comes from a business strategy that offloads the costs and risks onto suppliers, bottlers, and taxpayers. Yes, taxpayers. We subsidize soda companies' use of city water supplies. We, not the companies, recycle discarded cans and bottles and pay for dealing with containers that are not recycled. We pay for the health care of the overweight and diabetic. The public, he says, should be setting and collecting the price for use of public resources, rather than "accepting the bill for corporate waste."

Personal Accounts

Enrico, Roger, and Jesse Kornbluth. *The Other Guy Blinked: How Pepsi Won the Cola Wars.* Bantam, 1986. At the time he wrote this book, Enrico was president and CEO of PepsiCo USA and later of PepsiCo Worldwide Beverages. From him, you will learn more than you ever wanted to know about the Pepsi Challenge (to Coca-Cola), the advertisements featuring Michael Jackson, and Pepsi's role in inducing Coca-Cola to change its formula and introduce the ill-fated Classic Coke. In his view, the rivalry between the two companies is good for both: "At Pepsi, we *like* the Cola Wars. We know they're good for business—for *all* soft drink brands. . . . Everybody in the business wins" (p. 15).

Isdell, Neville, with David Beasley. *Inside Coca-Cola: A CEO's Life Story of Building the World's Most Popular Brand.* St. Martin's Press, 2011. Isdell is of Northern Irish origins, grew up in Zambia, began his career with Coca-Cola in Africa, and spent thirty years as an executive supervising the company's international bottling operations. Retired in Barbados, he was called back and served as Coca-Cola's chairman and CEO from 2004 to 2009. This is his version of how he turned the company around after his predecessors made a mess of things. Most of the book deals with the ways he solved management problems, but it ends with his idealistic vision of Coca-Cola as an exemplar of what he calls "connected capitalism"—boosting private-sector profits by fighting disease and poverty, healing the planet, and improving education. Contrast his view with that of Elmore's "Coca-Cola capitalism" in *Citizen Coke.*

List of Tables

List of Figures

Acknowledgments

I have many colleagues, friends, acquaintances, as well as people I've not yet met to thank for help with this book. Let me begin with Lydia Wills, the literary agent I've worked with since *Food Politics,* who along with Neal Baer suggested that I write about the soda industry as a means to encourage advocacy for food issues. Neal also gets my thanks for arranging with the Robert Wood Johnson Foundation to fund my purchase of the industry research report, for commenting on an early draft of the manuscript, and for his gracious Afterword.

Much of the inspiration for this book comes from the soda advocacy work of Harold Goldstein of the California Center for Public Health Advocacy, Michael Jacobson and Margo Wootan at the Center for Science in the Public Interest, and Lori Dorfman of the Berkeley Media Studies Group. Kelly Brownell and Marlene Schwartz at the Rudd Center for Food Policy and Obesity set an example of how research can be used to inform policy. Michele Simon of Eat, Drink, Politics, and Andy Bellatti of Small Bites provided much critical insight.

For materials and insight into the Mexican soda tax, I thank Mireia Vilar from Universidad Iberoamericana, and the remarkable staff of El Poder del Consumidor: Rebecca Berner, Alejandro Calvillo, Xaviera Cabada Barrón, and Katia Garcia Maldonado.

I am deeply grateful to a long list of additional people who provided documents, articles, or photographs to which I might not otherwise have had access: Kate Adamick, Tatiana Andreyeva, Elinor Blake, Marie Bragg, Wendel Brunner, David Clark, Olivier de Schutter, Richard Daynard, Kathryn Diaz, Yoni Freedhoff, Trace George, Corinna Hawkes, Nancy Huehnergarth, David Johns, Andrew Lim, Lauren Lindstrom, Patricia Martz, Michael Moss, Cathy Nonas, Megan Orciari, Pilar Parra, Mark Pendergrast, Robert Pincus, John Rankin, Jeff Ritterman, Ray Rogers, Barry Rossnick, Lisa Sasson, Daniel Schultz, Rachel Silverman, Diane Sokal, Karen Sokal-Gutierrez, Hans Taparia, Anne Traver, Fred Tripp, Claire Wang, Elaine Watson, Cara Wilking, and Lisa Young. If I inadvertently omitted someone from this list, please forgive.

My special thanks go to Declan Conroy of Food Chemical News and Jason Huffman of Politico Pro for daily access to the wealth of information on their sites.

During the course of writing the book, several NYU students helped with research: Samvida Patel, Reina Podell, and Eleanor Talbot West. Others, the exceptionally talented Elizabeth Krietsch and Caitlin Crowley, created the charts illustrating trends in use and consumption of sodas and sugars and how consumption increases with income in a country.

Diana Caley, George Flowers, Loma Flowers, Sara Flowers, and Daniel Bowman Simon read and commented on early drafts of some of the more sensitive chapters. I especially thank Daniel Bowman Simon for his ability to find anything online, his sense of just what I need to know, and his diligence in making sure I get the facts right. Daniel also contributed some of the photographs in this book, as did my geologist-photographer son, Charles Nestle (thanks Charlie).

Earning my version of hero medals are the truly extraordinary people who volunteered to read page proofs: Joanne Csete, Maya Joseph, Mal Nesheim, Esther Trakinski, Victoria Woollard, and my daughter Rebecca Nestle who has the gift, clearly not inherited from me, of spotting bloopers missed by everyone else.

At NYU, Keith Olsen and Ben Vien made sure my computers were in good working order. I am ever thankful for the unflappable daily support I get from colleagues and staff of the Department of Nutrition, Food Studies, and Public Health, particularly Stephen Ho, Kelli Ranieri, Tara Tempone, and Christina Waite. I am everlastingly grateful to my department chair, Krishnendu Ray, to former Steinhardt School deans Ann Marcus and Mary Brabeck, and to my current Steinhardt School dean Dominic Brewer for giving so much support to my work.

I want to mention how much I enjoyed working with the team at Oxford University Press, and to particularly thank senior production editor Joellyn Ausanka for her warmth and infinite patience, and my wonderful editor Max Sinsheimer for being a joy to work with and for his unfailing support at difficult moments.

Last, but never least, I thank my partner and occasional co-author, Mal Nesheim, for reading every chapter, making sure that everything in the text "sounded" right, and holding my hand through the highs and lows of this project and much else.

Notes

Much of the research in *Soda Politics* is based on print sources, but more derives from materials found online from 2012 to 2015. Online sources, alas, must be considered ephemeral. Soda companies and government agencies are constantly tinkering with their websites, and sources available when I started the research often disappeared soon after. A surprising number of links that were functional in January 2015, for example, no longer worked in April. Consequently, these reference notes provide only basic web addresses. Documents are best located by typing their titles into search engines. To save space, the notes use abbreviations of frequently cited sources. I list those here with their current web addresses.

ABBREVIATIONS

Ad	Advertising
Am	American
ABA	American Beverage Association, at www.ameribev.org
AJCN	American Journal of Clinical Nutrition, at http://ajcn.nutrition.org/
AJPH	American Journal of Public Health, at http://ajph.aphapublications.org/
AP	Associated Press
Assoc	Association
CDC	Centers for Disease Control and Prevention, at www.cdc.gov
Clin	Clinical
CSPI	Center for Science in the Public Interest, at www.cspinet.org
EPA	Environmental Protection Agency, at www.epa.gov
ERS	Economic Research Service of the USDA, at www.ers.usda.gov
FAO	Food and Agriculture Organization of the United Nations, at www.fao.org
FDA	U.S. Food and Drug Administration, at www.fda.gov
FNS	Food and Nutrition Service of USDA, at www.fns.usda.gov
FTC	Federal Trade Commission, at www.ftc.gov
GAO	Government Accountability Office (until 2004, General Accounting Office), at www.gao.gov

HHS	U.S. Department of Health and Human Services
Int	International
IOM	Institute of Medicine of the National Academies, at www.iom.edu
J	Journal, journal of
JADA	Journal of the American Dietetic Association (now JAND), at www.andjrnl.org
JAND	Journal of the Academy of Nutrition and Dietetics (formerly JADA), at www.andjrnl.org
JAMA	Journal of the American Medical Association, at http://jama.jamanetwork.com/journal.aspx
Med	Medicine
NCHS	National Center for Health Statistics of the CDC, at www.cdc.gov/nchs
N.d.	No date
NEJM	New England Journal of Medicine, at www.nejm.org
Nutr	Nutrition
NYC	New York City
NYT	New York Times, at www.nytimes.com
Prev	Prevention, Preventive
Res	Research
Rev	Review
Suppl	Supplement
U	University
USDA	U.S. Department of Agriculture, at www.usda.gov
WHO	World Health Organization of the United Nations, at www.who.int
WSJ	Wall Street Journal, at http://online.wsj.com

CHAPTER 1. SODAS: INSIDE THOSE CONTAINERS

1. For discussions of soda names: Carbonated Beverages in the United States: Historical Review. American Can Company, 1972; von Schneidemeister L. Soda or pop? J English Linguistics, 1996;24:270–87; The Soda vs. Pop Map. NYT, Sept 11, 2008.

2. FDA. Proposed changes to the Nutrition Facts label. Mar 3, 2014.

3. PepsiCo. The facts about your favorite beverage. www.pepsicobeveragefacts.com. Figures for Coca-Cola come from its package labels and information provided online in 2013. CDC. Americans consume too much sodium (salt). Feb 24, 2011.

4. Kahn EJ. The Big Drink: The Story of Coca-Cola. Random House, 1960.

5. Wise PM, et al. The influence of bubbles on the perception carbonation bite. PLoS ONE, 2013;8(8):e71488 USDA. National Nutrient Data Base for Standard Reference, Release 26. Basic report 14148: Carbonated beverage: cola. http://ndb.nal.usda.gov.

6. In 2002, Mexico imposed a 20 percent "soda tax" on beverages not sweetened with Mexican cane sugar. This ended the use of American HFCS in Mexican sodas. Following U.S. complaints to the World Trade Organization, which ruled in its favor, the countries agreed that bilateral free trade in sweeteners would take effect in 2008. See North American Free Trade Agreement (NAFTA). American Sugar Beet Association, 2008. www.americansugarbeet.org.

7. USDA/ERS. Sugars and sweeteners. Policy.

8. Holsendolph E. Big sugar users study substitutes. NYT, Aug 13, 1974. Daniels LA. Coke, Pepsi to use more corn syrup. NYT, Nov 7, 1984. Ricks TE, Flores D. Pepsi, Coke raise to 100% the corn syrup bottlers can use to sweeten cola drinks. WSJ, Nov 7, 1984.

9. Horovitz B. Pepsi plans "made with real sugar" offering. USA Today, Apr 8, 2014. www.usatoday.com.

10. Walker RW, et al. Fructose content in popular beverages made with and without high-fructose corn syrup. Nutr, 2014;30:928–35.

11. PepsiCo. The facts about your favorite beverages. Colors FAQs. www .pepsicobeveragefacts.com/colors.php. Coca-Cola. The Beverage Institute for Health and Wellness. Beverage ingredient glossary. http://beverageinstitute.org.

12. Coca Cola Journey. Coca-Cola statement regarding caramel in our beverages. Mar 9, 2012. www.coca-colacompany.com. AP. Coke and Pepsi change recipe to avoid cancer warning. Guardian, Mar 9, 2012. www.theguardian.com. PepsiCo. Policies. Caramel coloring. Aug 22, 2012. www.pepsico.com/company/Policies. Consumer Rep. Caramel color: The health risk that may be in your soda. Feb 10, 2014. www .consumerreports.org. Smith TJS, et al. Caramel color in soft drinks and exposure to 4-methylimidazole: A quantitative risk assessment. PLoS ONE, 2015;10(2):e0118138. Watson E. PepsiCo and Goya Foods targeted in lawsuit over 4-MEI. FoodNavigator-USA, Feb 5, 2014. www.foodnavigator-usa.com.

13. Pendergrast M. For God, Country & Coca-Cola, 3rd ed. Basic Books, 2013. May CD. How Coca-Cola obtains its coca. NYT, Jul 1, 1988.

14. Bouckley B. US class action slams "chemical Coke" for phosphoric acid use. Beverage Daily, Mar 21, 2014. www.beveragedaily.com

15. Carpenter M. Caffeinated: How Our Daily Habit Helps, Hurts, and Hooks Us. Hudson Press, 2014:71.

16. Allen F. Secret Formula: How Brilliant Marketing and Relentless Salesmanship Made Coca Cola the Best-Known Product in the World. HarperBusiness, 1994.

17. Committee on Nutrition and the Council on Sports Medicine and Fitness. Clinical report—sports drinks and energy drinks for children and adolescents: Are they appropriate? Pediatrics, 2011;127:1182–89. AP. Coca-Cola to put caffeine content information on U.S. labels. NYT, Feb 22, 2007.

18. Coca-Cola. Explore inside the vault of the secret formula. www.worldofcoca-cola.com. The Sacred Formula is given in Pendergrast, Appendix 1:487–94. Pepsi's is in Stoddard B. Pepsi-Cola: 100 Years. General Publishing Group, 1997:last (unnumbered) page.

19. The science fair project is reviewed in Nestle M. Food Politics, rev. ed., 2013:180. The brain scan study is McClure SM, et al. Neural correlates of behavioral preference for culturally familiar drinks. Neuron, 2004;44(2):379–87. Also see Blakeslee S. If you have a "buy button" in your brain, what pushes it? NYT, Oct 19, 2004:F5. The CU cola challenge. Consumer Rep. Feb 1984:66–70. Kühn S, Gallinat J. Does taste matter? How anticipation of cola brands influences gustatory processing in the brain. PLoS ONE, 2013;8(4):e61569.

20. The quote is attributed to an unnamed sheik in Cairo by E. J. Kahn Jr., in his book based on articles written for the New Yorker, The Big Drink: The Story of Coca-Cola, Random House, 1960.

21. Coca-Cola Customer Communications Center. Valves of gold: check these 5 steps to quality, 2012. www.cokesolutions.com.

22. Marburger W. Costing out soda & free refills—how to price soda. Pate Dawson Company, 2009. www.pdco.com.

23. Totten M. Why drinks are the most profitable item for fast food restaurants, Oct 2, 2012. www.helium.com.

24. National Library of Med. Sweeteners—artificial. Jan 23, 2012. www.nlm.nih. gov. Swithers SE. Artificial sweeteners produce the counterintuitive effect of inducing metabolic derangements. Trends in Endocrinology and Metabolism, 2013;24(9):431–41. Suez J, et al. Artificial sweeteners induce glucose intolerance by altering the gut microbiota. Nature, 2014;514:181–86. Bleich SN, et al. Diet-beverage consumption and caloric intake among US adults, overall and by body weight. AJPH, 2014;104:e72–e78.

25. Terhune C. In switch, Pepsi makes diet cola its new flagship. WSJ, Mar 16, 2005. Macarthur K. Sweet nothings. Ad Age, Mar 28, 2005. For an overview of artificial sweeteners see Schardt D. Sweet nothings: not all sweeteners are Equal. Nutr Action Healthletter, May 2004.

CHAPTER 2. SODA DRINKERS: FACTS AND FIGURES

1. Beverage Digest reports sales figures by brand in annual reports. See, for example, Special issue: US beverage business results for 2014, Mar 26, 2015.

2. USDA explains: "Data from carbonated soft drinks (1947–2003) are from the Census of Manufactures, replacing data previously provided by the Beverage Marketing Corporation of New York. At their request, ERS [USDA's Economic Research Service] has removed the Beverage Marketing Corporation's data series on carbonated soft drinks, bottled water, fruit drinks, and vegetable juices from the website and thus no longer provides this data in the Food Availability (Per Capita) Data System." USDA/ERS. Carbonated soft drinks: per capita availability. Feb 1, 2012.

3. Beverage Marketing Corporation. Carbonated Soft Drinks in the U.S., 2013 ed., Oct 2013.

4. Standard & Poor's provides a table of the U.S. population on Jul 1 from 1900 to the present at http://www.multpl.com/united-states-population/table. The figures for diet sodas in Table 2.3 in the previous reference are calculated from per capita production data in Exhibit 1.2 corrected by the annual percentages of diet soda given in Exhibit 3.20. Percentages for 1980–1983 are estimated based on extrapolation from those in the USDA's data set.

5. Ferdman RA. The soda industry is discovering what the future of Diet Coke looks like (and it isn't pretty). Washington Post, Mar 23, 2015.

6. Euromonitor International. Passport database. Statistics: market sizes/historic/ total volume/litres per capita, 2013.

7. Euromonitor International. Carbonates: can new markets keep growth fizzing? Dec 2013. Credit Suisse Research Institute. Sugar consumption at a crossroads. Credit Suisse, Sept 2013.

8. Ervin RB, Ogden CL. Consumption of added sugars among U.S. adults, 2005–2010. NCHS Data Brief No. 122. May 2013.

9. New methods using isotopes to measure sugar carbon may be useful for improving the accuracy of self-reports of soda consumption. Davy BM, et al. Association

of δ¹³C in fingerstick blood with added-sugar and sugar-sweetened beverage intake. JADA, 2011;111:874–78.

10. CDC. National Health and Nutrition Examination Survey. Hsiao A, Wang YC. Reducing sugar-sweetened beverage consumption: evidence, policies, and economics. Current Obesity Rep, 2013;2:191–99.

11. Ogden CL, et al. Consumption of sugar drinks in the United States, 2005–2008. NCHS Data Brief, No. 17, Aug 2011.

12. Han E, Powell LM. Consumption patterns of sugar-sweetened beverages in the United States. JAND, 2013;113:43–53.

13. Kit BK, et al. Trends in sugar-sweetened beverage consumption among youth and adults in the United States: 1999–2010. AJCN, 2013;98(1):180–88.

14. USDA and USDHHS. Dietary guidelines for Americans, 2010. Sodas are the fourth-largest source of calories for adults after "grain-based desserts," yeast breads, and chicken dishes. For children, sodas are third after desserts and pizza.

15. Park S, et al. Consumption of sugar-sweetened beverages among US adults in 6 states: Behavioral Risk Factor Surveillance System, 2011. Prev Chronic Disease, 2014;11:130304. Wang YC, Vine SM. Caloric effect of a 16-ounce (473-mL) portion-size cap on sugar-sweetened beverages served in restaurants. AJCN, 2013;98(2):430–35. Bleich SN, et al. Diet-beverage consumption and caloric intake among US adults, overall and by body weight. AJPH, 2014;104:e72–e78.

CHAPTER 3. THE SUGAR(S) PROBLEM: MORE FACTS AND FIGURES

1. Te Morenga L, et al. Dietary sugars and body weight: systematic review and meta-analyses of randomised controlled trials and cohort studies. BMJ, 2012;346:e7492. Bray GA, Popkin BM. Dietary sugar and body weight: have we reached a crisis in the epidemic of obesity and diabetes? Diabetes Care, 2014;37:950–56.

2. Ervin RB, Ogden CL. Consumption of added sugars among U.S. adults, 2005–2010. NCHS data brief n. 122. May 2013. Yang Q, et al. Added sugar intake and cardiovascular diseases mortality among US adults. JAMA Intern Med, 2014;174(4):516–24. Lustig RH, et al. Public health: The toxic truth about sugar. Nature, 2012;482:27–29. Lustig RH. Fat Chance: Beating the Odds Against Sugar, Processed Food, Obesity, and Disease. Hudson Street Press, 2012.

3. IOM. Dietary Reference Intakes for Energy, Carbohydrate, Fiber, Fat, Fatty Acids, Cholesterol, Protein, and Amino Acids. National Academies Press, 2002.

4. Pendergrast M. For God, Country & Coca-Cola, 3rd ed. Basic Books, 2013.

5. Rampersaud GC, et al. Knowledge, perceptions and behaviors of adults concerning non-alcoholic beverages suggest some lack of comprehension related to sugars. Nutr Res, 2014;34(2):134–42. FDA. Proposed changes to the Nutrition Facts label. Mar 7, 2014.

6. Coca-Cola. Spark C-Store Purchases with New 19.2-oz. Can. 2014. www.cokesolutions.com.

7. Flood JE, et al. The effect of increased beverage portion size on energy intake at a meal. JADA, 2006;106:1984–90. Wansink B, Cheney MM. Super bowls: serving bowl size and food consumption. JAMA, 2005;293(14):1727–28.

8. Ng SW, et al. Use of caloric and noncaloric sweeteners in US consumer packaged foods, 2005–2009. JAND, 2012;112:1828–34. Johnson RK, et al. Dietary sugars

intake and cardiovascular health: a scientific statement from the American Heart Association. Circulation, 2009;120(11):1011–120. USDA. Food availability (per capita) data system, 2013.

9. The calculation is 132 pounds × 454 grams/pound × 4 calories/gram divided by 365 days. USDA. What we eat in America: nutrient intakes from food and beverages: mean amounts consumed per individual by gender and age in the United States, 2011–2012.

10. CDC. Prevalence of overweight, obesity and extreme obesity among adults: United States, trends 1960–62 through 2005–2006. Flegal KM, et al. Prevalence and trends in obesity among US adults, 1999–2008. JAMA, 2010;303(3):235–41. Ogden CL, et al. Prevalence of obesity in the United States, 2009–2010. NCHS Data Brief No. 82, Jan 2012. Wang H, et al. Consistency between increasing trends in added-sugar intake and body mass index among adults: The Minnesota Heart Survey, 1980–82 to 2007–2009. AJPH, 2013;103:501–7.

11. Bray GA, et al. Consumption of high-fructose corn syrup in beverages may play a role in the epidemic of obesity. AJCN, 2004;79:537–43.

12. Lowndes J, et al. The effects of four hypocaloric diets containing different levels of sucrose or high fructose corn syrup on weight loss and related parameters. Nutr J, 2012;11:55.

13. USDA. Loss-adjusted food availability documentation. Mar 11, 2014. USDA. Food availability documentation: added sugar and sweeteners. The tables used to construct Figure 3.4 are at: Refined Sugar, Corn Syrup, Other Sweeteners.

14. Strom S. U.S. cuts estimate of sugar intake. NYT, Oct 26, 2012.

15. CSPI. Liquid Candy: How Soft Drinks are Harming Americans' Health, 1998 and 2005.

16. Mattes RD. Fluid energy—where's the problem? JADA, 2006;106;1956–1961. Wang JW, et al. Consumption of added sugars from liquid but not solid sources predicts impaired glucose homeostasis and insulin resistance among youth at risk of obesity. J Nutr, 2014;144:81–86. Kant AK, et al. Association of food form with self-reported 24-h energy intake and meal patterns in US adults: NHANES 2003–2008. AJCN, 2012;96:1369–68. DiMeglio DP, Mattes RD. Liquid versus solid carbohydrate: effects on food intake and body weight. Int J Obesity, 2000;24:794–800. Mattes RD. Fluid energy—where's the problem? JADA, 2006;106;1956–1961. CSPI. In the drink: When it comes to calories, solid is better than liquid. Nutr Action Healthletter. Nov 2009;7–9.

17. The ABA-sponsored review is Drewnowski A, Bellisle F. Liquid calories, sugar, and body weight. AJCN, 2007;85:651–61. Report of the Dietary Guidelines Advisory Committee on the Dietary Guidelines for Americans, 2010. USDA, 2010.

18. Carden TT, Carr TP. Food availability of glucose and fat, but not fructose, increased in the US between 1970 and 2009: analysis of the USDA food availability data system. Nutr J, 2013;12:130. Kelishadi R, et al. Association of fructose consumption and components of metabolic syndrome in human studies: A systematic review and meta-analysis. Nutr, 2014;30(5):503–10.

19. Malik VS, et al. Sugar-sweetened beverages and risk of metabolic syndrome and type 2 diabetes. Diabetes Care, 2010;33;2477–83. Lustig RH. Fructose: It's "alcohol without the buzz." Advances in Nutr, 2013;4:226–35.

20. Kanerva N, et al. Higher fructose intake is inversely associated with risk of nonalcoholic fatty liver disease in older Finnish adults. AJCN, 2014;100:1133–38. Chung M, et al. Fructose, high-fructose corn syrup, sucrose, and nonalcoholic fatty liver disease or indexes of liver health: a systematic review and meta-analysis. AJCN, 2014;100(3):833–49.

21. Johnston RD, et al. No difference between high-fructose and high-glucose diets on liver triacylglycerol or biochemistry in healthy overweight men. Gastroenterology, 2013;145(5):1016–25.e2. Chiu S, et al. Effect of fructose on markers of non-alcoholic fatty liver disease (NAFLD): a systematic review and meta-analysis of controlled feeding trials. European J Clin Nutr, 2014;doi:10.1038/ejcn.2014.8.

22. Tasevska N, et al. Sugars and risk of mortality in the NIH-AARP Diet and Health Study. AJCN, 2014;99:1077–88.

23. Stice E, et al. Relative ability of fat and sugar tastes to activate reward, gustatory, and somatosensory regions. AJCN, 2013;98(6):1377–84.

24. Brownell KD, Gold MS, eds. Food and Addiction: A Comprehensive Handbook. Oxford U Press, 2012.

25. Keast RS, Riddell LJ. Caffeine as a flavor additive in soft-drinks. Appetite, 2007;49:255–59. Keast RSJ, et al. Caffeine increases sugar-sweetened beverage consumption in a free-living population: a randomised controlled trial. British J Nutr, 2015.

26. Smith A. Effects of caffeine on human behavior. Food Chemistry and Toxicology, 2002;40:1231–55. Castellanos FX, Rapoport JL. Effects of caffeine on development and behavior in infancy and childhood: a review of the published literature, Food Chemistry and Toxicology, 2002;40:1235–42. Evatt DP, Griffiths RR. Caffeine, addiction, and food consumption. In: Brownell KD, Gold MS. Food and Addiction: A Comprehensive Handbook. Oxford U Press, 2012:238–43.

27. Meier B. Caffeinated drink cited in reports of 13 deaths. NYT, Nov 14, 2012. FDA. Voluntary and mandatory reports on 5-hour Energy, Monster Energy, and Rockstar energy drink, January 1, 2004, through October 23, 2012. FDA. Added caffeine in gum, May 8, 2013.

28. Bailin D, Goldman G, Phartiyal P. Sugar-coating science: How the food industry misleads consumers on sugar. Union of Concerned Scientists, May 2014.

29. Moss M. Sugar, Salt, Fat: How the Food Giants Hooked Us. Random House, 2013.

CHAPTER 4. DIETARY ADVICE: SUGARS AND SUGARY DRINKS

1. Council on Food and Nutr. Some nutritional aspects of sugar, candy and sweetened carbonated beverages. JAMA, 1942;120:763–65.

2. Reynolds LM, Finke MS. The influence of sweetened drink consumption on the likelihood of meeting the Recommended Daily Allowance for vitamins and minerals. Family and Consumer Sciences Res J, 2002;31:195–205.

3. Select Committee on Nutrition and Human Needs. United States Senate. Dietary Goals for the United States, 2nd ed. Government Printing Office, 1977. Although the first edition of the goals, published in February, elicited widespread protest from producers of foods high in sugar, salt, and fat, its sugar recommendation was rather generous. The first edition called only for a 40 percent sugar reduction to only 15 percent of total calories. The soft drink recommendation remained the same in both editions.

4. USDA and USDHHS. Dietary Guidelines for Americans, 2010.

5. USDA, HHS. Scientific Report of the 2015 Dietary Guidelines Advisory Committee. Feb 2015.

6. USDA. The Food Guide Pyramid. Home and Garden Bulletin No. 252, Aug 1992.

7. USDA. Tips for using the food guide pyramid for young children 2 to 6 years old (program aid 1647). Washington, DC: Center for Policy and Promotion, 1999.

8. USDA. Getting started with MyPlate, 2011. Cut back on your kids' sweet treats. www.choosemyplate.gov.

9. USDA and HHS. Dietary Guidelines for Americans, 2010:29. USDA, HHS. Scientific Report of the 2015 Dietary Guidelines Advisory Committee. Feb 2015.

10. See, for example, Northrup T. Truth, lies, and packaging: How food marketing creates a false sense of health. Food Studies, 2014;3(1):9–18. Pirotin S, et al. Looking beyond the marketing claims of new beverages. U of California Berkeley, Atkins Center for Weight and Health, Aug 2014. Munsell CR, et al. Parents' beliefs about the healthfulness of sugary drink options: opportunities to address misperceptions. Public Health Nutr, 2015;Mar 11, 2015:1–9.

11. Am Academy of Pediatrics. Fruit juice and your child's diet. May 11, 2013. www .healthychildren.org.

12. Cannon G. Food and Health: The Experts Agree. London: Consumers' Association, 1992.

13. IOM. Dietary Reference Intakes: Energy, Carbohydrates, Fiber, Fat, Fatty Acids, Cholesterol, Protein, and Amino Acids. National Academies Press, 2002. USDA. Is intake of added sugars associated with diet quality? Nutr Insights, Insight 21, Oct 2000. Gibson SA. Dietary sugars intake and micronutrient adequacy: a systematic review of the evidence. Nutrition Res Rev, 2007;20:121–31.

14. WHO. Diet, Nutrition, and the Prevention of Chronic Disease (WHO Technical Rep Series 916), Geneva, 2003. WHO. Global Strategy on Diet, Physical Activity, and Health, May 2004. Also see Waxman A. The WHO Global Strategy on Diet, Physical Activity and Health: the controversy on sugar. Development, 2004;47:75–82. Zarocostas J. WHO waters down draft strategy on diet and health. Lancet, 2004;363:1373.

15. WHO. Sugars intake for adults and children, 2015.

16. Te Morenga L, et al. Dietary sugars and body weight: systematic review and meta-analyses of randomised controlled trials and cohort studies. BMJ, 2012;346:e7492. Moynihan PJ, Kelly SAM. Effect on caries of restricting sugars intake. Systematic review to inform WHO guidelines. J Dental Res, 2014;93:8–18. Sheiham A, James WPT. A new understanding of the relationship between sugars, dental caries and fluoride use: implications for limits on sugars consumption. Public Health Nutr, 2014;17(10):2176–84.

17. Johnson RK, et al. Dietary sugars intake and cardiovascular health: a scientific statement from the American Heart Association. Circulation, 2009;120(11):1011–120. Heart & Stroke Foundation, Canada. Sugar, heart disease and stroke, position statement, Aug 2014.

18. Glickman D, et al., eds. Accelerating Progress in Obesity Prevention: Solving the Weight of the Nation. IOM, National Academies Press, 2012. Thow AM, Hawkes C. Global sugar guidelines: an opportunity to strengthen nutrition policy. Public Health Nutr, 2014;17(10):2151–55.

CHAPTER 5. THE HEALTH ISSUES: OBESITY, DIABETES, AND MORE

1. Lesser LI, et al. Relationship between funding source and conclusion among nutrition-related scientific articles. PLoS Med, 2007;4(1):e5. Massougbodji J, et al. Reviews examining sugar-sweetened beverages and body weight: correlates of their quality and conclusions. AJCN, 2014;99:1096–104.

2. CDC. Prevalence of overweight, obesity and extreme obesity among adults: United States, trends 1960–62 through 2005–2006. The CDC defines obesity as a body mass index (BMI) of 30 or more. Flegal KM, et al. Prevalence and trends in obesity among US adults, 1999–2008. JAMA, 2010;303(3):235–41. Ogden CL, et al. Prevalence of Obesity in the United States, 2009–2010. NCHS data brief no 82, Jan 2012. Ogden CL, et al. Prevalence of obesity among adults: United States, 2011–2012. NCHS data brief, no 131, 2013. Ogden CL, et al. Consumption of sugar drinks in the United States, 2005–2008. NCHS data brief, no 17, Aug 2011. Nestle M, Nesheim M. Why Calories Count: From Science to Politics. U of California Press, 2012.

3. Piernas C, et al. Low-calorie- and calorie-sweetened beverages: Diet quality, food intake, and purchase patterns of US household consumers. AJCN, 2014;99(3):567–77. USDA and HHS. Report of the Dietary Guidelines Advisory Committee on the Dietary Guidelines for Americans, 2010, May 2010. Ruff RR, et al. Calorie intake, sugar-sweetened beverage consumption, and obesity among New York City adults: findings from a 2013 population study using dietary recalls. J Community Health, 2014;39(6):1117–23. Kant AK, et al. Association of food form with self-reported 24-h energy intake and meal patterns in US adults: NHANES 2003–2008. AJCN, 2012;96:1369–68.

4. USDA and HHS. Report of the Dietary Guidelines Advisory Committee on the Dietary Guidelines for Americans, 2010. USDA, May 2010:405–6.

5. Examples of studies finding an effect: Striegel-Moore RH, et al. Correlates of beverage intake in adolescent girls: the National Heart, Lung, and Blood Institute Growth and Health Study. J Pediatrics, 2006;148:183–87. Pan L, et al. A longitudinal analysis of sugar-sweetened beverage intake in infancy and obesity at 6 years. Pediatrics, 2014;134:S29. Examples of studies finding no effect: Newby PK, et al. Beverage consumption is not associated with changes in weight and body mass index among low-income preschool children in North Dakota. JADA, 2004;104:1086–94. Hasnain SR, et al. Beverage intake in early childhood and change in body fat from preschool to adolescence. Childhood Obesity 2014 Feb;10(1):42–49. This last study, funded by the National Dairy Council, found milk and juices to protect against obesity.

6. Martin-Calvo N, et al. Sugar-sweetened carbonated beverage consumption and childhood/adolescent obesity: a case-control study. Public Health Nutr, 2014;17(10):2185–93.

7. Ludwig DS, et al. Relation between consumption of sugar-sweetened drinks and childhood obesity: a prospective, observational analysis. Lancet, 2001;357:505–8.

8. DeBoer MD, et al. Sugar-sweetened beverages and weight gain in 2- to 5-year-old children. Pediatrics, 2013;132(3):1–8.

9. de Ruyter JC, et al. The effect of sugar-free versus sugar-sweetened beverages on satiety, liking and wanting: an 18 month randomized double-blind trial in children. PLoS ONE, 2013;8(10):e78039.

10. de Ruyter JC, et al. A trial of sugar-free or sugar-sweetened beverages and body weight in children. NEJM, 2012;367:1397–406. Ebbeling CB, et al. Effects of decreasing sugar-sweetened beverage consumption on body weight in adolescents: a randomized, controlled pilot study. Pediatrics, 2006;117:673–80. James J, et al. Preventing childhood obesity by reducing consumption of carbonated drinks: cluster randomised controlled trial. BMJ, 2004;328:1237. Malik VS, et al. Sugar-sweetened beverages and weight gain in children and adults: A systematic review and meta-analysis. AJCN, 2013;98(4):1084–102.

11. The Obesity Society. Reduced consumption of sugar-sweetened beverages can reduce total caloric intake: position statement, Apr 2014. James J, Kerr D. Prevention of childhood obesity by reducing soft drinks. Int J Obesity, 2005;29:s54–s57. Pérez-Morales

E, et al. Sugar-sweetened beverage intake before 6 years of age and weight or BMI status among older children; systematic review of prospective studies. Nutrición Hospitalaria, 2013;28:47–51. Marr L. Soft drinks, childhood overweight, and the role of nutrition educators: let's base our solutions on reality and sound science. J Nutr Education and Behavior, 2004;36:258–65 (Coca-Cola funded this study).

12. Gibson S. Sugar-sweetened soft drinks and obesity: a systematic review of the evidence from observational studies and interventions. Nutr Res Rev, 2008; 21:134–47.

13. Malik VS, et al. Intake of sugar-sweetened beverages and weight gain: a systematic review. AJCN, 2006;84:274–88. Woodward-Lopez G, et al. To what extent have sweetened beverages contributed to the obesity epidemic? Public Health Nutr, 2011;14(3):499–509. Te Morenga L, et al. Dietary sugars and body weight: systematic review and meta-analyses of randomised controlled trials and cohort studies. BMJ, 2012;346:e7492. Basu S, et al. Relationship of soft drink consumption to global overweight, obesity, and diabetes: a cross-national analysis of 75 countries. AJPH, 2013;103:2071–77. Vartanian LR, et al. Effects of soft drink consumption on nutrition and health: a systematic review and meta-analysis. AJPH, 2007;97:667–75. Zheng M, et al. Substitution of sugar-sweetened beverages with other beverage alternatives: a review of long-term health outcomes. JAND, 2015;Mar 4 (epub ahead of print). Hu FB. Resolved: there is sufficient scientific evidence that decreasing sugar-sweetened beverage consumption will reduce the prevalence of obesity and obesity-related diseases. Obesity Rev, 2013;4:606–19.

14. Dhingra R, et al. Soft drink consumption and risk of developing cardiometabolic risk factors and the metabolic syndrome in middle-aged adults in the community. Circulation, 2007;116:480–88. Malik VS, et al. Sugar-sweetened beverages and risk of metabolic syndrome and type 2 diabetes. Diabetes Care, 2010;33;2477–83. Ma J, et al. Sugar-sweetened beverage consumption is associated with abdominal fat partitioning in health adults. J Nutr, 2014;144:1283–90. Welsh JA, et al. Caloric sweetener consumption and dyslipidemia among US adults. JAMA, 2010;303:1490–97. Hernández-Cordero S, et al. Substituting water for sugar-sweetened beverages reduces circulating triglycerides and the prevalence of metabolic syndrome in obese but not in overweight Mexican women in a randomized controlled trial. J Nutr, 2014;144:1742–52.

15. County of Los Angeles Public Health. Trends in diabetes: a reversible public health crisis. LA Health, Nov 2009. Reis JP, et al. Lifestyle factors and risk for new-onset diabetes a population-based cohort study. Annals of Internal Med, 2011;155:292–99.

16. Gross LS, Li L, Ford ES, Liu S. Increased consumption of refined carbohydrates and the epidemic of type 2 diabetes in the United States: an ecologic assessment. AJCN, 2004;79:774–79. Basu S, et al. Nutritional determinants of worldwide diabetes: an econometric study of food markets and diabetes prevalence in 173 countries. Public Health Nutr, 2013;16(1):179–86. Gorana MI, et al. High fructose corn syrup and diabetes prevalence: A global perspective. Global Public Health, 2013;8(1):55–64. Basu S, et al. The relationship of sugar to population-level diabetes prevalence: an econometric analysis of repeated cross-sectional data. PLoS ONE 2013;8(2):e57873. de Koning L, et al. Sugar-sweetened and artificially sweetened beverage consumption and risk of type 2 diabetes in men. AJCN, 2011;93:1321–27. Schulze MB, et al. Sugar-sweetened beverages, weight gain, and incidence of type 2 diabetes in young and middle-aged women. JAMA, 2004;292:927–34. The InterAct consortium. Consumption of sweet beverages and type 2 diabetes incidence in European adults: results from EPIC-InterAct. Diabetologia, 2013;56(7):1520–30.

17. ABA. Myth vs. Fact: Sugar-sweetened beverages and diabetes. Jul 28, 2014. Bray GA, Popkin BM. Dietary sugar and body weight: have we reached a crisis in the epidemic of obesity and diabetes? Diabetes Care, 2014;37:950–56.

18. Malik AH, et al. Impact of sugar-sweetened beverages on blood pressure. Am J Cardiology, 2014;113:1574–80. Fung TT, et al. Sweetened beverage consumption and risk of coronary heart disease in women. AJCN, 2009;89:1037–42. De Koning L, et al. Sweetened beverage consumption, incident coronary heart disease, and biomarkers of risk in men. Circulation, 2012;125:1735–41. Eshak ES, et al. Soft drink intake in relation to incident ischemic heart disease, stroke and stroke subtypes in Japanese men and women: the Japan Public Health Centre-based study cohort. AJCN, 2012;96:1390–97. Bernstein AM, et al. Soda consumption and the risk of stroke in men and women. AJCN, 2012;95:1190–99. Te Morenga LA, et al. Dietary sugars and cardiometabolic risk: systematic review and meta-analyses of randomized controlled trials of the effects on blood pressure and lipids. AJCN, 2014;100(1):65–79. Larsson SC, et al. Sweetened beverage consumption is associated with increased risk of stroke in women and men. J Nutr, 2014;144:856–60. Johnson RK, et al. Dietary sugars intake and cardiovascular health: a scientific statement from the American Heart Association. Circulation, 2009;120:1011–20.

19. Larsson SC, et al. Consumption of sugar and sugar-sweetened foods and the risk of pancreatic cancer in a prospective study. AJCN, 2006;84:1171–76. Choi M, et al. Sugar-sweetened beverage intake and the risk of type I and type II endometrial cancer among postmenopausal women. Cancer Epidemiology Biomarkers & Prevention, 2013;22(12):2384–94. Boyle P, et al. Sweetened carbonated beverage consumption and cancer risk: meta-analysis and review. European J Cancer Prev, 2014;23(5):481–90.

20. FDA. High intensity sweeteners. May 19, 2014. National Cancer Institute. Artificial sweeteners and cancer. www.cancer.gov. American Cancer Society. Aspartame. www.cancer.org. World Cancer Research Fund/American Institute for Cancer Research. Food, Nutrition, Physical Activity, and the Prevention of Cancer: a Global Perspective. AICR, 2007.

21. Ruff JS, et al. Human-relevant levels of added sugar consumption increase female mortality and lower male fitness in mice. Nature Communications, 2013;4:2245.

22. Tasevska N, Park Y, Jiao L, et al. Sugars and risk of mortality in the NIH-AARP Diet and Health Study. AJCN, 2014;99:1077–88.

23. Singh G, et al. Abstract MP22: mortality due to sugar-sweetened beverage consumption: a global, regional, and national comparative risk assessment. Am Heart Assoc Scientific Sessions, 2013.

24. Amato D, et al. Acute effects of soft drink intake on calcium and phosphate metabolism in immature and adult rats. La Revista de Investigación Clínica, 1998;50:185–89. Mazariegos-Ramos E, et al. Consumption of soft drinks with phosphoric acid as a risk factor for the development of hypocalcemia in children: a case-control study. J Pediatrics, 1995;126;940–42. Wyshak G. Teenaged girls, carbonated beverage consumption, and bone fractures. Archives of Pediatrics and Adolescent Med, 2000;154:610–13. Tucker KL, et al. Colas, but not other carbonated beverages, are associated with low bone mineral density in older women: The Framingham Osteoporosis Study. AJCN, 2006;84:936–42.

25. Ferraro PM, et al. Soda and other beverages and the risk of kidney stones. Clinical J Am Society of Nephrology, 2013;8(8):1389–95. Park S, et al. Regular-soda intake independent of weight status is associated with asthma among US high school students. JAND, 2013;113:106–11. Choi HK, et al. Fructose-rich beverages and risk of gout

in women. JAMA, 2010;304:2270–78. Hu Y, et al. Sugar-sweetened soda consumption and risk of developing rheumatoid arthritis in women. AJCN, 2014;100:959–67. Am Academy of Neurology. Hold the diet soda? Sweetened drinks linked to depression, coffee tied to lower risk, Jan 9, 2013. Suglia SF, et al. Soft drinks consumption is associated with behavior problems in 5-year-olds. J Pediatrics, 2013;163(5):1323–28. Carwile JL, et al. Sugar-sweetened beverage consumption and age at menarche in a prospective study of US girls. Human Reproduction, 2015;30(3):675–83.

26. Leung CW, et al. Soda and cell aging: associations between sugar-sweetened beverage consumption and leukocyte telomere length in healthy adults from the National Health and Nutrition Examination Surveys. AJPH, 2014;104(12):2425–31. Oaklander M. Soda may age you as much as smoking, study says. Time, Oct 17, 2014. Engber D. Does drinking soda really age your cells? Slate, Oct 27, 2014.

27. Ambrosini GL, et al. Prospective associations between sugar-sweetened beverage intakes and cardiometabolic risk factors in adolescents. AJCN, 2013;98(2):327–34. Hert KA, et al. Decreased consumption of sugar-sweetened beverages improved selected biomarkers of chronic disease risk among US adults: 1999 to 2010. Nutr Res, 2014;34(1):58–65.

28. Beverage industry addresses sugar-sweetened beverages and obesity articles in the New England J Med., Sept 21, 2012.

29. Coca-Cola. Annual report to the United States Securities and Exchange Commission, Dec 31, 2014:11.

CHAPTER 6. ADVOCACY: SODA-FREE TEETH

1. Marcenes W, et al. Global burden of oral conditions in 1990–2010: A systematic analysis. J Dental Res, 2013;92:592–97. Benzian H, et al. Political priority of global oral health: an analysis of reasons for international neglect. Int Dental J, 2011;61(3):124–30. CDC. Chronic diseases and health promotion. CDC. Oral health resources. WHO. Preventing chronic diseases: a vital investment, 2013. WHO. Marketing of food and non-alcoholic beverages to children: Set of recommendations. 21 May 2010. Institute for Health Metrics and Evaluation. The Global Burden of Disease: Generating Evidence, Guiding Policy. Mar 4, 2013. www.healthmetricsandevaluation.org.

2. Lula ECO, et al. Added sugars and periodontal disease in young adults: an analysis of NHANES III data. AJCN, 2014;100:1182–87. Mishu MP, et al. Relationship between untreated dental caries and weight and height of 6- to 12-year-old primary school children in Bangladesh. Int J Dentistry, 2013;2013:629675. Tang R-S, et al. Relationship between dental caries status and anemia in children with severe early childhood caries. Kaohsiung J Med Science, 2013;29(6):330–36.

3. Dye BA, Beltrán-Aguilar ED. Selected oral health indicators in the United States, 2005–2008. NCHS data brief no. 96, May 2012. National Institute of Dental and Craniofacial Research. Dental caries (tooth decay) in children (age 2 to 11). Dental caries (tooth decay) in adults (age 20 to 64). Updated Mar 25, 2011. www.nidcr.nih.gov. da Silveira Moreira R. Epidemiology of dental caries in the world, oral health care—pediatric, research, epidemiology and clinical practices. In: Virdi M, ed. InTech, 2012. www.intechopen.com. Bagramian RA, et al. The global increase in dental caries. A pending public health crisis. Am J Dentistry, 2009;22:3–8. Sheiham A, James WPT. A new understanding of the relationship between sugars, dental caries and fluoride use: implications for limits on sugars consumption. Public Health Nutr, 2014;17(10):2176–84. Sheiham A, James WPT. A reappraisal of the quantitative relationship between sugar intake and dental

caries: the need for new criteria for developing goals for sugar intake. BMC Public Health, 2014;14:863.

4. Ross WD, ed. The Works of Aristotle, Vol. VII. Problemata, Book XXII. Oxford U Press, 1927.

5. Gustafsson BE, et al. The Vipeholm dental caries study; the effect of different levels of carbohydrate intake on caries activity in 436 individuals observed for five years. Acta Odontologica Scandinavia, 1954;11:232–64. Newbrun E. Dietary carbohydrates: their role in cariogenicity. Med Clinics of North America, 1979;63:1069–86. Burt BA, Ismail AI. Diet, nutrition, and food cariogenicity. J Dental Res, 1986; 65:1475–84. Newbrun E. Sugar and dental caries: a review of human studies. Science, 1982;217:418–23.

6. Stomach acid is about pH 3. The pH value of 2.6 was obtained from a freshly opened bottle of Coca-Cola using a Cornell laboratory pH meter as well as pH paper on Jun 24, 2013.

7. Needleman I, et al. Oral health and impact on performance of athletes participating in the London 2012 Olympic Games: a cross-sectional study. British J Sports Med, 2013;47(16):1054–8. Kelleher O. Athletes suffer tooth decay due to sugar in sports drinks. Irish Times, Apr 18, 2015.

8. Cheng R, et al. Dental erosion and severe tooth decay related to soft drinks: a case report and literature review. J Zhejiang U—Science B. 2009;10(5):395–99. Al-Malik MI, et al. The relationship between erosion, caries and rampant caries and dietary habits in preschool children in Saudi Arabia. Int J Paediatric Dentistry, 2001;11(6):430–39. Li H, Zou Y, Ding G. Dietary factors associated with dental erosion: a meta-analysis. PLoS ONE, 2012;7(8):e42626. Sohn W, et al. Carbonated soft drinks and dental caries in the primary dentition. J Dental Res, 2006;85:262–68. Bassiouny MA. Dental erosion due to abuse of illicit drugs and acidic carbonated beverages. General Dentistry, 2013;61(2):38–44. Armfield JM, et al. Water fluoridation and the association of sugar-sweetened beverage consumption and dental caries in Australian children. AJPH, 2013;103:494–500. Ismail AI, et al. Current trends of sugar consumption in developing societies. Community Dental and Oral Epidemiology, 1997;25:438–43. Marshall TA, et al. Dental caries and beverage consumption in young children. Pediatrics, 2003;112:3 Sept:e184–e191. Minnesota Dental Association. The hard facts. www.sipallday.org.

9. Am Dental Assoc. Mouth healthy: Baby bottle tooth decay, 2013. www.mouthhealthy .org. Dew mouth and the luxury of dental hygiene. HuffPostLive, Sept 24, 2013.

10. Am Dental Assoc. Diet and tooth decay. J Am Dental Assoc, 2002;133;527. Moynihan P, Petersen PE. Diet, Nutrition and the prevention of dental diseases. Public Health Nutr, 2004;7:201–26. Puska P, et al. Dental diseases and oral health: Facts. WHO, 2003. Moynihan PJ, Kelly SAM. Effect on caries of restricting sugars intake: systematic review to inform WHO Guidelines. J Dent Res, 2014;93:8–18. Whitehead RJ. Researchers call for tooth-decay warnings on soft drinks. Food Navigator—Asia. Jan 31, 2013.

11. ABA. Oral Health: Beverages & Oral Health.

12. CDC. Trends in oral health status: United States, 1988–1994 and 1999–2004. Vital Health Statistics, Apr 2007.

13. Am Academy of Pediatric Dentistry. Policy on dietary recommendations for infants, children, and adolescents, revised 2012. www.aapd.org. M. Dental group is under fire for Coke deal. NYT, Mar 4, 2003.

14. Ness C. Prof takes on a global health crisis, one toothbrush at a time. U of California, Berkeley, News Center, Jun 15, 2012. http://newscenter.berkeley.edu.

Dr. Sokal-Gutierrez describes the project in a TEDx video on YouTube: "Trick or treat? The new child health pandemic," May 12, 2013. PBS NewsHour described the program in a video, "In El Salvador, tooth decay epidemic blamed on junk food, lack of information," Jun 8, 2012.

15. See, for example, Indiana Dental Association: Drinks destroy teeth. http://drinksdestroyteeth.org. Wisconsin Dental Association: Sip all day, get decay. www.wda.org. Australian Dental Association: FAQ. www.ada.org.au.

CHAPTER 7. MEET BIG SODA: AN OVERVIEW

1. Williams JD, Goldsworthy P. Breaking down the chain: a guide to the soft drink industry. National Policy and Legal Action Network and Public Health Law and Policy, 2011. http://changelabsolutions.org. Euromonitor International. Passport: Soft Drinks in 2013: Products, Performance, Prospects. Apr 2013.

2. Prendergrast M. For God, Country & Coca-Cola, 2nd ed. New York: Basic Books, 2000:462.

3. IBISWorld. Global Soft Drink & Bottled Water Manufacturing. IBISWorld Industry Report C1124-GL, Jan 2013. Although the higher estimate also includes fruit and vegetable juices and ready-to-drink coffees and teas, sales of these products can hardly be great enough to explain a $600 billion discrepancy.

4. ABA. History. Accessed Apr 13, 2015.

5. Howard P, et al. The illusion of diversity: visualizing ownership in the soft drink industry. Michigan State U, Aug 2010. www.msu.edu. Beverage Marketing Corporation. Carbonated Soft Drinks in the U.S., Sept 2012. Coca-Cola. Press release: The Coca-Cola Company and Monster Beverage Corporation enter into long-term strategic partnership. August 14, 2014.

6. Special Issue: U.S. Beverage Business Results for 2014. Beverage Digest, Mar 26, 2015.

7. Dant A, Russell K. The pay at the top. NYT, Apr 12, 2014. Information about current stock prices, market capitalization, and major holders is available from Yahoo at http://finance.yahoo.com. The New York Stock Exchange indicates Coca-Cola by KO, PepsiCo by PEP, and Dr Pepper Snapple by DPS.

8. Apple Insider Staff. Apple ends Coca-Cola's 13-year reign as world's most valuable brand. Sept 30, 2013. http://appleinsider.com.

9. Coca-Cola's website lists its registered brands and explains its system. www.coca-colacompany.com. Wikipedia lists Fanta flavors.

10. Thomas M. Belching Out the Devil. Nation Books, 2009.

11. PepsiCo. Carbonated soft drinks—per serving. www.pepsicobeveragefacts.com.

12. Choi C. PepsiCo CEO Indra Nooyi gets 2013 pay bumped 5 percent to $13.2 million. Daily Reporter, Mar 21, 2014. www.greenfieldreporter.com.

13. PepsiCo, Inc. United States Securities and Exchange Commission, Form 10-K, Dec 29, 2012. www.sec.gov. Louis JC, Yazijian HZ. The Cola Wars. Everett House, 1980:252.

14. Fun + Flavor + Innovation: A Formula for Growth. Dr Pepper Snapple Group, 2012. www.dpsgannualreport.com. Information about stock prices and trends are available from Google at www.google.com/#q+stock+prices. DuBois S. The last big all-American soda company. CNN Money, May 8, 2013.

15. ABA. Board of Directors (undated).

16. Elmore BJ. Citizen Coke: The Making of Coca-Cola Capitalism. Norton, 2015.

17. See interactive data base: Bostock M, et al. Across US companies, tax rates vary greatly. NYT Sunday Review, May 26, 2013. Hickey W. 17 great American companies that keep mountains of cash overseas just like Apple does. Business Insider, May 21, 2013.

18. Levy J. Wake up Coke and Pepsi: SodaStream is declaring a cola war. Business Community, Mar 8, 2014. Taube A. Corporate executives think these are the 10 best brands in America. Business Insider, Aug 24, 2013. Bouckley B. "Rumble in the snack soda jungle": Peltz v. PepsiCo. Beverage Daily, Feb 20, 2014. Calvert Investments. Is the Coca-Cola Company (KO) a sustainable and responsible investment? Oct 22, 2013. www.calvert.comwww.business2community.com. Scanlon J. Dean Kamen reinvents Coke's soda fountain. Bloomberg BusinessWeek, Oct 7, 2009. Zmuda N. In-Spired: Pepsi lets drinkers mix the flavor they favor. Ad Age, Jul 28, 2014:28.

CHAPTER 8. OBESITY: BIG SODA'S RESPONSE

1. Louis JC, Yazijian HZ. The Cola Wars. Everest House, 1980:252–62.

2. Also see Brownell KD, et al. Personal responsibility and obesity: A constructive approach to a controversial issue. Health Affairs, 2010;29(3):379–87.

3. US Public Health Service. The Surgeon General's Call to Action to Prevent and Decrease Overweight and Obesity, 2001.

4. Streets J, et al. Absolute risk of obesity. London: UBS Warburg Global Equity Research, Nov 27, 2002, and Mar 4, 2003. Massot S, Fujimori R. Obesity: a lingering concern. London: Morgan Stanley Global Equity Research, Oct 31, 2003. Langlois A, et al. Food manufacturing: obesity: the big issue. London: JP Morgan European Equity Research, Apr 16, 2003. Langlois A, et al. Obesity: re-shaping the food industry, Jan 24, 2006. Thompson S. Obesity fear frenzy grips food industry. Ad Age, Apr 23, 2007.

5. Coca-Cola. Annual Report to United States Securities and Exchange Commission, Form 10-K, Dec 31, 2013:33. Such reports are archived online from 2003 on.

6. Koplan JP, Brownell KD. Response of the food and beverage industry to the obesity threat. JAMA, 2010;304:1487–88. Are all calories created equal? An analysis of the Coca-Cola company's communication in the fight against obesity: 2014 case study competition. Arthur W. Page Society, Jan 16, 2014. Simon M. PepsiCo and public health: Is the nation's largest food company a model of corporate responsibility or a master of public relations? City U of New York Law Review 2012;15(1):9–26. Also see Simon M. Appetite for Profit: How the Food Industry Undermines our Health and How to Fight Back. Nation Books, 2006.

7. Brownell KD, Warner KE. The perils of ignoring history: Big Tobacco played dirty and millions died. How similar is Big Food? Milbank Quarterly, 2009;87:259–94. The playbook is summarized at Yale Rudd Center. Food industry playbook.

8. ABA. Obesity.

9. ABA. Let's clear it up. Obesity.

10. AP. Coca-Cola ad banned in UK for misleading consumers [video]. Huffington Post, Jul 18, 2013. The ad was also banned in Mexico.

11. Euromonitor International. The Coca-Cola Co in health and wellness, Jul 2013. PepsiCo Inc in Health and Wellness, Jun 2013. Hudson Institute. Better-for-you foods: It's just good business. Obesity Solutions Initiative, Oct 2011.

12. Coca-Cola. Advertisement, NYT, May 30, 2013:A9.

13. Coca-Cola. Home page. Ciccone A. Coca-Cola gets cute with latest anti-obesity installment. BrandChannel, Aug 20, 2013. The CSPI video, Coming Together, Translated, and the original Coca-Cola commercial are available at www.youtube.com.

14. Are all calories created equal? An analysis of the Coca-Cola Company's communication in the fight against obesity. Arthur W. Page Society, 2014 Case Study Competition, Jan 16, 2014.

15. PepsiCo, Inc. United States Securities and Exchange Commission, Form 10-K, Dec 28, 2013:17. Nooyi IK. Annual letter to shareholders. PepsiCo, Annual Report, 2012.

16. Morris B. What makes Pepsi great? Fortune, Mar 3, 2008:54–58.

17. Seabrook J. Snacks for a fat planet. New Yorker, May 16, 2011:54–71.

18. Strom S. Pepsi chief shuffles management to soothe investors. NYT, Mar 13, 2012.Esterl M, Bauerlein V. PepsiCo wakes up and smells the cola. WSJ, Jun 28, 2011.

19. Brown A. PepsiCo's CEO earned breathing room in 2012. Q4 profit rises 17 percent. Forbes, Feb 14, 2013.

20. Sharma LL, Teret SP, Brownell KD. The food industry and self-regulation: standards to promote success and to avoid public health failures. AJPH, 2010;100(2):240–46. ABA. All the ways we deliver, Apr 5, 2012.

21. Harris JL, et al. Sugary drink facts: evaluating sugary drink nutrition and marketing to youth. Yale Rudd Center, Oct 2011. www.sugarydrinkfacts.org.

22. Rudd Center for Food Policy & Obesity. Sugary drink facts: food advertising to children and teens score, 2014.

23. Healthy Weight Commitment Foundation. Press release: Food and beverage companies surpass 2015 goal of reducing calories in the U.S. three years ahead of schedule, May 30, 2013.

24. Coca-Cola. Statement on support for HWCF, May 30, 2013. Gold M, Hennessey K. Michelle Obama's nutrition campaign comes with political pitfalls. Los Angeles Times, Jul 20, 2013. Cardello H, Wolfson J. Lower-calorie foods and beverages drive Healthy Weight Commitment Foundation companies' sales growth: Interim report, May 2013. www.obesity-solutions.org.

CHAPTER 9. MARKETING SUGARY DRINKS: SEVEN BASIC PRINCIPLES

1. Warhol A. The Philosophy of Andy Warhol (From A to B and Back Again). Penguin, 1975.

2. Allen F. Secret Formula: How Brilliant Marketing and Relentless Salesmanship Made Coca-Cola the Best-Known Product in the World. HarperBusiness, 1994. In one year in the 1920s, according to Allen, Coca-Cola gave away 1 million calendars, 17 million paper napkins, 75,000 "ice cold" signs, 6,000 gross of pencils, 50,000 oval serving trays, 15,000 oilcloth signs, 100,000 streetcar signs, and 3 million blotters.

3. Carbonated Beverages in the United States: Historical Review. American Can Company, 1972. The jingle is available on YouTube.

4. Pendergrast M. For God, Country, and Coca-Cola, 3rd ed. Basic Books, 2013:151–53, 170–71. Waters P. Coca-Cola: An Illustrated History. Doubleday, 1978.

5. Aizenman NC. Former Coke executive slams "share of stomach" marketing campaign. Washington Post, Jun 7, 2012. Moss M. Salt, Sugar, Fat: How the Food Giants Hooked Us. Random House, 2013:110.

6. Enrico R, Kornbluth J. The Other Guy Blinked. How Pepsi Won the Cola Wars. Bantam, 1986:15.

7. Ad Age. 100 Leading advertisers, 2013. Jun 22, 2014. Choi C. Coca-Cola sells more drinks but soda dips. ABC News, Apr 15, 2014. World Bank. Gross domestic product, 2012.

8. Beverage Marketing Corporation. Carbonated Soft Drinks in the U.S., 2013.

9. U of Pennsylvania School of Design and Philadelphia Department of Public Health. Retail advertising for tobacco products and sugary beverages in Philadelphia, Aug 2013. National Association for Convenience & Fuel Retailing. NACS/Coca-Cola Retailing Research Council releases "Playbook for Success." Feb 13, 2013.

10. Coca-Cola. #OpenUp: Coke's new Ramadan campaign encourages an open mind. Coca-Cola Journey, Jul 11, 2014.

11. Williams JD, Goldsworthy P. Breaking down the Chain: A Guide to the Soft Drink Industry. National Policy and Legal Action Network and Public Health Law and Policy, 2011. http://changelabsolutions.org.

12. Darzi A. Sugar high on the London Eye: Coca-Cola sponsorship should make us weep. Guardian, Jan 27, 2015.

13. Major brands recognize the new heartland consumer in national ad campaigns. MarketWire, Aug 14, 2012. Leschin-Hoar C. Does the American heartland need more soda? PepsiCo thinks so. Take Part, Jul 31, 2012.

14. Bragg MA, et al. Athlete endorsements in food marketing. Pediatrics, 2013;132(5):1–5.

15. Pollack J. Coca-Cola's Joe Tripodi at the ANA conference: how we market to millennials. Ad Age, Oct 4, 2013.

16. Totten M. Why drinks are the most profitable item for fast food restaurants. Helium.com, Oct 2, 2012. Andreyeva T, Brownell KD. The impact of food prices on consumption: a systematic review of research on the price elasticity of demand for food. AJPH, 2010;100:216–22. Block JP, et al. Point-of-purchase price and education intervention to reduce consumption of sugary soft drinks. AJPH, 2010;100(8):1427–33. Zmuda N. In-Spired: Pepsi lets drinkers mix the flavor they favor. Ad Age, Jul 28, 2014:28.

17. Beverage Marketing Corporation. Carbonated Soft Drinks in the U.S., 2013: Exhibit 9.84.

18. Nestle M. What to Eat. North Point Press, 2006.

19. Beverage Marketing Corporation. Carbonated Soft Drinks in the U.S., 2013: Exhibit 9.85. Totten M. Why drinks are the most profitable item for fast food restaurants. Helium.com, Oct 2, 2012.

20. USDA. Sugar and Sweeteners: Policy.

21. Point Foundation. 2012–13 Annual Report. Coca-Cola's donation was in the $10,000-to-$24,999 category. Knight H. Milk club Dems line up with soda industry on sugary-drink tax. San Francisco Chronicle, Aug 23, 2014. Rodriguez JF. Big Soda spends $9 million in SF Election: Did a progressive political club sell out to the beverage industry? SF Weekly, Nov 3, 2014.

22. Peeples J. LGBT organization plans protest of Coca Cola Olympic sponsorship. Advocate, Aug 24, 2013.

23. Queer Nation's remix parody of "I'd like to buy the world a Coke," which depicts LGBT protests at the Sochi Olympics, is available on YouTube. Shayon S. Coke quietly responds to Sochi social protests with LGBT-friendly ad. BrandChannel, Feb 4, 2014.

24. Griner D. Coca-Cola drops gay wedding from Irish version of heartwarming new ad. Adweek, Jan 2, 2014.

25. Coca-Cola. Our company. Our progress. PepsiCo. PepsiCo receives perfect score in the 2014 Corporate Equality Index. Dec 9, 2013.

CHAPTER 10. STARTING EARLY: MARKETING TO INFANTS, CHILDREN, AND TEENS

1. National Council of La Raza. 2013 Event Sponsors. www.nclr.org The White House. Remarks by the First Lady to the National Council of La Raza. Jul 23, 2013.

2. The White House, Office of the First Lady. Remarks by the First Lady at a Grocery Manufacturers Association Conference, Mar 16, 2010.

3. USDA. Getting started with MyPlate, 2011. Dodd AH, et al. Disparities in consumption of sugar-sweetened and other beverages by race/ethnicity and obesity status among United States schoolchildren. J Nutr Education and Behavior, 2013;45(3):240–9. Harris JL, et al. Sugary Drink Facts: Food Advertising to Children and Teens Score. Rudd Center for Food Policy & Obesity, 2014.

4. Siener K, et al. Soft drink logos on baby bottles: do they influence what is fed to children? J Dentistry for Children, 1977;64(1)55–60. Diet Pepsi, 100 percent uh huh. On the Fridge. Washington Post, Aug 4, 1993. Robinson TN, et al. Effects of fast food branding on young children's taste preferences. Archives of Pediatric and Adolescent Med, 2007;161(8):792–97.

5. Batada A, Seitz MD, Wootan MG, Story M. Nine out of 10 food advertisements shown during Saturday morning children's television programming are for foods high in fat, sodium, or added sugars, or low in nutrients. JADA, 2008;108:673–78. Grimm GC, et al. Factors associated with soft drink consumption in school-age children. JADA, 2004;104;1244–49. Olafsdottir S, et al. Young children's screen habits are associated with consumption of sweetened beverages independently of parental norms. Int J Public Health, 2014;59(1):67–75.

6. Andreyeva T, et al. Exposure to food advertising on television: Associations with children's fast food and soft drink consumption and obesity. Economics and Human Biology, 2011;9:221–33. Zimmerman FJ, Bell JF. Associations of television content type and obesity in children. AJPH, 2010;100:334–40.

7. American Academy of Pediatrics. Policy statement—children, adolescents, obesity, and the media. Pediatrics, 2011;128:201–8.

8. Ustjanauskas AE, et al. Food and beverage advertising on children's websites. Pediatric Obesity, 2013. Brogan C. Fishing where the fish are: mapping social media to the buying cycle. Undated slide presentation. Montgomery K, Chester J. Digital food marketing to children and adolescents: problematic practices and policy interventions. Public Health Law & Policy, Oct 2011. http://changelabsolutions.org.

9. Wilking C, et al. State law approaches to address digital food marketing to youth. Public Health Advocacy Institute, Berkeley Media Studies Group, and Center for Digital Democracy, Dec 2013. Demissie Z, et al. Electronic media and beverage intake among States high school students—2010. J Nutr Education and Behavior, 2013;45:756–60.

10. FTC. Marketing food to children and adolescents: a review of industry expenditures, activities, and self-regulation, Jul 2008.

11. FTC. A review of food marketing to children and adolescents: follow-up report. Dec 2012. Powell LM, et al. Food marketing expenditures aimed at youth: putting the numbers in context. Am J Prev Med, 2013 Oct;45(4):453–61.

12. Internal Revenue Service. Publication 535 (2012), Business Expenses, Section 11: Other expenses, 2012. Thorndike JJ. Should we tax advertising? TaxAnalysts, Aug 8, 2013. http://taxhistory.tax.org.

13. Aizenman NC. Former Coke executive slams "share of stomach" marketing campaign. Washington Post, Jun 7, 2012. A video of Putman's speech is at ABC News. Former Coca-Cola executive Todd Putman confesses to targeting kids, Jun 8, 2012.

14. Scheer R. The doctrine of multinational sell: an essential lesson in the new free enterprise from Don Kendall and Pepsi-Cola. Esquire, 1975;83(4):124–27, 160–64.

15. Harris JL, et al. Monitoring food company marketing to children to spotlight best and worst practices. In: Williams JD, et al, eds. Advances in Communication Research to Reduce Childhood Obesity. Springer Science+Business Media, 2013:153–75. Dembeck CR, et al. Trends in television food advertising to young people: 2013 update. Yale Rudd Center for Food Policy and Obesity, May 2014.

16. Coca-Cola Canada. Open Happiness project, Toronto soccer video. YouTube, Oct 9, 2013. Freedhoff Y. Coca-Cola never, ever markets to kids. Weighty Matters, Aug 28, 2014.

17. Lukovitz K. Coke ends "American Idol" sponsorship. Marketing Daily, Dec 16, 2014. Cheyne A, et al. Food and beverage marketing to children and adolescents: An environment at odds with good health. Berkeley Media Studies Group, Apr 1, 2011.

CHAPTER 11. ADVOCACY: STOPPING SODA MARKETING TO KIDS

1. Simon M. Can food companies be trusted to self-regulate—an analysis of corporate lobbying and deception to undermine children's health. Loyola Los Angeles Law Review, 2006;169(1). Wilking C, et al. State law approaches to address digital food marketing to youth. Public Health Advocacy Institute, Berkeley Media Studies Group, and Center for Digital Democracy, Dec 2013.

2. Children's Advertising Review Unit (CARU). Self-Regulatory Program for Children's Advertising, 9th ed., 2009. Its parent organization is the Advertising Self-Regulatory Council (ASRC) of the Better Business Bureau. See Rudd Center for Food Policy and Obesity. Industry self-regulation.

3. Beales JH. Advertising to kids and the FTC: A regulatory retrospective that advises the present. FTC, Mar 2, 2004.

4. Dietz WH. New strategies to improve food marketing to children. Health Affairs, 2013;32(9):1652–58. Also see an account by a former FTC official: Westen T. Government regulation of food marketing to children: The Federal Trade Commission and the Kid-Vid controversy. Loyola of Los Angeles Law Review, 2006;39:79–92. Foote SB, Mnookin RH. The "Kid Vid" Crusade. Public Interest, 1980;61:90–105.

5. IOM. Food Marketing to Children and Youth: Threat or Opportunity? Washington, DC: National Academies Press, 2005. Am Academy of Pediatrics. Children, adolescents, and advertising. Pediatrics, 2006;118:2563–69.

6. FTC and HHS. Perspectives on Marketing Self-Regulation & Childhood Obesity. Washington, DC, Apr 2006. FTC. Marketing Food to Children and Adolescents: A Review of Industry Expenditures, Activities, and Self-Regulation. Washington, DC, 2008. The House inserted the provision for the Interagency Working Group in its Omnibus Appropriations Act, 2009 (H.R. 1105; Public Law 111-8).

7. What the candidates had to say. Washington Post, May 18, 2008.

8. FTC, CDC, FDA, USDA. Interagency Working Group on Food Marketed to Children: Tentative Proposed Nutrition Standards, Dec 15, 2009. Watzman N. Food and media companies lobby to weaken guidelines on marketing food to children. Sunlight Foundation Reporting Group, Dec 14, 2011.

9. White House Task Force on Childhood Obesity. Report to the President: Solving the Problem of Childhood Obesity Within a Generation, May 2010.

10. House Committee on Energy and Commerce. Internal memorandum. Oct 7, 2011. Eggerton J. Legislators say food marketing guidelines need study. Broadcasting & Cable, Oct 12, 2011.

11. Vladeck DC. Prepared statement of the Federal Trade Commission on the Interagency Working Group on Food Marketed to Children, House Energy and Commerce Committee, Subcommittee on Commerce, Manufacturing, and Trade and the Subcommittee on Health, Oct 12, 2011.

12. Wilson D, Roberts J. Food fight: How Washington went soft on childhood obesity, Reuters special report, Apr 27, 2012.

13. American Academy of Pediatrics. Policy statement—children, adolescents, obesity, and the media. Pediatrics, 2011;128:201–8. IOM. Challenges and Opportunities for Change in Food Marketing to Children and Youth—Workshop Summary, Mar 4, 2013. National Academies Press, 2013.

14. International Council of Beverages Associations. International Council of Beverages Associations Guidelines on Marketing to Children, 2008.

15. Accenture. Compliance Monitoring of Global Advertising for Television, Print, and Internet for the International Council of Beverages Associations, Nov 10, 2009. Accenture. 2012 Compliance Monitoring Report for the International Council of Beverages Associations: On Global Advertising in Television, Print and Internet, Mar 2013.

16. CSPI. Report card on food-marketing policies, Mar 2010. Galbraith-Emami S, Lobstein T. The impact of initiatives to limit the advertising of food and beverage products to children: a systematic review. Obesity Rev, 2013;14:960–74. Kunkel DL, et al. Evaluating industry self-regulation of food marketing to children. Am J Prev Med, 2015.

17. Pomeranz JL. Television food marketing to children revisited: the federal trade commission has the constitutional and statutory authority to regulate. J Law, Med & Ethics, 2010;Spring:98–116. Graff S, et al. Government can regulate food advertising to children because cognitive research shows it is inherently misleading. Health Affairs, 2012;31(2):392–98. Wilking C. Issue brief: reining in pester power, food and beverage marketing. Public Health Advocacy Institute, 2011.

18. De Lauro R. DeLauro introduces bill ending subsidy for marketing unhealthy foods to children. Jul 25, 2013.

19. WHO. Set of recommendations on the marketing of foods and non-alcoholic beverages to children. Resolution of the Sixty-third World Health Assembly adopted 21 May 2010: WHA63.14 Marketing of food and non-alcoholic beverages to children, 2010.

CHAPTER 12. ADVOCACY: GETTING SODAS OUT OF SCHOOLS

1. Taber DR, et al. Association between state laws governing school meal nutrition content and student weight status: implications for new USDA school meal standards. JAMA Pediatrics, 2013;167(6):513–19.

2. Food Research and Action Center. How competitive foods in schools impact student health, school meal programs, and students from low-income families: issue briefs for child nutrition reauthorization #5, Jun 2010. USDA. Child nutrition programs.

3. Terry-McElrath YM, et al. Commercialism in US elementary and secondary school nutrition environments: trends from 2007 to 2012. JAMA Pediatrics, 2014.

4. Much of this history is drawn from Nestle M. Food Politics: How the Food Industry Influences Nutrition and Health. U of California Press, 10th anniversary ed., 2013:197–246, 402–5. Other sources: Martin J, Oakley C. Managing Child Nutrition Programs: Leadership for Excellence. Jones & Bartlett, 2007. Poppendieck J. Free for All: Fixing School Food in America. U of California Press, 2011.

5. The National School Lunch Act. P.L. 396, 79th Congress, Jun 4, 1946, 60 Stat. 231. See Gunderson GL. National School Lunch Program (NSLP): Background and development. In: www.fns.usda.gov/nslp/history.

6. Salisbury CG. Make an investment in our school children: increase the nutritional value of school lunch programs. Brigham Young U Education and Law J, 2004;331–52. GAO. School lunch program: role and impacts of private food service companies (GAO/RCED-96-217), Aug 1996.

7. Nestle M. Soft drink "pouring rights": marketing empty calories. Public Health Rep, 2000;115:308–19. McGeehan P. Pepsi wins battle in Cola wars: $21 million CUNY deal. NYT, Aug 13, 2013. Coca-Cola signs $15.4M pouring rights deal with UCLA. AJC .com, Oct 17, 2013.

Hignite K. Human resources enterprise: health as a social movement. Business Officer Magazine, Jan 2014. See, for example, U of Arkansas. Sponsorship and beverage pouring rights proposal. N.d., but probably 2011. Easley JA. Pepsi outs Coke at UC Davis in sweet $10M deal. DailyDemocrat.com, Sept 11, 2014.

8. Wiecha JL, et al. School vending machine use and fast-food restaurant use are associated with sugar-sweetened beverage intake in youth. JADA, 2006;106:1624–30. Finkelstein DM, et al. School food environments and policies in US public schools. Pediatrics, 2008;122:e251-e259.

9. Park S, et al. The impact of the availability of school vending machines on eating behavior during lunch: The Youth Physical Activity and Nutrition Survey. JADA, 2010;110:1532–6. Editorial: School district now frowns on Coke and a smile. Tampa Bay Times, May 1, 2014.

10. School Nutrition Association. Competitive foods guidelines by state, as of Sept 2013. www.schoolnutrition.org. Mayor Menino's speech was to the annual meeting of the American Public Health Association in Boston, Nov 3, 2013. Cradock AL, et al. Effect of school district policy change on consumption of sugar-sweetened beverages among high school students, Boston, Massachusetts, 2004–2006. Preventing Chronic Disease, 2011;8(4):A74.

11. Terhune C. Coke's guidelines for soft drinks in schools faces some criticism. WSJ, Nov 17, 2003.

12. Mello MM, Pomeranz J, Moran P. The interplay of public health law and industry self-regulation: the case of sugar-sweetened beverage sales in schools. AJPH, 2008;98:595–604.

13. ABA. School Beverage Guidelines, 2005. Burros M, Warner M. Bottlers agree to a school ban on sweet drinks. NYT, May 4, 2006. McKay B. Soda makers support tougher curbs. WSJ, Jun 9, 2007.

14. Martin A. Sugar finds its way back to the school cafeteria. NYT, Sept 16, 2007. The Alliance for a Healthier Generation is at www.healthiergeneration.org. Its webpage, "Drop Liquid Calories," advises, "Remove all sweet drinks from your home." USDA. School Nutrition Dietary Assessment Study IV: Summary. Nov 2012. Wescott RF, et al. Industry self-regulation to improve student health: quantifying changes in beverage shipments to schools. AJPH, 2012 Oct;102(10):1928–35. Turner L, Chaloupka FJ. Wide availability of high-calorie beverages in US elementary schools. Archives of Pediatric and Adolescent Med, 2011;165(3):223–28.

15. IOM. Nutrition Standards for Foods in Schools: Leading the Way Toward Healthier Youth, 2007; IOM. School Meals: Building Blocks for Healthy Children, 2009; and IOM. Nutrition Standards and Meal Requirements for National School Lunch and Breakfast Programs: Phase I. Proposed Approach for Recommending Revisions, 2008, all from National Academies Press. And see: USDA. Nutrition standards in the National School Lunch and School Breakfast Programs: final rule. Federal Register, 2012;77(17): 4088–167. Kohan EG. Congress thwarts Obama administration's plans for healthier school meals. Obama Foodorama, Nov 15, 2011.

16. USDA. National School Lunch Program and School Breakfast Program: nutrition standards for all foods sold in school as required by the Healthy, Hunger-Free Kids Act of 2010. Federal Register, 2013;78(125):39068–120. USDA. Smart snacks in school: USDA's "All Foods Sold in Schools" standards.

17. Bridging the Gap. State laws for school snack foods and beverages. Jan 21, 2014. http://foods.bridgingthegapresearch.org/#.

18. Smith LH, Holloman C. Piloting "Sodabriety": A school-based intervention to impact sugar-sweetened beverage consumption in rural Appalachian high schools. J School Health, 2014;84(3):177–84. Bishop K, Wootan MG. Estimating the economic impact of national school nutrition standards on schools and the beverage industry. CSPI, May 2013. AP. Portland schools bar soda sales on grounds. Bangor Daily News, Aug 3, 2013.

19. Jacobson J. USDA releases rules for competitive beverages in schools. Beverage Industry, Aug 12, 2013.

20. Evich HB. Behind the school lunch fight. PoliticoPro, Jun 4, 2014.

21. School Nutrition Association. 2014 position paper talking points. http://docs. schoolnutrition.org. USDA. Press release: support for healthy meals standards continues to grow. Jul 9, 2014. USDA reported 95% compliance, May 6, 2015. Siegel BE. House committee approves healthy school meals waiver; 19 past presidents break with School Nutrition Association. The Lunch Tray, May 30, 2014.

22. Probart C, et al. Existence and predictors of soft drink advertisements in Pennsylvania high schools. JADA, 2006;106:2052–6. Polacsek M, et al. Examining compliance with a statewide law banning junk food and beverage marketing in Maine schools. Public Health Reports, 2012;127(2):216–23.

23. Molnar A, et al. Promoting consumption at school: health threats associated with schoolhouse commercialism—the fifteenth annual report on schoolhouse commercializing trends: 2011–2012. Boulder, CO: National Education Policy Center, 2013.

24. Coca-Cola. Responsible Marketing Policy. Coca-Cola Journey, Jan 1, 2012.

25. PepsiCo. Responsible Marketing & Advertising. The quotation is from PepsiCo policy on responsible advertising to children, 2012.

26. The White House, Office of the First Lady. Press release: The White House and USDA announce School Wellness Standards. Feb 25, 2014.

27. CSPI. Support nutrition and physical activity in schools! www.cspinet.org/takeaction/#/26. Campaign for a Commercial-Free Childhood. Tell the USDA: Schools should be commercial-free.

28. Gentzel TJ, National School Boards Association. Letter to the Honorable Tom Vilsack, Secretary, USDA. Apr 28, 2014.

29. The National Alliance for Nutrition and Activity (NANA) is at www.cspinet .org/nutritionpolicy/nana.html.

30. The Food Marketing Workgroup is at www.foodmarketing.org. See U.S. Senate, Committee on Appropriations. Departments of Labor, Health and Human Services, and Education, and Related Agencies Appropriation Bill. Report. Jul 11, 2013.

31. Berkeley Media Studies Group. Issue 15: Obesity crisis or soda scapegoat? The debate over selling sodas in schools. Jan 1, 2005.

CHAPTER 13. ADVOCACY: GETTING KIDS INVOLVED

1. Kids finally speak on celebrity-based ads for food and beverages. PR Newswire, Dec 4, 2013.

2. Wang YC, et al. Increasing caloric contribution from sugar-sweetened beverages and 100 percent fruit juices among US children and adolescents, 1988–2004. Pediatrics, 2008;121:e1604–e1614. Kit BK, et al. Trends in sugar-sweetened beverage consumption among youth and adults in the United States: 1999–2010. AJCN, 2013;98:180–88. Babey SH, Wolstein J, Goldstein H. Still bubbling over: California adolescents drinking more soda and other sugar-sweetened beverages. Oct 2013. www .publichealthadvocacy.org.

3. Reedy J, Krebs-Smith SM. Dietary sources of energy, solid fats, and added sugars among children and adolescents in the United States. JADA, 2010;110:1477–84. USDA and HHS. Dietary Guidelines for Americans, 2010. Kosova EC, et al. The relationships between sugar-sweetened beverage intake and cardiometabolic markers in young children. JADA, 2013;113:219–27.

4. Briefel RR, et al. Reducing calories and added sugars by improving children's beverage choices. JAND, 2013;113:269–75.

5. Committee on Nutrition, American Academy of Pediatrics. The use and misuse of fruit juice in pediatrics. Pediatrics, 2001;107:1210–13. This policy was reaffirmed in Aug 2013.

6. What it costs. Ad Age, April 6, 2015:14–17.

7. King County. Public health data watch: youth consumption of sugary drinks in King County, Sept 2012.

8. American Heart Association. Voices for Healthy Kids: Sugar-Sweetened Beverages Toolkit. Rudd 'Roots Parents. Advocacy 101. www.ruddrootsparents.org/advocacy-101. U of California, San Francisco, Center for Vulnerable Populations, and Youth Speaks. The Bigger Picture Toolkit. http://youthspeaks.org.

CHAPTER 14. MARKETING TO AFRICAN AND HISPANIC AMERICANS:
A COMPLICATED STORY

1. The Hispanic Institute. Obesity, Hispanic America's Big Challenge, Apr 2013. www.thehispanicinstitute.net.

2. De La Isla J. Latina obesity exacerbated by food industry. The Republic, May 29, 2013.

3. Lopez MH. Hispanic or Latino? Many don't care, except in Texas. Pew Research Center, Oct 28, 2013. www.pewresearch.org.

4. Mintel. Carbonated Soft Drinks—US—Feb 2012. This survey polled nearly 25,000 consumers, of which 1,700 were black and 7,800 Hispanic.

5. Dodd AH, et al. Disparities in consumption of sugar-sweetened and other beverages by race/ethnicity and obesity status among United States schoolchildren. J Nutr Education and Behavior, 2013;45:240–49. Flegal KM, et al. Prevalence of obesity and trends in the distribution of body mass index among US adults, 1999–2010. JAMA, 2012;307(5):491–97.

6. National Diabetes Clearinghouse. National Diabetes Statistics, 2011.

7. Capparell S. The Real Pepsi Challenge: How One Pioneering Company Broke Color Barriers in 1940s American Business. Wall Street Books, 2007. Goldstein W. The color of cola. NYT Book Review, Feb 4, 2007.

8. Hale GE. When Jim Crow drank Coke. NYT, Jan 29, 2013. Mooney P. Setting the record straight: Coke, racism, and civil rights. Coca-Cola Company, Jan 29, 2013.

9. Ryan T. Stepping up to the plate: When Coca-Cola owned a baseball team...and went to bat for Atlanta's first integrated sporting event. Coca-Cola, Oct 7, 2013.

10. The Museum of Public Relations. Moss Kendrix: A retrospective. www .prmuseum.com. The history of African Americans on Madison Avenue is discussed in Chambers J. Madison Avenue and the Color Line: African Americans in the Advertising Industry. U of Pennsylvania Press, 2009. Also see Pollack M. An early history of blacks on Madison Avenue. NYT, Mar 13, 2015.

11. Pendergrast M. For God, Country & Coca-Cola, 3rd ed. Basic Books, 2013:253.

12. Weiner M. Consumer culture and participatory democracy: the story of Coca-Cola during World War II. In: Counihan C, ed. Food in the USA: A Reader. Routledge, 2002:123–41.

13. Booker J. Fighting for civil rights at the soda fountain. Coca-Cola, Jan 14, 2013. Hale S. An award for all mankind, a dinner for one—the Atlanta Nobel Prize party for MLK, given by the city's image-conscious white leadership. Saporta Report, Jan 19, 2015.

14. Martin Luther King Jr. I've been to the mountaintop. Mason Temple (Church of God in Christ Headquarters), Memphis, TN, Apr 3, 1968.

15. Roberts JL. Threatening boycotts, Jesse Jackson's PUSH wins gains for blacks. WSJ, Jul 21, 1982. Foust D. Coke: Say good bye to the good ol' boy culture. BusinessWeek (archives), May 28, 2000.

16. Coca-Cola. Hispanic Business Agenda. Ogilvy & Mather, 1984.

17. Cola wars take aim at minority markets: Coke and Pepsi both try to grab share among blacks, Hispanics. Milwaukee J, Feb 17, 1992.

18. Harvey CP. What Happened at Coca-Cola? In: Harvey CP, Allard MJ. Understanding & Managing Diversity: Readings Cases & Exercises, 4th ed. Prentice Hall, 2009:305–13. Hays CL. The Real Thing: Truth and Power at the Coca-Cola

Company. Random House, 2004. Winter G. Coca-Cola settles racial bias case. NYT, Nov 17, 2000. Girard R. Corporate Profile: Inside the Real Thing. Polaris Institute, Aug 2005:41.

19. Post C. It's the real thing: Activists push Coca-Cola boycott despite $1 billion diversity plan. Atlanta Daily World, May 18, 2000:1.

20. Maharaj D. Coca-Cola to settle racial bias lawsuit. Los Angeles Times, Nov 17, 2000. Herman AM, et al. Fifth annual report of the task force, Dec 1, 2006. Marzulli J. Coke's not it: 16 workers sue, call giant "cesspool" of racial discrimination. New York Daily News, Mar 16, 2012.

21. U.S. Equal Opportunity Employment Commission. Press release: Pepsi to pay $3.13 million and make major policy changes to resolve EEOC finding of nationwide hiring discrimination against African Americans, Jan 11, 2012. Latino 100. Latino Magazine, Spring 2013:27–36.

22. 11th Annual Hispanic Fact Pack. Ad Age, Jul 28, 2014:28. Kunkel D, et al. Food marketing to children on U.S. Spanish-language television. J Health Communication 2013:1–13. Fleming-Milici F, et al. Amount of Hispanic youth exposure to food and beverage advertising on Spanish- and English-language television. JAMA Pediatrics, 2013;167(8):723–30. Grier SA, Kumanyika SK. The context for choice: health implications of targeted food and beverage marketing to African Americans. AJPH, 2008;98:1616–29. Sugary drink targeted marketing. Rudd Center for Food Policy & Obesity, 2014.

23. Lowe AP, Hacker G. Selfish giving: how the soda industry uses philanthropy to sweeten its profits. CSPI, 2013.

24. Coke pledges $50 million for minorities. Chronicle of Philanthropy, Jun 1, 2000:13. Coca-Cola. The Coca-Cola Foundation: 2011 grants. Coca-Cola. The Coca-Cola Foundation gives back $36 million to raise living standards worldwide. Jun 20, 2013.

25. Quintero F. What is PepsiCo buying with donations to communities of color? Berkeley Media Studies Group blog, Aug 20, 2012. PepsiCo. Press release: PepsiCo contributes $50,000 to the National Association of Hispanic Journalists (NAHJ) for scholarships and internships, Jun 16, 2011. Coca-Cola Company. Surprise $1 million grant awarded to the National Council of Negro Women, May 2, 2013.

26. Liptak A. Justice's plans for event tied to Pepsi stir outcry by Yale alumni. NYT, Feb 7, 2013:A16. See discussion in Chapter 19.

27. Robertson I. A history of Beyoncé's relationship with Pepsi. Vibe, Dec 12, 2012. Sisario B. In Beyoncé deal, Pepsi focuses on collaboration. NYT, Dec 9, 2012. Kohan EG. White House takes down petition calling for Beyoncé to be "disinvited" from inauguration due to PepsiCo deal. Obama Foodorama, Jan 16, 2013.

28. Heine C. Mountain Dew pulls "most racist commercial in history." Adweek, May 1, 2013. Vega T. Lil Wayne puts Mountain Dew in crisis mode. NYT, May 7, 2013. Elliott S, Vega T. Trying to be hip and edgy, ads become offensive. NYT, May 11, 2013. For the offending words, see Dabitch. Mountain Dew drops DeWeezy Lil Wayne for offensive lyrics. Adland, May 4, 2013. Bouckley B. Coke 2013 Super Bowl ad draws Arab-American race criticism. BeverageDaily.com, Jan 13, 2013.

29. Morse D. Hats off to the soft-drink industry for giving attention to Hispanics and blacks. Ad Age, Jun 15, 2012. Morse's book is Multicultural Intelligence: Eight Make-or-Break Rules for Marketing to Race, Ethnicity, and Sexual Orientation. Paramount Market Publishing, 2009.

30. Wentz L. Rising Hispanic artists to watch: marketers should know these hot acts with crossover appeal. Ad Age, Oct 1, 2013.

31. Aizenman NC. Former Coke executive slams "share of stomach" marketing campaign. Washington Post, Jun 7, 2012.

32. Berkeley Media Studies Group. Target marketing soda & fast food: problems with business as usual. Dec 7, 2010. www.bmsg.org.

CHAPTER 15. SELLING TO THE DEVELOPING WORLD

1. The first quotation is from Scheer R. The doctrine of multinational sell: an essential lesson in the new free enterprise from Don Kendall and Pepsi-Cola. Esquire, 1975;83(4):124–27, 160–64. The next two are from Cohen R. Coke's World View—a special report: For Coke, world is its oyster. NYT, Nov 21, 1991.

2. Giebelhaus AW. The pause that refreshed the world: The evolution of Coca-Cola's global marketing strategy. In: Jones G, Morgan NJ, eds. Adding Value: Brands and Marketing in Food and Drink. Routledge, 1994:191–214. Pendergrast M. For God, Country & Coca-Cola, 3rd ed. Basic Books, 2013. Meitar A. An Unimaginable Journal: How Pepsi Beat the Odds in Romania. BookSurge, 2009. Coca-Cola. Coca-Cola (volume published to celebrate the company's 125th anniversary). Assouline Publishing, 2011. Stanley A. Clinton chooses Coke in Russia's cola war. NYT, May 11, 1995.

3. Gelski J. Coke sees $300 billion international opportunity. Food Business News, Sept 5, 2014. Euromonitor International. Passport: Soft Drinks in 2013: Products, Performance, Prospects. Apr 2013.

4. Coca-Cola. Per capita consumption of company beverage products, 2012. Hebblethwaite C. Who, what, why: In which countries is Coca-Cola not sold? BBC News, Sept 11, 2012. Note that when Coke and Pepsi say they sell in more than 200 countries, they use that number as a figure of speech. In 2013, geographers identified only 196 countries. Oddly, Coca-Cola's list includes places like Puerto Rico that are not independent countries, but does not include places like Kosovo, Somalia, or Sudan, which are.

5. PepsiCo. 2012 PepsiCo Annual Report.

6. Rabobank International. Global Beverage Outlook—2013. Rabobank Industry Note #357, Jan 2013.

7. Bhargava Y. Coca Cola's 58th bottling plant in India commences operations. The Hindu, Oct 25, 2013. Cavale S, Jourdan A. Small is beautiful for Coca-Cola as volumes soar in China. Asian Age, Apr 24, 2014. Zacks Equity Research. Coca Cola pushes into China. Nov 8, 2013. Bhargava Y. Coca-Cola's 58th bottling plant in India commences operations. The Hindu, Oct 25, 2013. Shirland Ventures Ltd. Understanding shopper loyalty within different retail formats in Eurasia & Africa. Coca-Cola Retailing Research Councils, Aug 2012. McGroarty P. In Swaziland, Coke holds sway with the king. WSJ, Nov 18, 2013. PepsiCo. PepsiCo announces plans for $5 billion investment in Mexico. Jan 24, 2014.

8. Srivastava A. India should limit foreign investment in junk food. Economic Times, Nov 30, 2013. Ramachandran A, Snehalatha C, Shetty AS, Nandita A. Trends in prevalence of diabetes in Asian countries. World J Diabetes 2012;3(6):110–17. Mullaney L. Top 10 emerging markets for food and drink manufacturers. Food and Drink Europe, May 28, 2013. Flores LS, Anelise R. Gaya, Ricardo DS, Petersen AG. Trends of underweight, overweight, and obesity in Brazilian children and adolescents. J Pediatria, 2013;89:456–61.

9. Terhune C, Kahn G. Coke lures Japanese customers with cellphone come-ons. WSJ, Sept 8, 2003:B1.

10. Wilson D, Kerlin A. Special report: food, beverage industry pays for seat at health-policy table. Reuters, Oct 19, 2012.

11. PepsiCo and the Asian Football Development Project (AFDP) sign strategic partnership agreement. Al Bawaba Business, Apr 8, 2013.

12. Shepp J. Creepy Ad Watch, May 19, 2014.

13. Consultant survey finds Coke's brand image in top 10 in 6 markets. Nation Multimedia, Jun 14, 2013.

14. Shamah D. Sharing a Coke using Israeli tech. Times of Israel, May 26, 2013. Bouckley B. Bittersweet Coke taste in Israel as personalized cans stoke controversy. Beverage Daily, May 24, 2013.

15. Clark M. French deputies pass bill to curb sale of Coca-Cola. NYT, Mar 1, 1950.

16. Palast G. A Marxist threat to cola sales? Pepsi demands a US coup. Goodbye Allende. Hello Pinochet. Guardian, Nov 8, 1998. Louis JC, Yazijian HZ. The Cola Wars. Everest House, 1980. Coca-Cola Journey. The Facts: The Coca-Cola Company and Colombia. Jan 25, 2006. Fromson D. The pause that represses? Coca-Cola's controversies. Atlantic, Oct 18, 2010.

17. On the "Killer Coke" campaign: Blanding M. The Coke Machine. Avery, 2010. Thomas M. Belching Out the Devil. Nation Books, 2008.

18. LaFranchi H. Iran sanctions kick in, and Ahmadinejad says he'll ban Coca-Cola. Christian Science Monitor, Jul 1, 2010. AP. Hugo Chávez tells Venezuelans to drink juice not Coke. Guardian, Jul 23, 2012. Niazi S. India Muslims boycott Coke, Pepsi over Gaza. On Islam, Aug 2, 2014. Bouckley B. "Profits are sent to the corrupt West!" Russian Communists push for Coke, Pepsi sanctions. Beverage Daily, Aug 11, 2014 (quote edited from Google Translate). Iyer B. Why consumers in Vietnam are calling for a ban on Coke. Campaign Asia-Pacific, May 28, 2013.

19. Thai Health Promotion Foundation. Sweet Enough Network persuades schools to avoid risk of "obesity." Dec 15, 2010.

20. CSPI and the International Association of Consumer Food Organizations. The Global Dump Soft Drinks Campaign. www.dumpsoda.org.

21. WHO. Sixty-third World Health Assembly. Agenda item 11.9. Prevention and control of noncommunicable diseases: implementation of the global strategy: report by the Secretariat, Apr 1, 2010. Marketing of food and non-alcoholic beverages to children. In: 3rd World Health Assembly, Geneva, 17–21 May 2010. Geneva, WHO, 2010. WHO. Population-based Approaches to Childhood Obesity Prevention, 2012. De Schutter O. Report submitted by the Special Rapporteur on the Right to Food, United Nations General Assembly, Human Rights Council, Dec 26, 2011.

22. Hawkes C. The worldwide battle against soft drinks in schools. Am J Prev Med, 2010;38(4):457–61. Hawkes C. Regulations, guidelines and voluntary initiatives on soft drink availability in schools around the world. World Heart Federation, Geneva. WHO. Global nutrition policy review: what does it take to scale up nutrition action? WHO, 2013.

23. Natti S. India thinks healthy, drinks healthy. New Indian Express, Jun 9, 2013. PepsiCo. PepsiCo policy on responsible advertising to children, Sept 2014.

CHAPTER 16.   ADVOCACY: EXCLUDING SODAS FROM SNAP

1. Center for Budget and Policy Priorities. Policy basics: introduction to SNAP, Mar 28, 2013.

2. Poppendieck J. Breadlines Knee Deep in Wheat: Food Assistance in the Great Depression, 2nd ed. U of California Press, 2014. Center for the Study of the Presidency

and Congress. SNAP to Health: A Fresh Approach to Strengthening the Supplemental Nutrition Assistance Program. Washington, DC, Jun 2012. www.snaptohealth.org. Simon D. Soda, surplus, and food stamps: a short history. Huffington Post, Jun 24, 2012.

3. DeVault ML, Pitts JP. Surplus and scarcity: hunger and the origins of the food stamp program. Social Problems, 1984;31(5):545–57.

4. USDA/FNS. Supplemental Nutrition Assistance Program (SNAP): participation and costs, Jul 11, 2014. Johnson R, Monke J. What Is the Farm Bill? Congressional Research Service, Oct 3, 2012.

5. Bleich SN, Vine S, Wolfson JA. American adults eligible for the Supplemental Nutritional Assistance Program consume more sugary beverages than ineligible adults. Prev Med, 2013;57:894–899. Leung CW, et al. Dietary intake and dietary quality of low-income adults in the Supplemental Nutrition Assistance Program. AJCN, 2012;96:977–88. Leung CW, et al. Low-income Supplemental Nutrition Assistance Program participation is related to adiposity and metabolic risk factors. AJCN, 2012;95:17–24. Condon E, et al. Diet quality of Americans by SNAP participation status. Data from NHANES, 2007–2012. USDA/FNS, May 2015.

6. Ver Ploeg M, Mancino L, Lin B-H. Food stamps and obesity: ironic twist or complex puzzle? Amber Waves, Feb 2006. Leung CW, et al. Associations of food stamp participation with dietary quality and obesity in children. Pediatrics, 2013;131:463–72.

7. Congressional Record. U.S. Senate, 1964;110(Jun 30):15441.

8. USDA/FNS. Supplemental Nutrition Assistance Program. Eligible food items.

9. Shenkin JD, Jacobson MF. Using the food stamp program and other methods to promote healthy diets for low-income consumers. AJPH, 2010;100:1562–64. Brownell KD, Ludwig DS. The Supplemental Nutrition Assistance Program, soda, and USDA policy: who benefits? JAMA, 2011;306:1370–71. Fernandes MM. Effect of Supplemental Nutrition Assistance Program (SNAP) on frequency of beverage consumption among youth in the United States. JAND, 2012;112;1241–46. Andreyeva T, et al. Grocery store beverage choices by participants in federal food assistance and nutrition programs. Am J Prev Med, 2012;43(4):411–18.

10. New York State Department of Taxation and Finance. Beverages sold by food stores, beverage centers, and similar establishments. Tax Bulletin ST-65 (TB-ST-65), Apr 13, 2011. New York State Department of Taxation and Finance. Coupons and Food Stamps, Tax Bulletin ST-140 (TB-ST-140), Mar 26, 2010.

11. Andrews M, et al. An alternative to developing stores in food deserts: can changes in SNAP benefits make a difference? Applied Economic Perspectives and Policy, 2013;35(1):150–70. USDA/FNS SNAP Benefit Redemption Division. We welcome SNAP: putting healthy food within reach. 2010 Annual Report, 2010. Coleman-Lochner L, Patton L. Supervalu-led stores chasing $55 billion in food stamps: retail. Bloomberg News, Jan 17, 2012. Statement of Steven S. Fishman, chair, CEO, and president of Big Lots. Big Lots management discusses Q4 2012 results—earnings call transcript, Mar 6, 2013.

12. USDA/FNS. Retail store eligibility: USDA Supplemental Nutrition Assistance Program.

13. Monster Beverage management discusses Q4 2012 results—earnings call transcript, Feb 27, 2013. Also see Meier B. In a new aisle, energy drinks sidestep rules. NYT, Mar 20, 2013.

14. Wilde PE. The new normal: the Supplemental Nutrition Assistance Program (SNAP). Am J Agricultural Economics May 16, 2012. Simon M. Food Stamps: Follow the Money. Eat Drink Politics, Jun 2012.

15. This saying is attributed to the essayist and editor Charles Dudley Warner (1829–1900), who adapted it from a line in Shakespeare's The Tempest, "Misery acquaints a man with strange bedfellows." Also see Ludwig DS, Blumenthal SJ, Willett WC. Opportunities to reduce childhood hunger and obesity: restructuring the Supplemental Nutrition Assistance Program (the Food Stamp program). JAMA, 2012;308:2567–68.

16. Oliveira V, et al. The WIC Program: Background, Trends, and Issues. Food Assistance and Nutrition Research Rep No (FANRR-27), USDA/ERS, Oct 2002. WIC food packages—regulatory requirements for WIC-eligible foods. Nov 11, 2014. USDA/ERS. The food assistance landscape: FY 2012 annual report, Mar 2013.

17. Sheehan A, Sykes B. HRA research notes, results from a survey of food stamp recipients' food shopping and eating habits. Human Resources Administration, Office of Evaluation and Research, 2011. Long MW, et al. Public support for policies to improve the nutritional impact of the Supplemental Nutrition Assistance Program (SNAP). Public Health Nutr, 2014;17(1):219–24.

18. AP. Slay, 17 other mayors: limit use of food stamps to buy soda. Jun 19, 2013. Mayors of Baltimore, Boston, Chicago, Los Angeles, et al. Letter to the Honorable John Boehner and the Honorable Nancy Pelosi, Jun 18, 2013. American Medical Association. AMA announces new policy on final day of annual meeting, Jun 19, 2013. National Center for Public Policy Research. Press release: Big Soda SNAPping up welfare dollars. Apr 26, 2013.

19. National Center for Public Policy Research. Press release: Pepsi CEO responds to questions about company's food stamp lobbying, May 1, 2013.

20. ABA. Worth a read: why SNAP restrictions don't work. May 13, 2013.

21. Levin R. Beverage association on guard against limits to food stamp use. The Hill Healthwatch, May 17, 2012. Merlin M. Farm bill still hanging: more than 70 groups lobby on food stamps. Open Secrets, Dec 3, 2012. Eggleston E. The state's broken record: food stamp policy waivers, Apr 4, 2012. See Influence Explorer for lobbying details at http://influenceexplorer.com.

22. USDA/FNS: Implications of restricting the use of food stamp benefits—summary, Mar 1, 2007. But see Jessica E. Todd JE, Ver Ploeg M. Restricting sugar-sweetened beverages from SNAP purchases not likely to lower consumption. Amber Waves, USDA, March 2, 2015.

23. Food Research and Action Center. Coalition statement on preserving food choice in SNAP/Food Stamps, Jul 25, 2011. An earlier version of the statement is at www.frac.org/pdf/foodchoicemay10final.pdf.

24. Congressional Hunger Center. Major donors, 2009–2011. Black J. SNAP judgment. Slate, Aug 6, 2013.

25. Food Resource and Action Center. Report and financial statements, Dec 31, 1994 and 1993. These are available at http://legacy.library.ucsf.edu/tid/ery36c00/pdf. Also see: Hunger and nutrition among Hispanics focus of FRAC's annual dinner. Democracy in Action, Jun 8, 2011. Feeding America. Leadership partners, and supporting partners. CSPI. Selfish Giving: How the Soda Industry Uses Philanthropy to Sweeten Its Profits, 2013.

26. Meriwether K. Health Bucks expands to all NYC farmers markets: EBT participants will get extra $2 for every $5 spent. Epoch Times, Jul 2, 2012. W. K. Kellogg Foundation. W. K. Kellogg Foundation provides $1.2 million for healthy food by doubling food stamp benefits at Michigan farmers' markets, Feb 9, 2011. USDA. Letter to state SNAP-Ed cooperators, Mar 26, 2013. USDA. Dietary guidelines consumer brochure and Selected messages for consumers. www.choosemyplate.gov. SNAP Nutrition Education

is available on the USDA website. USDA/FNS. Research: Nutrition education studies, Jan 2012.

27. USDA/FNS. SNAP: Healthy incentives pilot. Feb 25, 2014.

28. USDA/FNS. Supplemental Nutrition Assistance Program: feasibility of implementing electronic benefit transfer systems in farmers' markets: rep to Congress. Jun 24, 2010. USDA. SNAP Retailer Management 2013 Annual Rep.

29. Wholesome Wave. Programs. http://wholesomewave.org/program. Double Up Food Bucks is at www.doubleupfoodbucks.org. Charles D. How "double bucks" for food stamps conquered Capitol Hill. The Salt, NPR, Nov 10, 2014.

30. SNAP Gardens. www.snapgardens.org.

31. Basu S, et al. Ending SNAP subsidies for sugar-sweetened beverages could reduce obesity and type 2 diabetes. Health Affairs, 2014;33(6):1032–9.

32. The New York State Office of Temporary and Disability Assistance. A proposal to create a demonstration project in New York City to modify allowable purchases under the Federal Supplemental Nutrition Assistance Program. This unsigned and undated document is available on blog sites that uploaded it at the time (www.foodpolitics.com, for example). New York City's Human Resources Administration tracks numbers of SNAP recipients at Supplemental Nutrition Assistance Program (SNAP) Participation Rates,www.nyc.gov/html/hra/html/facts/snap_stats.shtml.

33. Farley T, Daines RF. No food stamps for sodas. NYT, Oct 7, 2010.

34. Skorburg J. Feds deny Minnesota request for ban on junk food purchases with food stamps. Heartland Institute, Aug 1, 2004. Barnhill A. Impact and ethics of excluding sweetened beverages from the SNAP program. AJPH, 2011;101:2037–43.

35. Hartocollis A. New York asks to bar use of food stamps to buy sodas. NYT, Oct 6, 2010. Congressional Black Caucus Foundation, Inc. Development, 2013. www.cbcfinc.org. Pear R. Soft drink industry fights proposed food stamp ban. NYT, Apr 29, 2011.

36. Shahin J, associate SNAP administrator. Letter to Elizabeth R. Berlin, executive deputy commissioner, New York State Office of Temporary and Disability Assistance. Aug 19, 2011.

37. Bloomberg M. Statement of Mayor Michael R. Bloomberg on USDA's denial of Supplemental Nutrition Assistance (SNAP) waiver, Aug 19, 2011.

38. Eggleston E. The state's broken record: food stamp policy waivers. Curious Terrain, Apr 4, 2012. Williams M. USDA says SC faces uphill battle to change SNAP. ABC Columbia, Mar 27, 2013.

39. Guthrie JF, et al. Can food stamps do more to improve food choices? Economic Information Bulletin No. 29-1, USDA/ERS, Sept 2007. Barnhill A, King KF. Evaluating equity critiques in food policy: the case of sugar-sweetened beverages. J Law Med Ethics, 2013;41(1):301–9. Leung CW, et al. A qualitative study of diverse experts' views about barriers and strategies to improve the diets and health of Supplemental Nutrition Assistance Program (SNAP) beneficiaries. JAND, 2013;113:70–76. Guthrie JF, et al. Improving food choices—can food stamps do more? Amber Waves, Apr 2007:23–28.

CHAPTER 17. MARKETING CORPORATE SOCIAL RESPONSIBILITY

1. Coca-Cola. Coca-Cola releases 2011–2012 Global Sustainability Report, Nov 7, 2012.

2. PepsiCo. Performance with purpose: sustainability summary 2010. Dr Pepper Snapple. Our values: corporate philanthropy. Foundation Center. Top funders. 2014. http://foundationcenter.org.

3. Fisher A, Gottlieb R. Who benefits when Walmart funds the food movement? Civil Eats, Dec 18, 2014.

4. Lowe AP, Hacker G. Selfish Giving: How the Soda Industry Uses Philanthropy to Sweeten Its Profits. CSPI, 2013. ABA. Beverage industry is a good part of America. Press release, Oct 24, 2011.

5. Peloza J, Ye C, Montford WJ. When companies do good, are their products good for you? How corporate social responsibility creates a health halo. J Public Policy & Marketing, Jul 2014.

6. IEG Consulting Group. Soft drinks: a sponsorship category update, 2014.

7. Ludwig DS, Nestle M. Can the food industry play a constructive role in the obesity epidemic? JAMA, 2008;300(15):1808–11.

8. Yach D, et al. The role and challenges of the food industry in addressing chronic disease. Globalization and Health, 2010;6:1–10. Pepsi. Strategic grants. 2012 global citizenship giving. http://www.pepsico.com/Purpose/Global-Citizenship/Strategic-Grants.

9. Strom S. In ads, Coke confronts soda's link to obesity. NYT, Jan 15, 2013. The Coca-Cola Company. Our position on obesity. Dec 2013.

10. ABA. Press release: Six U.S. cities win grant awards to support childhood obesity prevention initiatives. Jan 22, 2015.

11. Calvert Investments. Is the Coca-Cola Company (KO) a sustainable and responsible investment? Oct 22, 2013. www.calvert.com.

12. Coca-Cola. 2011/2012 Sustainability Report. Dr Pepper Snapple. Our values: health and wellness. www.drpeppersnapplegroup.com.

13. PepsiCo. Performance with a purpose. Human sustainability. PepsiCo. Nutrition: Defining. Guiding. Leading. Energy balance. Undated pamphlet (probably 2010). Johnston CA, et al. The role of low-calorie sweeteners in diabetes. US Endocrinology, 2013;9(1):13–15.

14. Horowitz B. Coca-Cola ad to defend artificial sweeteners. USA Today, Aug 14, 2013. ABA. Thirsty for facts: setting the record straight on low- and no-calorie sweeteners. Am Society of Nutrition, Advances and Controversies in Clinical Nutrition meeting, Dec 7, 2013.

15. Esterl M. Diet sodas' glass is half empty; sales of low-cal carbonated drinks falling faster than other types. WSJ, Dec 8, 2013. Truong A. Green Coke? In Argentina, Coca-Cola Life features green label, bottle, and ingredients. Fast Company, Jul 22, 2013. Coke Life's possible U.S. debut should bolster Coca-Cola and Stevia sales. Seeking Alpha, Dec 15, 2013. The FDA has not approved the use of extracts of whole *Stevia rebaudiana* leaves as sweetener additives to food, but has allowed chemically extracted Rebiana (rebaudioside A) to be considered generally recognized as safe. Jennings K. Here's why Coke Life and Pepsi NEXT will never take off in the US. Business Insider, Aug 19, 2014.

16. Esteril M. Coke tailors its soda sizes. WSJ, Sept 19, 2011. Suddath C. Coke confronts its big fat problem. Bloomberg BusinessWeek, Jul 31, 2014.

17. Byrne J. Coca-Cola gives $3M to city for anti-obesity, diabetes efforts. Chicago Tribune, Nov 12, 2012. Coca-Cola. 2011/2012 GRI Report, Oct 7, 2012.

18. Coca-Cola. 2011/2012 Sustainability Report. Active healthy living.

19. Choi C. Coke ad: It takes 23 minutes to burn off a soda. Chicago Sun-Times, Jun 6, 2014.

20. Nestle M, Nesheim M. Why Calories Count: From Science to Politics. U of California Press, 2012.

21. Coca-Cola. 2011/2012 Sustainability Report: Nutrition.

22. Coca-Cola. Annual report to the stockholders. Atlanta, 1922:16. American Bottlers of Carbonated Beverages. Liquids for Living (undated, but circa 1962).

23. Bartrina JA, Majem LS. Hydration at the Workplace. Madrid, 2012. PepsiCo. HydrateNow: Your informative guide and tracker, 2014.

24. ABA. America's beverage companies launch New Calories Count™ Vending Program, Oct 8, 2012. Dr Pepper Snapple. Health & wellness: doing good things with flavor. www.dpsgsustainability.com.

25. Ciccone A. Coca-Cola gets cute with latest anti-obesity installment. BrandChannel, Aug 20, 2013. de Sá TH. Can Coca Cola promote physical activity? Lancet, 2014:383:2041. Coca-Cola. 2011/2012 Sustainability Report: Charitable Contributions. CSR Wire. CSR profile of Coca-Cola. The World (fizzy drink) Cup 2014 [editorial]. Lancet, 2014;383:2020.

26. KaBOOM! Let's Play. http://kaboom.org.

27. NYC Department of Health and Mental Hygiene. Health Department launches campaign showing how drinking just one soda a day equals 50 pounds of sugar a year, Oct 24, 2011.

28. Wells R. Wells R. Experts slam Coca-Cola's obesity "weight-wash." Canberra Times, Jul 24, 2013.

29. Gómez L, et al. Sponsorship of physical activity programs by the sweetened beverages industry: public health or public relations? Revista de Saúde Pública, 2011;45(2):423–27.

30. Seabrook J. Snacks for a fat planet. New Yorker, May 16, 2011.

31. Ken I. A healthy bottom line: obese children, a pacified public, and corporate legitimacy. Social Currents, 2014;1:130–48. Hopkins M. Corporate Social Responsibility & International Development: Is Business the Solution? Earthscan, 2007. Vogel D. The Market for Virtue: The Potential and Limits of Corporate Social Responsibility. Brookings Institution Press, 2005. Strom S. Pepsi chief shuffles management to soothe investors. NYT, Mar 12, 2012.

32. Karnani A. The case against corporate social responsibility. WSJ, Jun 14, 2012. Karnani echoes Milton Friedman's classic essay, The social responsibility of business is to increase its profits. NYT Magazine, Sept 13, 1970.

33. Moodie R, et al. Profits and pandemics: prevention of harmful effects of tobacco, alcohol, and ultra-processed food and drink industries. Lancet, 2013; 381: 670–679. Dorfman L, et al. Soda and tobacco industry corporate social responsibility campaigns: how do they compare? PLoS Med, 2012;9(6):e1001241.

CHAPTER 18. INVESTING IN SPONSORSHIP AND COMMUNITY PARTNERSHIPS

1. IEG Consulting Group. Soft Drinks: A Sponsorship Category Update, 2014.

2. Lefton T. Sports sponsor of the year: Pepsi Beverages Co. Sports Business, May 22, 2014.

3. Bartell Drugs. Bartell Drugs and Coca-Cola invite you to live positively at Seattle Center's Winterfest. Business Wire, Dec 18, 2012.

4. PepsiCo. Strategic grants. 2012 global citizenship giving. www.pepsico.com/Purpose/Global-Citizenship/Strategic-Grants.

5. Coca-Cola's website has a page describing the Coca-Cola Foundation. www.coca-colacompany.com. Coca-Cola. The Coca-Cola Foundation awards $8.1 million in 3rd quarter benefitting 3.8 million people worldwide. Market Watch, Oct 18, 2013.

6. Coca-Cola. 2013/2014 Sustainability Report.

7. PepsiCo. Performance with a purpose: sustainability report 2011/2012. Dr Pepper Snapple. Dr Pepper Snapple Group launches ACTION Nation corporate philanthropy program, Aug 9, 2010. Dr Pepper Snapple Philanthropy is at www.drpepper snapplegroup.com/values/philanthropy.

8. In mid-2015, Pepsi Refresh commercials could be viewed at www.nbcnews .com/video/nbcnews.com/37277514#37277514. Goldhirsh B. Progress report: GOOD and the Pepsi Refresh Project. GOOD Magazine, September 26, 2010.

9. Norton MI, Avery J. Case study: the Pepsi Refresh project: a thirst for change. Harvard Business Rev, Aug 26, 2013.

10. Zmuda N. A teaching moment: professors evaluate Pepsi Refresh project. Ad Age, Oct 8, 2012. (This article contains a useful timeline of the Pepsi Refresh project.) Bida C. Why Pepsi canned the Refresh project. MediaPost, Oct 29, 2012.

11. Lowe AP, Hacker G. Selfish Giving: How the Soda Industry Uses Philanthropy to Sweeten Its Profits. CSPI, 2013.

CHAPTER 19. SUPPORTING WORTHY CAUSES: HEALTH PROFESSIONALS AND RESEARCH

1. Allen F. Secret Formula. HarperBusiness, 1994. It is ironic that the Fred Stare Chair at the Harvard School of Public Health is currently held by Dr. Walter Willett, whose research consistently links sodas to poor health. Stare FJ, Shea JA. Teenagers do not eat right. McCall's, Mar 1954:100. Pendergrast M. For God, Country & Coca-Cola, 3rd ed. Basic Books, 2013:251f.

2. Wojcicki JM, Heyman MB. Malnutrition and the role of the soft drink industry in improving child health in Sub-Saharan Africa. Pediatrics, 2010;126(6):e1617–21.

3. Huston L. Newly elected president of Institute of Medicine is on the PepsiCo board of directors. Forbes, Feb 19, 2014. Armstrong D. PepsiCo director quitting to lead health institute that touted soda tax. Bloomberg BusinessWeek, Feb 21, 2014.

4. Ungoed-Thomas J, Mansey K. Sugar watchdog works for Coca-Cola. Sunday Times (UK), Jan 19, 2014. Harrison-Dunn AR. Conflict of interest? On the sugar payroll. Food Navigator, Jan 20, 2014. The fee was worth $9,350 in 2015.

5. Simon M. How did PepsiCo's CEO infiltrate the Robert Wood Johnson Foundation's annual report on obesity? Appetite for Profit, Jul 1, 2010.

6. Evich HB. Pepsi CEO fires back at calorie cut skeptics. PoliticoPro, Sept 24, 2014.

7. Choi C. Coke as a sensible snack? Coca-Cola works with dietitians who suggest cola as snack. Star-Tribune, Mar 16, 2015.

8. Rippe JM, Saltzman E. Sweetened beverages and health: current state of scientific understandings. Advances in Nutr, 2013;4:527–529. Similar sessions were held in 2014 and 2015. Corn Refiners Association. Sweetener studies: http://sweetenerstudies .com.

9. Simon M. And Now a Word from Our Sponsors: Are America's Nutrition Professionals in the Pocket of Big Food, Jan 2013. www.eatdrinkpolitics.com. Butler K. I went to the nutritionists' annual confab. It was catered by McDonald's. Mother Jones, May 12, 2014.

10. The academy lists industry partners at www.eatright.org/corporatesponsors. Coca-Cola. Beverage Institute for Health and Wellness. http://beverageinstitute .org/us.

11. The origins of the parody ad are explained in Dryznar J. Favor from clever dudes. Live Journal, Mar 4, 2004. The "not parody" image was constructed from information from AND at www.eatright.org/corporatesponsors. The parody ad was created by RJ White, as he explained in Fact-Checking on his blog, Ice Cream Motor. http://rjwhite.tumblr.com. Also see The City Desk: Fictional Urbanism. http://thecitydesk.net/baby_soda_ad.

12. E-mail from PepsiCoFNCE@pepsico.com to AND member Lisa Young, Oct 10, 2013. Used with permission. Coca-Cola. CPE Programs, webinars, and podcasts. http://beverageinstitute.org.

13. Reitshamer E, et al. Members' attitudes toward corporate sponsorship of the Academy of Nutrition and Dietetics. J Hunger & Environmental Nutr, 2012;7:149–64. Dietitians for Professional Integrity is at http://integritydietitians.org.

14. Am Academy of Family Physicians. Press release: American Academy of Family Physicians launches consumer alliance with first partner: The Coca-Cola Company, Oct 6, 2009. www.aafp.org. Nestle M. Family doctors resign from AAFP over coke partnership. FoodPolitics.com, Oct 29, 2009. Dr. Walker resigns membership in American Academy of Family Physicians to protest its partnership with Coca-Cola. Contra Costa Health Services, Oct 29, 2009. http://cchealth.org. Brody H. Professional medical organizations and commercial conflicts of interest: ethical issues. Annals of Family Med, 2010;8:354–58. Bruno R, Burns K. The not-so-sweet relief: how the soda industry is influencing medical organizations. The Equation, Union of Concerned Scientists, Oct 15, 2014. http://blog.ucsusa.org.

15. Roberts I. Corporate capture and Coca-Cola. Lancet, 2008;372:1934–35.

16. Lowe AP, Hacker G. Selfish Giving: How the Soda Industry Uses Philanthropy to Sweeten Its Profits. CSPI, 2013. Personal communication: E-mail from Fabio da Silva Gomes, Jul 12, 2012.

17. Lesser LI, et al. Relationship between funding source and conclusion among nutrition-related scientific articles. PLoS Med, Jan 9, 2007. Bes-Rastrollo M, et al. Financial conflicts of interest and reporting bias regarding the association between sugar-sweetened beverages and weight gain: a systematic review of systematic reviews. PLoS Med, 2013;10(12):e1001578. Massougbodji J, et al. Reviews examining sugar-sweetened beverages and body weight: correlates of their quality and conclusions. AJCN, 2014;99:1096–104.

18. Zachwieja J, et al. Public-private partnerships: the evolving role of industry funding in nutrition research. Advances in Nutr, 2013;4:570–572. SourceWatch tracks ILSI funding at www.sourcewatch.org.

19. Mitka M. Do flawed data on caloric intake from NHANES present problems for researchers and policy makers? JAMA, 2013;310(20):2137–38.

20. Cope MB, Allison DB. White hat bias: examples of its presence in obesity research and a call for renewed commitment to faithfulness in research reporting. Int J Obesity, 2010;34:84–88.

21. Allison DB, Mattes RD. Nutritively sweetened beverage consumption and obesity. JAMA, 2009;301:318–20. Harris D, Patrick M. Is "Big Food's" big money influencing the science of nutrition? ABC World News, Jun 21, 2011. This program elicited its own attacks. See Butterworth T. ABC News attacks scientist who exposed bias in obesity research. Forbes, Jun 22, 2011.

22. Krimsky S. Do financial conflicts of interest bias research? An inquiry into the "funding effect" hypothesis. Science Technology & Human Values, 2013;38:566–87. Marks JH. Toward a systemic ethics of public-private partnerships related to food and health. Kennedy Institute of Ethics J, 2014;24(3):267–99.

23. PepsiCo funds new fellowship in nutritional science. Yale News, Dec 11, 2009. Karlin M. A Pepsi nutrition fellowship at Yale, You got it! BuzzFlash, Mar 21, 2013.

24. Simon M. PepsiCo and public health: is the nation's largest food company a model of corporate responsibility or master of public relations? CUNY Law Review, Jul 22, 2012.

25. Nestle M. Food company sponsorship of nutrition research and professional activities: a conflict of interest? Public Health Nutr, 2001;4(5):1015–22.

26. Gomes F. Big Food Watch. Words for our sponsors [commentary]. World Nutr, 2013;4(8):618–44. www.wphna.org/worldnutrition.

27. Marks JH. What's the big deal? The ethics of public-private partnerships related to food and health. Edmond J. Safra Research Lab Working Papers, No. 11, Harvard University, May 23, 2013.

28. United Nations Standing Committee on Nutrition. SCN Private Sector Engagement Policy, Rule 20, revised June 19, 2006. www.unscn.org.

29. Freedhoff Y, Hébert PC. Partnerships between health organizations and the food industry risk derailing public health nutrition. Canadian Med Assoc J, 2011;183(3):291–92. Freedhoff Y. The food industry is neither friend, nor foe, nor partner. Obesity Rev, 2014;15:6–8.

CHAPTER 20. RECRUITING PUBLIC HEALTH LEADERS: WORKING FROM WITHIN

1. Coca-Cola. Meet our people. www.coca-colacompany.com. McPherson K. Can we leave industry to lead efforts to improve population health? No. BMJ 2013;346:f2426.

2. Waxman A. The WHO Global Strategy on Diet, Physical Activity and Health: the controversy on sugar. Development 2004;47:75–82.

3. Tackling big tobacco: the establishment of the Framework Convention on Tobacco Control: An interview with Derek Yach. Multinational Monitor, 2005;26(5). Beaglehole R, et al. A tobacco-free world: a call to action to phase out the sale of tobacco products by 2040. Lancet, 2015;385:1011–18 (Yach is a co-author). Yach D. The origins, development, effects, and future of the WHO Framework Convention on Tobacco Control: a personal perspective. Lancet 2014; 383:1771–79. Yach D, Bialous SA. Junking science to promote tobacco. AJPH. 2001;91(11):1745–48.

4. Olson E. Five questions for Derek Yach: fighting fat by going to the source. NYT, Nov 17, 2002. Hawkes C. Marketing food to children: changes in the global regulatory environment. WHO, 2004. The Treviso meeting was held at the headquarters of Benetton, the Italian clothing company known for its provocative advertising. In his comments on this chapter, Dr. Yach noted that "the US government formally complained about us holding that meeting and doing so with Benetton at the time they were running an ad campaign against the death sentence in the US." Email to author, May 30, 2014.

5. WHO. Diet, Nutrition, and the Prevention of Chronic Disease (WHO Technical Rep Series 916), Geneva, 2003. WHO. Global Strategy on Diet, Physical Activity, and Health, May 22, 2004. For an eyewitness account of the events, see Waxman A. The WHO Global Strategy on Diet, Physical Activity and Health: the controversy on sugar. Development 2004;47:75–82. Other accounts: Zarocostas J. WHO waters down draft strategy on diet and health. Lancet 2004;363:1373; Brownell KD, Nestle M. Op-ed: The sweet and lowdown on sugar. NYT, Jan 23, 2004:A23.

6. BBC One. The trouble with sugar (video), Oct 4, 2004. The unofficial transcript is at http://news.bbc.co.uk. In this chapter, it is edited slightly for clarity.

7. Yach D. Emailed comments to author, May 30, 2014, and Feb 8, 2015 All of his quotations not otherwise cited come from these messages.

8. PepsiCo. PepsiCo appoints Derek Yach as Director—Global Health Policy. RedOrbit, Feb 8, 2007.

9. Uauy R. Invited commentary to Yach editorial: Do we believe Derek's motives for taking his new job at PepsiCo? Public Health Nutr. 2008;11(2):111–112.

10. Byrnes N. Pepsi brings in the health police. Bloomberg BusinessWeek, Jan 14, 2010.

11. Yach D. Invited editorial: a personal view. Food companies and nutrition for better health. Public Health Nutr. 2008;11(2):109–111.

12. Martin A. Makers of sodas try a new pitch: they're healthy. NYT, Mar 7, 2007. Barnes B. Limiting ads of junk food to children. NYT, Jul 18, 2007. PepsiCo. Health and Wellness, 2007. http://dbuu.com/images/printed/PepsiCo_Brochure.pdf.

13. Powell K, et al. Letter to Dr. Margaret Chan, Director General World Health Organization. A Global Commitment to Action on the Global Strategy on Diet, Physical Activity and Health, May 13, 2008. www.ifballiance.org.

14. Bauerlein V. PepsiCo chief defends her strategy to promote "good for you" foods. WSJ, Jun 28, 2011. Strom S. Pepsi chief shuffles management to soothe investors. NYT, Mar 12, 2012.

15. International health policy analyst Derek Yach joins the Vitality Group. PR Newswire, Oct 23, 2012. Boseley S. The Shape We're In: How Junk Food and Diets Are Shortening Our Lives. Guardian Books, 2014:274.

16. Yach D, et al. Can the food industry help tackle the growing global burden of undernutrition? AJPH. 2010;100(6):974–980 Yach D, et al. The role and challenges of the food industry in addressing chronic disease. Globalization and Health. 2010;6:10. Yach D. Can we leave industry to lead efforts to improve population health? Yes. BMJ. 2013;346:f2279.

17. Brownell B, Yach D. Is there a seat at the table for the food and beverage industry in the global fight against obesity? Council on Foreign Relations, Nov 30, 2012.

18. Norum K. Invited commentary to Yach editorial: PepsiCo recruitment strategy challenged. Public Health Nutr. 2008;11(2):112–113.

19. Ludwig D, Nestle M. Can the food industry play a constructive role in the obesity epidemic? JAMA. 2008;300;1808–11.

CHAPTER 21. ADVOCACY: DEFENDING THE ENVIRONMENT

1. Coca-Cola. Building a Sustainable Tomorrow: Our Journey in 2012. Corporate Responsibility & Sustainability Report, 2012/2013.

2. Dr Pepper Snapple. Sustainability. www.drpeppersnapplegroup.com.

3. PepsiCo. Performance with a Purpose: Sustainability Report 2011/2012. Coca-Cola. Infographic: Our 2020 environmental goals.

4. EPA. Overview of greenhouse gases. http://epa.gov. Research on the carbon footprint of carbonated soft drinks. Beverage Industry Environmental Roundtable, Jun 2012. www.bieroundtable.com.

5. EPA. Greenhouse gas emissions from a typical passenger vehicle, Dec 2011. Sierra Club. Future fleet—why soda companies? Beyond Oil, 2012.

6. Coca-Cola. 2011/2012 Sustainability Report. EPA. Top 30 On-site Generation, Sept 19, 2013.

7. Walker A. Coke's "Downtown in a Box" delivers clean water and Wi-Fi to Africa. Gizmodo, Oct 10, 2013. Ungerleider N. Why Coke is bringing solar power to rural Kenya. CoExist, Jun 4, 2013. Gelski J. Food companies make Global 100 sustainability index. Food Business News, Jan 23, 2015.

8. Bouckley B. "Last year around 5bn PET bottles went to landfill, amazing isn't it?" Beverage Daily, Oct 15, 2014.

9. Elmore BJ. Citizen Coke: The Making of Coca-Cola Capitalism. Norton, 2015. Center for Responsive Politics. Influence and lobbying. www.opensecrets.org/influence.

10. Coca-Cola. 2013/2014 Sustainability Report.

11. The Coca-Cola Foundation gives $8.8 million to help develop sustainable communities. Market Watch, Aug 8, 2013. The Coca-Cola Foundation awards $8.1 million in 3rd quarter benefitting 3.8 million people worldwide. Market Watch, Oct 18, 2013.

12. Perkins M. NASCAR Green: A race worth leading. Coca-Cola Journey, Sept 17, 2013. Coca-Cola. How can a drink build a more sustainable tomorrow? Corporate responsibility & sustainability report, 2011/2012. Stones M. Coca-Cola Enterprises wins top environmental award—on film. FoodManufacture.co.uk, Nov 14, 2012. Coca-Cola rewards customers that pledge to recycle. GreenBiz.com, Aug 13, 2013. Bouckley B. Coca-Cola Enterprises adopts on-pack recycling label. Beverage Daily, Aug 23, 2013. Doland A. Coca-Cola turns empty bottles into paintbrushes, lamps, toys. Ad Age, May 28, 2014.

13. PepsiCo. PepsiCo and the Nature Conservancy partner to increase recycling and protect drinking water. Jul 31, 2014. ABA. How we support recycling efforts.

14. ABA. Recycling facts. 2014.

15. ABA. Questions & answers: beverage container deposits. 2014.

16. Herrick J. Coca-Cola officials claim bottle bill adds unneeded cost to recycling effort. VTDigger, Sept 12, 2013.

17. Barringer F. Parks chief blocked plan for Grand Canyon bottle ban. NYT, Nov 9, 2011.

18. Johnson R. Sale of plastic water bottles banned at Grand Canyon National Park. National Parks Traveler, Feb 6, 2012. Schwartz D. Grand Canyon to ban bottled water sales. Reuters, Feb 8, 2012.

19. PepsiCo. Our commitment to sustainable agriculture practices. N.d., but probably 2011.

20. WWF. Agriculture and Environment: Sugarcane. CABI-Bioscience and WWF. Sugar and the environment: encouraging better management practices in sugar production. 2005. http://wwf.panda.org. Cheesman OD. Environmental Impacts of Sugar Production: The Cultivation and Processing of Sugarcane and Sugar Beet. CABI, 2004. Clay J. World Agriculture and the Environment: A Commodity-by-Commodity Guide to Impacts and Practices. Island Press, 2004.

21. Coca-Cola. Sustainable agriculture guiding principles, Apr 2013. Coca-Cola. 2012/2013 GRI [Global Reporting Initiative] Report, 2013. Bonsucro. Production standard. http://bonsucro.com. Oxfam. Behind the Brands: Scorecard, Mar 2015. www.behindthebrands.org/scorecard.

22. Project Catalyst. http://projectcatalyst.net.au.

23. ABA. American Beverage Association celebrates America Recycles Day, Nov 14, 2013.

24. Lowe AP, Hacker G. Selfish Giving: How the Soda Industry Uses Philanthropy to Sweeten Its Profits. CSPI, 2013.

25. Container Recycling Institute. Bottle bill myths and facts. www.bottlebill.org.

26. Container Recycling Institute. Bottle Bill Resource Guide. www.bottlebill.org. Gitlitz J. Bottled Up: Beverage Container Recycling Stagnates (2000–2010): Container Recycling Rates & Trends. Container Recycling Institute, Oct 2013. www.container-recycling.org.

27. ABA. How we support recycling. ABA. Deposits & taxes: the beverage industry & beverage container deposits.

28. Herrick J. Coca-Cola officials claim bottle bill adds unneeded cost to recycling effort. VT-Digger, Sept 12, 2013. Shayon S. Greenpeace goes after Coca-Cola in ongoing recycling battle in Australia. BrandChannel, May 10, 2013.

29. Greenpeace. The benefits and, well, benefits! Your 11-step guide to effective recycling in Australia.

30. Greenpeace Australia. Coke Refunds. www.cokerefunds.org. Bouckley B. Greenpeace Australia attacks Coke with spoof recycling website. Beverage Daily, Aug 21, 2013. Lepitak S. Greenpeace to release spoof advert linking Coca-Cola packaging firm to death of sea birds. The Drum, May 6, 2013.

31. Galland A. Waste & opportunity: U.S. beverage container recycling scorecard and report. As You Sow, 2011. http://www.asyousow.org. Press release: Major beverage companies willing to take responsibility for post-consumer packaging, study finds. As You Sow, Aug 11, 2011.

32. Container Recycling Institute. Bottle bill toolkit: a resource for bottle bill activists. http://toolkit.bottlebill.org.

33. Sierra Club, ForestEthics, 350.org, et al. Open Letter to leading North American companies on tar sands—an extreme, dirty fuel source, Jul 2, 2013. ForestEthics, Sierra Club. Tar sands: why soda companies? ForestEthics, Sierra Club. Tastes like tar sands. http://action.sierraclub.org.

34. Oxfam. Behind the Brands: Food justice and the "Big 10" food and beverage companies. Oxfam Briefing Paper, Feb 26, 2013.

35. Oxfam. Sugar rush: Land rights and the supply chains of the biggest food and beverage companies. Oxfam Briefing Note, Oct 2, 2013.

36. Bouckley B. Coca-Cola vows to engage with Tate & Lyle Sugars over "land grabbing" controversy. Beverage Daily, Nov 8, 2013. Oxfam. Behind the Brands: Land. Oxfam. Behind the Brands: PepsiCo.

37. Grossman-Cohen. PepsiCo declares "zero tolerance" for land grabs in supply chain. Oxfam, Mar 18, 2014. PepsiCo. Performance with a purpose: policies. Pepsi joins Coke in support of UN-backed guidelines on local peoples' right to land, livelihoods. UN News Centre, Apr 15, 2014. Also see FAO voluntary guidelines on the responsible governance of tenure, at www.fao.org.

CHAPTER 22. ADVOCACY: PROTECTING PUBLIC WATER RESOURCES

1. PepsiCo wins the 2012 Stockholm Industry Water Award. Stockholm International Industry Water Institute, Jun 13, 2013.

2. Coca-Cola Enterprises. Coca-Cola Enterprises recognized for outstanding water management and reduction performance, Feb 19, 2013.

3. Coca-Cola. Annual Report to U.S. Securities and Exchange Commission, Form 10-K, Dec 31, 2013.

4. Watching water: a guide to evaluating corporate risks in a thirsty world. JP Morgan Global Equity Research, Mar 31, 2008.

5. Coca-Cola. 2011/2012 Sustainability Report: Water Stewardship. Coca-Cola. 2013/2014 Sustainability Report.

6. Coca-Cola Enterprises. Building a Sustainable Tomorrow: Our Journey in 2012. 2012/2013 Corporate Responsibility & Sustainability Report, 2013.

7. International Bottled Water Association (IBWA). Water Use Benchmarking Study: Executive Summary, Oct 21, 2013. www.bottledwater.org.

8. Ercin AE, et al. Corporate water footprint accounting and impact assessment: The case of the water footprint of a sugar-containing carbonated beverage. Water Resource Management, 2011;25:721–41. Also see Water Footprint Network. Product water footprints: soft drinks. The network provides assessments for other products as well. Hoekstra AY, et al. The water footprint assessment manual: setting the global standard, Earthscan, 2011.

9. Coca-Cola Europe. Toward sustainable water sourcing in Europe: water footprint sustainability assessment (WFSA), Aug 2011. www.waterfootprint.org.

10. The Coca-Cola Company and the Nature Conservancy. Product Water Footprint Assessments, Sept 2010. www.waterfootprint.org.

11. The Nature Conservancy. Working with companies: the Coca-Cola Company and the Coca-Cola Foundation. 2013. www.nature.org.

12. The Coca-Cola Company and the Nature Conservancy release water footprint report. PRWeb, Sept 8, 2010. See also, for example, World Wildlife Fund, Nature Conservancy receive $3 million in gifts. Philanthropy News Digest, May 16, 2013. 52 new sustainability grants from the Coca-Cola Foundation. Earth Protect, Dec 4, 2012.

13. Sarni W. Corporate Water Strategies. Routledge, 2011.

14. Bouckley B. Coke plans to roll-out "first of its kind" water recovery system from 2013. Beverage Daily, Jul 24, 2012. Rye C. Coca-Cola, Cargill monitor producers' efforts. The Messenger, Sept 15, 2013. Coca-Cola. Sustainability at Coca-Cola, Feb 2013.

15. PepsiCo, Inc. CEO Water Mandate Communication on Progress, Dec 10, 2009. PepsiCo. Environmental sustainability: water.

16. PepsiCo. United Nations CEO water mandate: 2012 communication on progress, Feb 2013. PepsiCo. Water stewardship: good for business. Good for society (n.d., circa 2010).

17. PepsiCo and the Nature Conservancy. Striving for positive water impact: lessons from a partnership approach in five watersheds. 2011. PepsiCo. PepsiCo and the Nature Conservancy partner to increase recycling and protect drinking water. Jul 31, 2014.

18. PepsiCo Foundation. Programs. Water/Environment. Pepsi-Co to deliver water dam in Amman. ConstructionWeek.com, Nov 13, 2013.

19. WaterAid joins forces with the Coca-Cola Africa Foundation to bring safe drinking water to Burkina Faso and Ethiopia. Water Aid, Apr 29, 2013. Dean Kamen's Slingshot aims to bring fresh water to the world. Huffington Post Green, Mar 25, 2013. Coca-Cola. Coca-Cola launches global EKOCENTER partnership to deliver safe drinking water and basic necessities to rural communities, Sept 24, 2013.

20. Brancaccio D, Bitker J. Coca-Cola CEO Muhtar Kent on water, obesity. Marketplace, Sept 27, 2013.

21. Walker A. Coke's "Downtown in a Box" delivers clean water and Wi-Fi to Africa. Gizmodo, Oct 20, 2013. Higginbotham A. Dean Kamen's mission to bring unlimited clean water to the developing world. Wired, Aug 13, 2013. Coca-Cola. EKOCENTER delivers safe access to water and other basic necessities to communities in need. Sept 24, 2013. McNeil DG. Coca-Cola plans kiosks with water and Internet. NYT, Sept 30, 2013.

22. Coca-Cola partners with WaterHealth International to bring clean water to a million students in developing countries under their "Child with Water" project. The Nation, May 18, 2014.

23. Coca-Cola. The water stewardship and replenish report, 2012.

24. Coca-Cola Africa Foundation. The Coca-Cola Africa Foundation broadens reach of Replenish Africa initiative, Apr 14, 2015.

25. Coca-Cola. The Coca-Cola Foundation gives $8.8 million to help develop sustainable communities, Aug 8, 2013. The Coca-Cola Foundation awards $8.1 million in 3rd quarter benefitting 3.8 million people worldwide. Market Watch, Oct 18, 2013.

26. Hunt L. Indian Valley meadow restoration project. The River Blog, Sept 20, 2012. www.americanrivers.org. Video: USDA Forest Service. Indian Valley restoration project. YouTube. Nov 2, 2012.

27. USDA. USDA and Coca-Cola partner to replenish one billion liters of water to nature: initial projects to improve water resources in five states. Sept 13, 2013.

28. Food Empowerment Project. Water usage & privatization, 2014. www .foodispower.org. Leith S. Coca-Cola's grip on water. Atlanta Journal-Constitution, Jun 11, 2003.

29. Choi C. America's new love: water. Associated Press, Mar 11, 2013.

30. Lovegrove N, Thomas M. Triple-strength leadership. Harvard Business Rev, Sept 2013. Coca-Cola. 2011/2012 Sustainability Report: Water Stewardship. Elmore BJ. Citizen Coke: The Making of Coca-Cola Capitalism. Norton, 2015.

31. Case against Coca-Cola Kerala State: India. The Rights to Water and Sanitation, n.d. (circa 2007).

32. Also see Food Empowerment Project. Water usage & privatization. www .foodispower.org/water-usage-privatization. Rai S. Protests in India deplore soda makers' water use. NYT, May 21, 2003.

33. Shiva V. Resisting water privatisation, building water democracy: paper for the World Water Forum, 2006. www.globalternative.org.

34. Srivastava A. Coca-Cola and water—an unsustainable relationship. India Resource Center, Mar 8, 2006. www.indiaresource.org.

35. Bouckley B. Coke's largest India bottler abandons 25 m bottle line, campaigners claim "colossal victory." Beverage Daily, Sept 10, 2014. Mehdiganj—The Issues. India Resource Center, Oct 26, 2014. www.indiaresource.org. Coca Cola stalls expansion plans in Varanasi. One India, Aug 30, 2014. http://news.oneindia.in. Arthur R. Coca-Cola India bottling plant halted—more water rows? Beverage Daily, Apr 22, 2015. Mitchell S. Coca-Cola denies allegations of illegal water use in Indonesia. Sydney Morning Herald, Apr 23, 2014.

36. Karnani A. Corporate social responsibility does not avert the tragedy of the commons—case study: Coca-Cola India. Ross School of Business Working Paper Series, U of Michigan, Feb 2014. Water studies. Times of India, May 12, 2014.

37. Bellatti A. Coca-Cola's assault on tap water. Huffington Post, Nov 13, 2013. Soon after appearance of this post, Coca-Cola removed information about the program from its website, as did graphic designer Pen Williamson, whose website had featured a poster for the

program. Gleick P. Bottled and Sold: The Story Behind Our Obsession with Bottled Water. Island Press, 2010. Also see summary at Circle of Blue, May 3, 2010. Coca-Cola Solutions. Cap the Tap. http://big.assets.huffingtonpost.com/CokeWebsiteScreenShot1.png.

38. Coca-Cola Foodservice. The Crew Review. Coke Solutions, fall 2009:1–2.

39. Dietz WH, Dorfman L. How far will Big Soda go to keep people from drinking water? Beyond Chron, Feb 2, 2014. Neporent L. Gatorade mobile game referred to water as "the enemy." ABC News, Jan 9, 2014. Huehnergarth N. Big Soda double-crosses Michelle Obama's "Drink Up" water program—in less than 3 months. Civil Eats, Nov 25, 2013. Partnership for a Healthier America. Drink Up: supporters. http://youarewhatyoudrink.org/supporters. The White House. First Lady Michelle Obama to ask everyone to "Drink Up" with more water. Press release, Sept 12, 2013.

40. Oxfam. Behind the Brands Scorecard, Mar 2015. www.behindthebrands.org/scorecard.

CHAPTER 23. LOBBYING, THE REVOLVING DOOR, CAMPAIGN CONTRIBUTIONS, AND LAWSUITS

1. Lofland CH. The National Soft Drink Association: A Tradition of Service. NSDA, 1986.

2. S. 1 (110th): Honest Leadership and Open Government Act of 2007. The act amends the Lobbying Disclosure Act of 1995. Fang L. The shadow lobbying complex: where have all the lobbyists gone? The Nation, Mar 10/17, 2014.

3. U.S. Senate. Query the Lobbying Disclosure Act Database. http://soprweb.senate.gov. Center for Responsive Politics. Open Secrets. Influence and lobbying. www.opensecrets.org/influence.

4. Spires S. Food and beverage background. Open Secrets, Oct 2010. www.opensecrets.org.

5. White House Office of Management and Budget. Meeting record regarding: National School Lunch and School Breakfast Programs: nutrition standards for all foods sold in school, as required by the Healthy, Hunger-Free Kids Act of 2010, Jun 29, 2012.

6. Federal workers with professional degrees earned about 23 percent less than their private-sector counterparts. Congressional Budget Office. Comparing the compensation of federal and private-sector employees. Jan 30, 2012.

7. Federal Election Commission. Quick answers to general questions. Contribution limits, 2013–14.

8. Supreme Court of the United States. McCutcheon et al. v. Federal Election Commission. Apr 2, 2014. Sullivan S. Everything you need to know about McCutcheon v. FEC. Washington Post, Apr 2, 2013. Gidfar M. McCutcheon one of the worst Supreme Court decisions of all time—here's what you need to know. Huffington Post, Apr 2, 2014.

9. Center for Responsive Politics, Open Secrets, 2013. www.opensecrets.org.

10. Center for Responsive Politics. Open Secrets, 2013. www.opensecrets.org.

11. Hightower J. Corporate largesse revealed. Holland Sentinal, Oct 20, 2014.

12. Center for Responsive Politics, Open Secrets, 2013. www.opensecrets.org.

13. The illustration comes from the Tucson Citizen, which ceased print May 16, 2009, but continued as TucsonCitizen.com until Jan 31, 2014 (though the website archive ends in 2009). The image was captured in a screenshot: Phillips RJ. Tucson Citizen takes on Supreme Court in wordless editorial. Donald W. Reynolds National Center for Business Journalism, Feb 2, 2010.

14. Blumenthal P. "Dark money" hits $172 million in 2012 election, half of independent group spending. Huffington Post, Jul 29, 2012. McGregor R. "Dark money" floods in to US election. Financial Times, May 19, 2014.

15. Cornfield J. State says grocers group broke law, must reveal donors. Herald Net, Oct 16, 2013. Cornfield J. Grocers group fighting I-522 reveals donors. Herald Net, Oct 17, 2013. Public Disclosure Commission. Cash contributions for: Grocery Manufacturers Assn against I-522, Oct 2013. www.pdc.wa.gov.

16. Connelly J. Big money helps defeat food labeling initiative, but fight not over. Seattle Post-Intelligencer, Nov 5, 2013. For election results, see Washington Secretary of State. Initiative to the Legislature 522 concerns labeling of genetically-engineered foods, Nov 26, 2013. http://vote.wa.gov.

17. Lifsher M. Food growers, beverage firms bolster effort against Prop. 37. Los Angeles Times, Aug 22, 2012. Organic Consumers Association. Organic Consumers Association calls for boycott of organic brand parent companies that helped defeat Prop 37. Nov 15, 2012. Strom S. Election day entailed casting votes for soda taxes and food issues too. NYT, Nov 5, 2014.

18. Alexander RM, Mazza SW, Scholz S. Measuring rates of return on lobbying expenditures: an empirical case study of tax breaks for multinational corporations. J Law Policy, 2009; 25:401.

19. Chen H, Parsley DC, Yang Y-W. Corporate lobbying and firm performance. Social Science Research Network, Jul 22, 2013. de Figueiredo RJ, Edwards G. Does private money buy public policy? Campaign contributions and regulatory outcomes in telecommunications. Institute of Governmental Studies, U of California, Berkeley, 2005.

20. Powell LW. The Influence of Campaign Contributions in State Legislatures: The Effects of Institutions and Politics. U of Michigan Press, 2012. U of Rochester. Press release: Campaign contributions influence public policy, finds study of 50 state legislatures, May 22, 2012.

21. ABA. Choice Prevails in NC! Oct 2, 2013.

22. The Food Revolution Network and the Center for Food Safety. Boycott Coca-Cola. http://cokeboycott.com.

23. See, for example, Public Citizen's Citizens United against Citizens United, Senator Al Franken's (D-IL) MoveOn.Org call for repeal of Citizens United, and Common Cause's election reform campaign in New York State.

CHAPTER 24. USING PUBLIC RELATIONS AND FRONT GROUPS

1. Basu A. Private and public linkages of soda. EpiAnalysis, Jan 24, 2013.

2. Barbaro M, Hartocollis A. As Bloomberg fought sodas, nominee sat on Coke board. NYT, Nov 16, 2010.

3. National Women's History Museum. Indra Krishnamurthy Nooyi (1955–). www.nwhm.org. Bloomberg BusinessWeek. PepsiCo: Indra K. Nooyi. The NYT tables of CEO pay (Business section, Jun 8, 2014:6–7) give Nooyi's compensation as $13.2 million in 2013, a 5 percent increase over 2012. Her additional compensation included $2.5 million in stock option gains, $7.5 million in stock award gains, $15.7 million in lump-sum pension, $10.5 million in deferred compensation, and $87.6 million in accumulated value of equity holdings.

4. Bloomberg BusinessWeek. Coca-Cola: Muhtar Kent. The precise amount of executive pay depends on how its various elements—base salary, bonuses, stock options,

and perquisites—are counted. The NYT tables of CEO pay (Business section, Jun 8, 2014:6–7) state that Kent's compensation was $18.2 million in 2013, a 16 percent decrease since 2012, and $2 million lower than the Bloomberg estimate. Mr. Kent also held $182 million in equity holdings, $33.6 million in lump-sum pension funds, and deferred compensation of another $2 million. The CEO of Coca-Cola Enterprises, John Brock III, had a salary of $17 million in 2013, an increase of 66 percent over the previous year; his accumulated holdings added up to another $200 million.

5. Shumate M. The Gates Foundation and Coca Cola at odds or legitimate bedfellows? Nonprofit Quarterly, Jan 31, 2013.

6. Ruskin G. Spooky business: corporate espionage against nonprofit organizations. Essential Information, Nov 20, 2013. www.corporatepolicy.org.

7. Rich F. The billionaires bankrolling the Tea Party. NYT, Aug 28, 2010. Froomkin D. American Legislative Exchange Council, ultra-conservative lobby, loses 2 major funders. Huffington Post, Apr 5, 2012. American Legislative Exchange Council. Resolution in opposition to discriminatory food and beverage taxes. www.alec.org. Wilce R. ALEC and Coca-Cola: A "classic" collaboration. PR Watch, Oct 12, 2011.

8. Merkelson S. Coca-Cola and Pepsi drop ALEC. The Nation, Apr 5, 2012.

9. Greely B. Why are McDonald's, Coca-Cola, and Intuit fleeing ALEC? Bloomberg BusinessWeek, Apr 13, 2012. Dem C. Grassley calls for boycott of Coca-Cola for ditching ALEC. Daily Kos, Apr 22, 2012. Grassley sent a tweet on April 21: "U might think abt not drinking Coca Cola since company sucombed [sic] to pressure fr Leftist not to support ALEC."

10. Simon M. Best public relations that money can buy: a guide to food industry front groups. Center for Food Safety, May 2013.

11. Kroll A, Schulman J. Leaked documents reveal the secret finances of a pro-industry science group. Mother Jones, Oct 28, 2013. American Council on Science and Health. Tag Archives: artificial sweetener. http://acsh.org. Savransky A. Attack on sugary drinks by the NYC Department of Health continues. American Council on Science and Health, Jun 11, 2013.

12. Coca-Cola. About the Beverage Institute for Health and Wellness.

13. Jilani Z. Big Soda hires PR flack behind "Harry and Louise" ad to fight Bloomberg soda ban. Republic Report, Jun 25, 2012. Goddard Gunster is at www.goddardgunster.com.

14. Huehnergarth N. The masterminds behind the phony anti-soda tax coalitions. Huffington Post, Jul 3, 2012.

15. The change of name certification was filed in the District of Columbia on Jan 28, 2014. Gerken J. "Environmental Policy Alliance," PR firm front group, targets LEED, green groups and EPA. Huffington Post, Mar 12, 2014.

16. Center for Consumer Freedom. About us. www.consumerfreedom.com.

17. Citizens for Responsibility and Ethics in Washington (CREW). Berman exposed. www.bermanexposed.org. Berman is sometimes referred to as "Dr. Evil," even by his own son. See Landman A. Front group king Rick Berman gets blasted by his son, David Berman. PRWatch, Jan 30, 2009.

18. Sargent G. Berman's battle. Prospect, Jan 3, 2005. Rampton S, Stauber J. & Co.: "Nonprofit" hustlers for the food & booze biz. PRWatch, 2001;8(1).

19. Shearn IT. Investigative Report: CCF's Richard Berman. Humane Society of the United States, n.d. (circa 2010). www.humanesociety.org.

20. Center for Media and Democracy. Source Watch: Center for Consumer Freedom. www.sourcewatch.org. Strom S. Nonprofit advocate carves out a for-profit

niche. NYT, Jun 17, 2010. The NYT article comes with an organizational chart of CCF enterprises. Lipton E. Hard-nosed advice from veteran lobbyist: "win ugly or lose pretty." NYT, Oct 31, 2014.

21. Stein S, Terkel A. Private documents show Coca-Cola played both sides of the drunk driving debate. Huffington Post, May 13, 2014.

22. Warner M. Striking back at the food police. NYT, Jun 12, 2005.

23. Waters R, Haar WL. Coca-Cola's "frank statement" a slick move to stave off regulation. Forbes, May 21, 2013.

CHAPTER 25. ADVOCACY: CAPPING SODA PORTION SIZES

1. NYC Obesity Task Force. Reversing the epidemic: The New York City Obesity Task Force plan to prevent and control obesity. May 31, 2012.

2. The city's soda cap campaign materials and documents in the court case are available from Orbach B. Regulation: the portion cap rule. http://regulationonline.com/drink-size. Citron R. The soda ban or the portion cap rule? Litigation over the size of sugary drink containers as an exercise in framing. Verdict, Jun 3, 2014.

3. Riley JJ. A History of the American Soft Drink Industry: Bottled Carbonated Beverages, 1807–1957. American Bottlers of Carbonated Beverages, 1958. Coca-Cola. Coca-Cola bottles: The history of our iconic bottle, 2010. www.coca-cola.co.uk.

4. Young LR. The Portion Teller. Morgan Road, 2005. McDonald's added 12-, 16-, and 21-ounce drinks in 1961, 1962, and 1974, respectively, a 32-ounce size in 1988, and a 42-ounce serving in 1999. See Young LR, Nestle M. Expanding portion sizes in the US marketplace: Implications for nutrition counseling. JADA, 2003;103:231–34.

5. Berger E. Why an effort to tax soda in Texas died yet again. Houston Chronicle, Jun 3, 2013.

6. Andreyeva T, Brownell KD. The impact of food prices on consumption: a systematic review of research on the price elasticity of demand for food. AJPH, 2010;100:216–22.

7. Young LR, Nestle M. The contribution of increasing portion sizes to the obesity epidemic. AJPH, 2002;92:246–49. Nielsen SJ, Popkin BM. Patterns and trends in food portion sizes, 1977–1998. JAMA, 2003;289:450–53. Young LR, Nestle M. Portion sizes and obesity: responses of the fast-food companies. J Public Health Policy, 2007;28:238–48. Rolls BJ, Morris EL, Roe LS. Portion size of food affects energy intake in normal-weight and overweight men and women. AJCN, 2002;76:1207–13. Wansink B, van Ittersum K. Portion size me: downsizing our consumption norms. JADA, 2007;107:1103–106. Wansink B, Chandon P. Meal size, not body size, explains errors in estimating the calorie content of meals. Annals of Internal Med, 2006:326–32. Diliberti N, et al. Increased portion size leads to increased energy intake in a restaurant meal. Obesity Res, 2004;12:562–68.

8. Just DR, Wansink B. Smarter lunchrooms: using behavioral economics to improve meal selection. Choices, 2009;24(3). CSPI. Literature review: defaults and choices, Feb 7, 2011. Surowieki J. The financial page: downsizing supersize. New Yorker, Aug 13/20, 2012:36. For a critique of the benefits of default options, see Salazar V, Alberto R. Libertarian paternalism and the dangers of nudging consumers. King's Law J, 2012; 23(1):51–67.

9. HHS. The Surgeon General's Call to Action to Prevent and Decrease Overweight and Obesity, 2001. HHS, USDA. Dietary Guidelines for Americans, 2005:15.

USDA, HHS. Dietary Guidelines for Americans, 2010.19. USDA. MyPlate. Washington, 2011. www.choosemyplate.gov.

10. White House Task Force on Childhood Obesity. Report to the President: Solving the Problem of Childhood Obesity Within a Generation, May 2010. USDA, HHS. Dietary Guidelines for Americans, 2010:58. Partnership for a Healthier America. In It for Good. 2013 Annual Report. See http://influenceexplorer.com. Search for Coca-Cola, PepsiCo, and the American Beverage Association.

11. Young LR, Nestle M. Reducing portion sizes to prevent obesity: A call to action. Am J Prev Med, 2012;43(5):565–68.

12. Some of this material in this section is reproduced from the afterword to Nestle M. Food Politics: How the Food Industry Influences Nutrition and Health, 10th anniversary ed. Berkeley: U of California Press, 2013. See also Grynbaum MM. New York plans to ban sale of big sizes of sugary drinks. NYT, May 30, 2012. In Aug 2012, the task force report and other documents related to the soda cap proposal were on the website of the NYC Department of Health and Mental Hygiene. www.nyc.gov.

13. NYC Department of Mental Health and Hygiene. Eating healthy initiatives. Also see NYC Department of Mental Health and Hygiene. Health department launches new initiatives to prevent childhood obesity. Nov 17, 2005. The ban on trans fats went relatively smoothly because restaurateurs had been unaware that their cooking oils contained trans fats, and they could easily substitute low-cost oils that had not been hydrogenated.

14. NYC Department of Mental Health and Hygiene. Health Department launches new ad campaign spotlighting increasing portion sizes and their devastating consequences, Jan 9, 2012. The city's anti-soda campaigns from 2007 to 2014 are described in Kansagra SM, et al. Reducing sugary drink consumption: New York City's approach. Am J Public Health, 2015;105(4):e61–64. The poster generated its own controversy when the supposedly diabetes-induced amputation turned out to have been Photoshopped. McGeehan P. Blame Photoshop, not diabetes, for this amputation. NYT, Jan 24, 2012.

15. NYC Department of Health and Mental Hygiene. Maximum size for a sugary drink—briefing document: from supersized to human-sized: reintroducing reasonable portions of sugary drinks in New York City, Jun 12, 2012.

16. Grynbaum MM. Soda makers begin their push against New York ban. NYT, Jul 2, 2012.

17. Hartocollis A. To gulp or to sip? Debating a crackdown on big sugary drinks. NYT, May 31, 2012. A ban too far [editorial]. NYT, May 31, 2012.

18. NYT reporter Kate Taylor tweeted the mayor's response. See @katetaylornyt, Jun 3, 2012.

19. Zmuda N, Morrison M. Sugary-drink ban would trim bottom lines. Ad Age, Jun 4, 2012:2–3,19.

20. The ABA website is www.letsclearitup.org.

21. Horovitz B. Coke executive answers questions about sugary drinks. USA Today, Jun 7, 2012.

22. Miet H. 40 Ounces of Freedom: Big Soda fights Bloomberg's ban. Atlantic Wire, Jul 2, 2012. Grynbaum MM. Fighting ban on big sodas with appeals to patriotism. NYT, Jul 23, 2012.

23. Severson K. "Anti-Bloomberg bill" in Mississippi bars local restrictions on food and drink. NYT, Mar 13, 2013:A16. Mississippi ranked 50th in overall health

outcomes in 2013. United Health Foundation. America's health rankings: Mississippi. www.americashealthrankings.org. State and city legislators call for new laws on sugar-sweetened beverages. National Restaurant Association, Mar 17, 2014.

24. Gostin JO, et al. The historic role of boards of health in local innovation: New York City's soda portion case. JAMA, 2014;312:1511–12. Pomeranz JL, Brownell KD. Can government regulate portion sizes? NEJM, 2014;371:1956–58.

25. Documents submitted in this case are available at Supreme Court Records On-Line Library, County Clerk and Superior Court of NY County, http://iapps.courts.state .ny.us/iscroll/index.jsp; enter case number 653584-2012. Other documents are at New York City Department of Health and Mental Hygiene: Physical Activity and Nutrition: Sugary Drinks.

26. Tingling MA. Supreme Court of the State of New York, New York Country. New York Statewide Coalition vs. New York City Department of Health and Mental Hygiene. Case disposition, Mar 11, 2013:34, 35. www.foodpolitics.com.

27. American Beverage Association reacts to NYC soda ban ruling. PRNewswire, Mar 11, 2013. Mayor Bloomberg discusses city's efforts to combat obesity and sugary beverage regulation, Mar 11, 2013. www1.nyc.gov.

28. Statements of Mayor Bloomberg and corporation counsel Cardozo on Appellate Division, First Department's decision on New York City's regulation limiting the portion size of sugary beverages. www1.nyc.gov. Jul 30, 2013.

29. Farley T. The precedent in regulating soda. Atlantic, Jun 3, 2014.

30. Court of Appeals, State of New York. No. 134: In the Matter of New York State-wide Coalition of Hispanic Chambers of Commerce v. The New York City Department of Health and Mental Hygiene. Jun 26, 2014.

31. The petition, filed Oct 12, 2012, is New York State Coalition vs. New York City Department of Health and Mental Hygiene, New York City Board of Health, and Dr. Thomas Farley.

32. Halloran DJ, Koppell O, Cabrera F, et al. Memorandum of Law of *Amici Curiae*. Supreme Court of the State of New York, County of New York, Nov 7, 2012. It and the NAACP and Hispanic Federation supporting brief are at https://iapps.courts. state.ny.us.

33. Confessore N. Bottlers and minority groups, soda war allies. NYT, Mar 13, 2013.

34. Dobnik V. New York soda ban: rally held against Bloomberg's proposal. Huffington Post, Jul 9, 2012. Federal Election Commission. Schedule A. Halloran 2012. Halloran was later caught attempting to bribe New York City political officials in a sting operation. See U.S.A. v. Malcolm A. Smith et al., Mar 29, 2013. New York City Campaign Finance Board. Searchable Database, Election Cycle 2013. www. nyccfb.info. Grynbaum MM. New York City soda fight, in court, tests agency's power. NYT, Jun 4, 2014.

35. Grynbaum M. Quinn, cool to Soda Ban, gets donations from Coke. NYT, Jan 25, 2013.

36. Goodman A. Lecture to New York University's Global Institute of Public Health, Nov 19, 2014. Saul MH. Forward push on soda ban. WSJ, Oct 15, 2014.

37. Grynbaum MM, Connelly. 60% in city oppose soda ban, calling it an overreach by Bloomberg, a poll finds. NYT, Aug 23, 2012. Opposition to soda ban sad proof that Americans still fight for what they believe in. The Onion, Mar 13, 2013.

38. Blain G. 7-Eleven's Big Gulps safe from Bloomberg's soda ban. New York Daily News, Feb 27, 2013.

39. Bloomberg appealing soda ban block. Health groups file friend of the court briefs for June hearing. CSPI, Mar 28, 2013.

40. Court of Appeals, State of New York. Brief of Amici Curiae, National Alliance for Hispanic Health, Association of Black Cardiologists, Harlem Health Promotion Center, et al. in support of respondents-appellants. Apr 24, 2014. National Alliance for Hispanic Health. National Alliance for Hispanic Health leads diverse "Friends of the Court" in support of NYC policy to reduce sugary drink portion size. Apr 28, 2014. Bassett MT, et al. Statements from Health Commissioner Mary T. Bassett and supporters of New York City's sugary drink portion rule. NYC Department of Health and Mental Hygiene, Jun 4, 2014.

41. Jealous B. Transcript: Up w/Chris Hayes. MSNBC, Mar 16, 2013.

42. Bellafonte G. In obesity epidemic, poverty is an ignored contagion. NYT, Mar 17, 2013.

43. Brown A. Americans reject size limit on soft drinks in restaurants. Gallup Well-Being, Jun 26, 2013. Public agrees on obesity's impact, not government's role. Pew Research, Nov 20, 2014.

44. The Hispanic Institute. Obesity, Hispanic America's big challenge, Apr 2013.

45. Hodgekiss A. "Some people don't realise how much sugar there is in Coca-Cola," admits the company's president. Daily Mail, Nov 29, 2013. Bouckley B. "Coke's Mini Can Can!" Muhtar Kent salutes small package "romance." Food Navigator, Jul 22, 2014.

CHAPTER 26. ADVOCACY: TAXING SUGARY DRINKS—EARLY ATTEMPTS

1. The Adam Smith quote is "Sugar, rum, and tobacco are commodities which are nowhere necessaries of life, which are become objects of almost universal consumption, and which are therefore extremely proper subjects of taxation." Smith A, Mazlish B. The Wealth of Nations: Representative Selections. Mineola, NY: Dover, 2002:294. For a brief review of the history of soda taxes from an anti-tax position, see Drenkard S. Special Report. Overreaching on obesity: Governments consider new taxes on soda and candy. Tax Foundation, Oct 2011.

2. Propose income and soft drink tax. NYT, Feb 12, 1919. Luxury tax test delayed by rain. NYT, May 2, 1919. Soda fountains protest. NYT, May 3, 1919. City's soda cost millions monthly. NYT, May 23, 1920. Pendergrast M. For God, Country & Coca-Cola, 3rd ed. Basic Books, 2013:102.

3. Bottlers oppose taxes. NYT, Nov 19, 1948. Riley JJ. A History of the American Soft Drink Industry: Bottled Carbonated Beverages, 1807–1957. American Bottlers of Carbonated Beverages, 1958. Kilborn PT. Soft-drink industry is fighting back over new taxes. NYT, Mar 24, 1993.

4. Brownell KD. Get slim with higher taxes. NYT, Dec 15, 1994. Jacobson MF, Brownell KD. Small taxes on soft drinks and snack foods to promote health. AJPH, 2000;90:854–57. Jacobson MF. Liquid Candy: How Soft Drinks Are Harming Americans' Health. CSPI, 2005. Vartanian LF, Schwartz MB, Brownell KD. Effects of soft drink consumption on nutrition and health: a systematic review and meta-analysis. AJPH, 2007;97(4):667–75.

5. Brownell KD, Frieden TR. Ounces of prevention—the public policy case for taxes on sugared beverages. NEJM, 2009;360:1805–808. Brownell KD, et al. The public health and economic benefits of taxing sugar-sweetened beverages. NEJM, 2009;361:1599–605. Waterlander WE, Mhurchu CN, Steenhuis IHM. Effects of a price increase on purchases of sugar sweetened beverages. Results from a randomized controlled trial. Appetite, 2014;78:32–39. For models, see Escobar MAC, et al. Evidence that a tax on sugar sweetened beverages reduces the obesity rate: a meta-analysis. BMC Public Health, 2013;13(1):1072. Liu Y, Lopez RA, Zhu C. The impact of four alternative policies to decrease soda consumption. Agricultural Resource Economics Rev, 2014;43(1):53–68. Thow AM, et al. A systematic review of the effectiveness of food taxes and subsidies to improve diets: understanding the recent evidence. Nutr Rev, 2014;72(9):551–65.

6. The Rudd Center provides a legislative database at www.yaleruddcenter.org/ legislation, along with an interactive map of sugar-sweetened beverage initiatives since 2009. DeLauro R. DeLauro introduces bill to tackle dual epidemics of obesity, diabetes, Jul 30, 2014. http://delauro.house.gov. Drake B. Tax sugary drinks? New Yorkers say "no" but leave some wiggle room. Politics Daily, Apr 4, 2013. Rivard C, et al. Taxing sugar-sweetened beverages: a survey of knowledge, attitudes, and behaviours. Public Health Nutr, 2012;15:1355–61. More than half of respondents to a poll in Kentucky said they would support a soda tax if the revenues were used for school nutrition and physical activity programs. Interact for Health and Foundation for a Healthy Kentucky. Kentuckians views on sodas and sugary drink policies. KHIP (Kentucky Health Issues Poll), Mar 2015.

7. CSPI. Key components of a soft drink tax. N.d.

8. Watts RA, et al. Tobacco taxes vs soda taxes: a case study of a framing debate in Vermont. Health Behavior & Policy Rev, 2014;1(3):191–96.

9. See http://influenceexplorer.com. Search for Coca-Cola, PepsiCo, and the American Beverage Association, Lobbying. The data on this site come from U.S. Senate, Office of Public Records.

10. These examples are reviewed in CSPI. Selfish Giving: How the Soda Industry Uses Philanthropy to Sweeten Its Profits. 2013. Also see Shields J. Heard in the hall: big beverage gives $10 million to CHOP. Philly.com, Mar 16, 2011.

11. Huehnergarth N. The masterminds behind the phony anti-soda tax coalitions. Huffington Post, Jul 3, 2012.

12. Americans Against Food Taxes is at www.nofoodtaxes.com.

13. Geiger K, Hamburger T. Soft drink tax battle shifts to states. Los Angeles Times, Feb 21, 2010.

14. Paterson D. Commentary: Why we need an obesity tax. CNN.com Health, Dec 18, 2008. Brownell K. Want a healthier state? Save Gov. Paterson's tax on sugar soda. New York Daily News, Feb 18, 2009:29.

15. Chan S. A tax on many soft drinks sets off a spirited debate. NYT, Dec 16, 2008. ABA. American Beverage Association statement in response to the New York governor's proposal to raise taxes. Dec 15, 2008. Confessore N. Paterson lowers expectations on soda tax, calling approval unlikely. NYT, Feb 13, 2009.

16. Wilson D, Roberts J. Food fight: How Washington went soft on childhood obesity. Reuters special report, Apr 27, 2012.

17. Berger J. New strategy for soda tax gives diet drinks a break. NYT, May 19, 2010. Hartocollis A. Failure of state soda tax plan reflects power of an antitax message. NYT, Jul 2, 2010.

18. Drake, Bruce. Tax sugary drinks? New Yorkers say "no" but leave some wiggle room. Politics Daily. Apr 14, 2010. Quinnipiac University. New Yorkers oppose fat-tax 2–1, Quinnipiac University poll finds; but split on tax if money is promised for health care. Apr 14, 2010.

19. Stanford DD. Anti-obesity soda tax fails as lobbyists spend millions: retail. Bloomberg BusinessWeek, Mar 13, 2012.

20. Drenkard S. Soda tax proposals bubbling up in California. Tax Foundation, Oct 25, 2012. Brown PL. Plan to tax soda gets a mixed reception. NYT, Jun 3, 2012.

21. Brunner W, et al. The impact of sugar-sweetened beverage consumption on the health of Richmond residents: A report prepared by Contra Costa Health Services for the Richmond City Council, Dec 9, 2011. http://cchealth.org.

22. Harless W. Beverage lobbyist funds "community" campaign against soda tax. California Watch, Jun 13, 2012. Rogers R. Soda tax debate pushes Richmond into national spotlight. San Jose Mercury News, Jul 4, 2012. Palmer C, Diaz R. New California Field Poll shows support for "soda tax." San Jose Mercury News, Feb 14, 2013.

23. Sheppard K. Beverage industry group bankrolls soda tax opposition. Mother Jones, Jul 25, 2012. Onishi N. Activist city savors role in fighting "big soda." NYT, Nov 5, 2012. The Community Coalition Against Beverage Taxes site was at www.norichmondbeveragetax.com. The coalition produced "No on N" materials in Spanish: "Vote NO en el impuesto sobre los refrescos en Richmond o este refresco va a costar más."

24. Jonassen W. Race-baiting in Richmond: How big business used race to drive a wedge through Richmond's progressive community—and why you should be concerned about it. East Bay Express, Jan 23, 2013. Nixon L, et al. Big Soda's long shadow: news coverage of local proposals to tax sugar-sweetened beverages in Richmond, El Monte and Telluride. Critical Public Health, 2015;25:333–47.

25. Rogers R. Richmond politics brimming with beverage industry dollars. Contra Costa Times, Oct 5, 2012.

26. Velazquez M. Voters overwhelmingly reject El Monte's "soda tax" measure. Pasadena Star News, Nov 7, 2012. Zingale D. Gulp! The high cost of big soda's victory. Los Angeles Times, Dec 9, 2012.

27. Rogers R. Richmond's progressive leaders look to future in wake of setbacks against Chevron, soda tax. Contra Costa Times, Nov 16, 2012.

28. Parts of this discussion are drawn from Nestle M. Denmark's "fat tax": what will it achieve? New Scientist, Oct 23, 2011. Buley J. Fat tax draws foreign attention. Copenhagen Post, Oct 4, 2010. Abend L. Beating butter: Denmark imposes the world's first fat tax. Time, Oct 6, 2011.

29. Denmark's food taxes: A fat chance. Economist, Nov 17, 2012.

30. Jensen JD, Smed S. The Danish tax on saturated fat: short run effects on consumption and consumer prices of fats. U of Copenhagen, Institute of Food and Resource Economics, 2012.

CHAPTER 27. ADVOCACY: TAXING SUGARY DRINKS—LESSONS LEARNED

1. Sparks I. France to impose fat tax on sugary drinks such as Coca-Cola and Fanta. Daily Mail, Oct 6, 2011. Taylor M. French soft drinks market lacks fizz: "Fat Tax" hits the French soft drinks industry hard. Canadean, Apr 23, 2013. Bouckley B. Coke

restates strong opposition to French soda tax that "stigmatizes our products and category." Beverage Daily, Oct 11, 2014.

2. FAO. The State of Food and Agriculture, 2013.

3. Rivera J, et al. Epidemiological and nutritional transition in Mexico: rapid increase of non-communicable chronic diseases and obesity. Public Health Nutr, 2013;5:113–22. Flannery NP. Why are Mexico and Mike Bloomberg battling Coca-Cola? Forbes, Oct 28, 2014. Stern D, et al. Caloric beverages were major sources of energy among children and adults in Mexico, 1999–2012. J Nutr, 2014;144 949–56. Table 15.2 gives a slightly lower estimate based on different sources of data.

4. Blanding M. The Coke Machine. Avery, 2010. Pendergrast M. For God, Country & Coca-Cola, 3rd ed. Basic Books, 2013. Boseley S. Mexico enacts soda tax in effort to combat world's highest obesity rate. Guardian, Jan 16, 2014.

5. Kearns R. The soft drink invasion on indigenous Chiapas; increased diabetes death. Indian Country Today, Jun 1, 2014. Mallén PR. Mexico, with world's top obesity rate, raises prices on soft drinks to fight it. Int Business Times, Sept 23, 2013. Pilcher J. Industrial tortillas and folkloric Pepsi: The nutritional consequences of hybrid cuisines in Mexico. In Belasco W, Scranton P, eds., Food Nations: Selling Taste in Consumer Societies, Routledge, 2002:222–39.

6. Guthrie A. Coca-Cola to Mexican school children: go ahead and drink the tap water. WSJ, Jun 20, 2014.

7. Malkin E. Mexico takes Bloomberg-like swing at soaring obesity. NYT, Oct 15, 2013. Bloomberg Philanthropies. Obesity prevention. www.bloomberg.org. The purposes of the grants were explained to me by Ch'uya Lane, the representative of Bloomberg Philanthropies in Mexico City.

8. World Health Organization supports Mexico's soda tax proposal. Banderas News, Aug 14, 2013. Rogers R. Richmond activists celebrate as Mexico passes soda tax similar to one that filed locally. Contra Costa Times, Nov 1, 2013.

9. Guthrie A. Health battle over soda flares in Mexico. WSJ, Aug 29, 2013. The film, produced by El Poder del Consumidor, is "Sweet Agony." The videos from El Poder del Consumidor in 2014 are "Make Someone Happy," an anti-commercial countering Coca-Cola's Christmas marketing campaign, and "Santa Claus Resigns," all available on www.youtube.com. The remaining text in the poster translates as "During the 2006–2012 presidency, 500,000 people died of diabetes. When will we act?"

10. Bittman M. ¡Viva México! NYT, Nov 29, 2013.

11. Fizzing with rage: A once-omnipotent industry fights what may be a losing battle. Economist, Oct 19, 2013. The Industria Refresquera Mexicana placed anti–"Bloomberg tax" ads—"he's trying to do in Mexico what he can't do in the U.S."—in newspapers such as Negocios, El Universal, and Reforma in October 2013. Guthrie A. Mexican nonprofit accuses Televisa, Azteca of avoiding anti-soft-drink ads. WSJ, Sept 30, 2013. The censored soda tax, "Anuncio censurado sobre impuesto al refresco para bebederos," is on YouTube, as is the ad attacking Alejandro Calvillo: "¿Quién está detrás de la campaña anti refresquera en México?" (Who is behind the anti-soft drink campaign in Mexico?).

12. Guthrie A. Mexico soda tax dents Coke bottler's sales. WSJ, Feb 26, 2014. Instituto Nacional de Salud Pública. Resultados preliminares sobre los efectos del impuesto de un peso a bebidas azucaradas en México (Preliminary results on the effects of a tax of one peso on sweetened beverages in Mexico), Sept 9, 2014. The English version is posted by U of North Carolina, Chapel Hill, Food Research Program. Choi C.

"Mexican Coke" in U.S. will still use cane sugar. AP, Oct 6, 2013. Khanh VT. Coca-Cola to invest $8.2 billion in Mexico by 2020. Beverage Manager, Jul 18, 2014. Esterl M, Revill J. PepsiCo, Nestlé to invest in Mexico. WSJ, Jan 24, 2014. Guthrie A. Survey shows Mexicans drinking less soda after tax. WSJ, Oct 13, 2014. Wilmore J. Just on call—Coca-Cola FEMSA cuts 1,300 jobs as Mexico soda tax bites. Just Drinks, Oct 23, 2014. Case B. Soft-drink thirst quenched by Pena Nieto tax. Bloomberg Business, Mar 27, 2014.

13. CSPI. National Soda Summit, 2014. www.cspinet.org/Soda-Summit-2014.html.

14. Editorial. Chronicle recommends S.F. soda-tax measure. San Francisco Chronicle, Oct 5, 2014.

15. Knight H. S.F. soda tax backers sweet on Mexico's sugar-fighting success. San Francisco Chronicle, Oct 11, 2014. City of San Francisco Sugary Drink Tax, Proposition E (Nov 2014). Results are at http://ballotpedia.org.

16. Much of this analysis is summarized by Dana Woldow in a series of articles in Beyond Chron, 2014. www.beyondchron.org/author/dana.

17. DiCamillo M, Field M. Most Californians see a direct linkage between obesity and sugary sodas. California Endowment, Feb 14, 2013. www.field.com.

18. Knight H. Why Berkeley passed a soda tax and S.F. didn't. San Francisco Chronicle, Nov 7, 2014. Knight H. Supervisors' soda tax vote isn't good omen for backers. San Francisco Chronicle, Jul 26, 2014.

19. Evich HB. Soda fight's last stand. Politico, Sept 24, 2014. Video: When grassroots protest rallies have corporate sponsors. ABC News Nightline, Nov 3, 2014.

20. Knight H. S.F. soda tax falls short; Berkeley's surges to victory. San Francisco Chronicle, Nov 5, 2014. Lagos M. S.F. soda-tax opponents pour in contributions. San Francisco Chronicle, Oct 24, 2014. Knight H. Why New York soda tax crusader passed on helping S.F.'s Prop. E. San Francisco Chronicle, Nov 15, 2014.

21. Press release: Statement by supervisors Scott Wiener, Eric Mar and Malia Cohen on Prop E results. Yes on E, Nov 4, 2014.

22. City of Berkeley sugary beverages and soda tax question, Measure D (Nov 2014). Results at http://ballotpedia.org.

23. Morales X. Behind Berkeley's efforts to pass Measure D, the soda tax. Jamie Oliver's Food Revolution, Oct 22, 2014.

24. Covarrubias A. Local measures against sugary-drink tax, fracking raise millions. Los Angeles Times, Nov 1, 2014. The independent newspaper Berkeleyside collected coverage of the events related to Measure D. Its articles include the photo essay by Gael McKeon, the source of Figures 7.1 and 8.2 in this book. Reich R. Berkeley vs. Big Soda. Sept 8, 2014. http://robertreich.org. Reich also appeared in a cartoon video on the politics of the Berkeley soda tax initiative: "Like Coke or Pepsi? Wait until you hear what they're doing," available on YouTube. Opponents proposed soda tax sue city allegedly biased ballot language. Daily Californian, Aug 14, 2014.

25. Nagourney A. Berkeley officials outspent but optimistic in battle over soda tax. NYT, Oct 7, 2014. Jacobson MF. Will Big Soda learn from election day 2014? Huffington Post, Nov 6, 2014.

26. Waters R. Soda battle by the bay: beverage industry opens its wallet but is $9 million enough to beat soda taxes in Berkeley and San Francisco? Forbes, Oct 10, 2014.

27. Evich HB. Soda fight's last stand. Politico, Sept 24, 2014.

28. Evich HB. Berkeley breaks through on soda tax. Politico, Nov 5, 2014. Garofoli J. Ex-NYC mayor Bloomberg buys World Series ad to push Berkeley soda tax. San Francisco Chronicle, Oct 24, 2014. Dinkelspiel F. Former NYC mayor Michael Bloomberg

donates $83,000 to support Berkeley's proposed soda tax. Berkeleyside, Oct 16, 2014. Lochner T. Former New York mayor Michael Bloomberg goes to bat in Berkeley soda tax effort. Contra Costa Times, Oct 24, 2014.

29. Email from Dr. Lynn Silver, senior advisor for chronic disease and obesity, Public Health Institute, Nov 6, 2014.

30. Tramutola L. Taking on Big Soda. Public CEO, Nov 25, 2014.

31. Fonseca F. Navajo Nation president approves junk-food tax. Santa Fe News, Nov 21, 2014. Renstrom E. This place just became the first part of the U.S. to impose a tax on junk food. Time, Mar 30, 2015. The tax went into effect Apr 1, 2015.

32. Heintz P. Beverage industry spends half a million to kill Vermont soda tax. Seven Days, Apr 27, 2015. Stuhldreher A. What Big Soda didn't buy. San Francisco Chronicle, Nov 14, 2014.

33. Friedman RR, Brownell KD. Sugar-sweetened beverage taxes: an updated policy brief. Rudd Center for Food Policy & Obesity, Oct 2012.

34. On the tax debate, see also Winkler JT. Why soft drink taxes will not work. British J Nutr, 2011;108:395–96. Yale Rudd Center. Sugar-sweetened beverage taxes and sugar intake: policy statements, endorsements, and recommendations, updated Nov 2012. Chokshi DA, Stine NW. Reconsidering the politics of public health. JAMA, 2013;310:1025–26. Quintero F. Media advocacy strategy for soda tax measures: Preparing for tough questions. Berkeley Media Studies Group, Dec 10, 2013. Niederdeppe J, et al. News coverage of sugar-sweetened beverage taxes: pro- and antitax arguments in public discourse. AJPH, 2013;103:e92.

CHAPTER 28. CONCLUSION: TAKING ACTION

1. WHO. Press release: WHO director-general addresses health promotion conference. Jun 10, 2013.

2. Freudenberg N. Lethal but Legal: Corporations, Consumption, and Protecting Public Health. Oxford U Press, 2014. Also see Ontario Medical Association. Applying lessons learned from anti-tobacco campaigns to the prevention of obesity. Ontario Med Rev, Oct 2012:12–15. Brownell KD, Warner KE. The perils of ignoring history: Big Tobacco played dirty and millions died. How similar is Big Food? Millbank Quarterly, 2009;87(1):259–94.

3. Coke and Pepsi lead list of most respected brands. Beverage World, Jul 14, 2014.

4. Michael Blanding. The Coke Machine, Avery, 2010. Thomas M. Belching Out the Devil, Nation Books, 2009. Garcia C, Gutiérrez G. The Coca-Cola Case: The Truth That Refreshes. National Film Board of Canada, 2009.

5. Coca-Cola. Human rights policy. N.d.

6. Killer Coke. Who we are. www.killercoke.org. Rogers R. Letter to Nicholas P. Panos, Senior Special Counsel, U.S. Securities and Exchange Commission. Corporate Crime Reporter, Apr 15, 2013.

7. SEC seeks to gag Ray Rogers on Coca-Cola. Corporate Crime Reporter, Apr 16, 2013.

8. McGeehan P. Pepsi wins battle in Cola wars: $21 million CUNY deal. NYT, Aug 13, 2013. Scandals and lack of ethics plague NYU. Killer Coke. N.d. Ambrosio J. University revisits past ban on Coca-Cola. Washington Square News, Feb 12, 2014. American Federation of Teachers. AFT Resolution. Stop Coca-Cola's abuse of children and violation of

human rights, 2014. AFT Ends four month old Coca-Cola boycott. Corporate Crime Reporter, Mar 31, 2015. Petition: Teaching does NOT go better with Coke. RootsAction. org (as of April 24, 2015, 14,364 people had signed on).

9. National Restaurant Association. Kids LiveWell Program. CSPI. Restaurant chains urged to dump soda from kids' menus. Jan 30, 2014. Bowerman M. Wendy's removes soda option from kids' meal. USA Today, Jan 15, 2015. The Davis, Calif., City Council banned sodas as the default in kids' meals in 2015.

10. Chou S-Y, et al. Fast-food restaurant advertising on television and its influence on childhood obesity. J Law and Economics, 2008;51(4):599–618. Blumenthal R. Statement: Stop subsidizing Childhood Obesity Act of 2014. May 18, 2014. The bills were introduced by Richard Blumenthal (D-Conn.), Tom Harkin (D-Iowa), and Rosa DeLauro (D-Conn.).

11. Capewell S. Sugar sweetened drinks should carry obesity warnings. BMJ, 2014;348:g3428. OMA policy paper: applying lessons learned from anti-tobacco campaigns to the prevention of obesity. Ontario Medical Rev, Oct 2012:12–15.

12. Morales X, Islas G. Diabetes and sugary soda. Fresno Bee, May 19, 2014. California Center for Public Health Advocacy. California-sweetened beverages safety warning bill (Monning). www.publichealthadvocacy.org. Californians for Beverage Choice. SB1000: What's In, What's Out. N.d.

13. Morales X. SB 1000 defeated, but we remain committed. Latino Coalition for a Healthy California, Jun 18, 2014. White JB. Field Poll: Californians broadly support soda tax, labeling. Sacramento Bee, Feb 19, 2014. White JB. California soda warning label bill stalls in committee. Sacramento Bee, Jun 17, 2014. New York State Assembly. Health Claims and Labels. NY A.B. 10172, introduced Aug 20, 2014. Colorado policy analysts track legislation relevant to soda consumption. See Ward T, Motika SM. Reducing sugar sweetened beverage consumption: A survey of legislation, policy and campaigns. Colorado Department of Public Health & Environment, Mar 2015. The California Center for Public Health Advocacy tracks legislation at www.kickthecan.info (see Campaigns).

14. Hodge JG, et al. A proposed ban on the sale to and possession of caloric sweetened beverages by minors in public. J Law, Med & Ethics, Spring 2014:110–14.

15. Evich HB. The plot to make Big Food pay. Politico, Feb 12, 2014.

16. Health Care Without Harm. Healthy beverages initiative. N.d. Healthier Hospitals Initiative. 2012 Milestone report. See, for example, Miels E. Baldwin Area Medical Center drops sugary and artificially sweetened beverages. Leader-Telegram (WI), Jun 4, 2014. Gunderman R. Does McDonald's belong in a children's hospital? Atlantic, Nov 13, 2013.

17. The Fed Up site is at http://fedupmovie.com/#/page/home. See Dargis M. Sugar, come out with your hands up: "Fed Up" descends on villains in the battle of the bulge. NYT, May 8, 2014.

18. Butler J. Mastering the Craft of Carbonation: Healthy Recipes You Can Make with or Without a Soda Machine. Quarry Books, 2014. Munarriz RA. Pepsi and SodaStream test-drive a new relationship. Daily Finance, Oct 31, 2014.

19. The CSPI video "Coming Together, Translated" is available on YouTube. Coca-Cola's heavily criticized "Coming Together" video is no longer available at the sites on which it was originally posted. Madrigal A. The new culture jamming: how activists will respond to online advertising. Atlantic, May 15, 2012. Boyd A, Mitchell DO, eds.

Beautiful Trouble: A Toolbox for Revolution. OR Books, 2012. http://beautifultrouble
.org.

20. Hawkes C. Promoting healthy diets through nutrition education and changes in the food environment: an international review of actions and their effectiveness. FAO, 2013. Thow AM, Hawkes C. Global sugar guidelines: an opportunity to strengthen nutrition policy. Public Health Nutr, 2014;17(10):2151–55.

21. The Berkeley Media Studies Group offers many resources on its website, for example, Handout: layers of strategy; Working upstream: skills for social change; and Resources: Media Advocacy 101. www.bmsg.org.

22. Horizon Foundation. Press release: Soda sales dropping faster in Howard County than nationally. Mar 30, 2015. Addy R. Sales of sports drinks and fruit juices are down 11% in Great Britain, where 60 percent of drinks contain no added sugar. Beverage Daily, Apr 8, 2015. Basu J. New campaign targets soft drink makers over health issues. Food and Drink Europe, Feb 23, 2015. Farand C. France to ban unlimited refills of soft drinks. The Local, Apr 2, 2015. Ng SW, et al. Turning point for US diets? Recessionary effects or behavioral shifts in foods purchased and consumed. AJCN, 2014;99:609–16.

23. Ferdman RA. The soda industry is discovering what the future of Diet Coke looks like (and it isn't pretty). Washington Post, Mar 23, 2015. Stanford D. Diet Pepsi dumps aspartame as consumer backlash hurts sales. Bloomberg News, Apr 24, 2015. Watson E. Pepsi exec: Aspartame is the #1 reason why US consumers say they are drinking less diet cola. Food Navigator-USA, Apr 27, 2015.

24. McCarthy J. Americans more likely to avoid drinking soda than before. Gallup Well-Being, Jul 28, 2014. Saad L. Nearly half of Americans drink soda daily. Gallup Well-Being, Jul 23, 2012. www.gallup.com/poll. CDC. Vital signs: obesity among low-income, preschool-aged children—United States, 2008–2011. Morbidity and Mortality Weekly Rep, 2013;62:1–6.

25. Bouckley B. Coke's capitulation to the 'new normal', and could a newly graduated MBA run the business? Beverage Daily, Oct 23, 2014. Coca-Cola. The Coca-Cola Company and Monster Beverage Corporation enter into long-term strategic partnership. Coca-Cola Journey, Aug 14, 2014. Esterl M. Coke pays $2 billion for stake in Monster Beverage. WSJ, Aug 15, 2014. Neate R. Coca-Cola enters dairy market with "Milka-Cola." Guardian, Nov 25, 2014. Video: "Fairlife cold filtration: the secret to nutrient-rich milk," available on YouTube. Douglas S. The Coca-Cola Company's (KO) presents at Morgan Stanley Global Consumer Conference (transcript). Seeking Alpha, Nov 18, 2014.

26. Esterl M. Soda producers set goals on cutting U.S. beverage calories. WSJ, Sept 23, 2014. RWJF statement regarding announcement by the Alliance for a Healthier Generation and American Beverage Association. Sept 23, 2014. Editorial Board. Soda giants' deal too sweet to buy: our view. USA Today, Sept 28, 2014.

27. Schultz EJ. Brita attacks big soda with sugar cube city ad [includes the video]. Ad Age, Oct 21, 2014. How Coca-Cola is trying to get its groove back. WSJ, Jul 30, 2014. Suddath C. Coke confronts its big fat problem. Bloomberg BusinessWeek, Jul 31, 2014.

28. Buffett pressures Coca-Cola over executive pay. WSJ, Apr 30, 2014. Calvert Investments. Is the Coca-Cola Company (KO) a sustainable and responsible investment? Oct 22, 2013. Winters DJ. Letter to fellow Coca-Cola shareholders. Wintergreen Advisers,

Jul 8, 2014. Streib L. Gates Foundation ditches McDonald's, Coca-Cola in fourth quarter. Bloomberg News, Feb 17, 2015.

29. Gallagher J. Mexico restricts soft drink TV ads to fight obesity. BBC News, Jul 16, 2014.

30. Bend D, King A. Why consider a benefit corporation? Forbes, May 30, 2014.

Index

Note: Page numbers in *italics* indicate photographs, illustrations, and tables.